An Illustrated Atlas of Tooth Carving and Wax-Up Techniques

An Illustrated Atlas of Tooth Carving and Wax-Up Techniques

Anil Bangalore Shivappa
King Faisal University
Al-Ahsa, Saudi Arabia

WILEY Blackwell

This edition first published 2021

Registered Office(s)
John Wiley & Sons, Inc., 111 River Street, Hoboken, NJ 07030, USA
John Wiley & Sons Ltd, The Atrium, Southern Gate, Chichester, West Sussex, PO19 8SQ, UK

Editorial Office
9600 Garsington Road, Oxford, OX4 2DQ, UK

For details of our global editorial offices, customer services, and more information about Wiley products visit us at www.wiley.com.

Wiley also publishes its books in a variety of electronic formats and by print-on-demand. Some content that appears in standard print versions of this book may not be available in other formats.

Library of Congress Cataloging-in-Publication Data

Names: Shivappa, Anil Bangalore, author.
Title: An illustrated atlas of tooth carving and wax-up techniques / Anil Bangalore Shivappa.
Description: Hoboken, NJ : Wiley-Blackwell, 2021. | Includes bibliographical references and index.
Identifiers: LCCN 2020030472 (print) | LCCN 2020030473 (ebook) | ISBN 9781119573586 (hardback) | ISBN 9781119573593 (adobe pdf) | ISBN 9781119573616 (epub)
Subjects: MESH: Tooth–anatomy & histology | Dental Prosthesis Design | Dental Models | Atlas
Classification: LCC RK305 (print) | LCC RK305 (ebook) | NLM WU 17 | DDC 617.6/3–dc23
LC record available at https://lccn.loc.gov/2020030472
LC ebook record available at https://lccn.loc.gov/2020030473

Cover Design: Wiley
Cover Images: Courtesy of Anil Bangalore Shivappa

Set in 9.5/12.5 STIXTwoText by SPi Global, Pondicherry, India

10 9 8 7 6 5 4 3 2 1

I dedicate this book to my parents, Smt. Mahadevamma and Shri. Shivappa B, for their endless encouragement, support, prayers, and love that enabled me to reach this stage.
I also dedicate this book to my family and my sisters for their boundless support in writing this book.

Contents

Preface

As a student and as a teaching faculty member for nearly six years in the course on dental anatomy, I perceived that students in this course found it difficult to understand the concept of carving and waxing in terms of cognitive and psychomotor skills even though they have better knowledge in related subjects.

According to German anatomist and physiologist, Friedrich Tiedemann (1781–1861), 'Doctors without anatomy are like moles. They work in the dark and the works of their hands are mounds'.

Dentistry, however, does not depend solely on knowledge but also on psychomotor skills. A successful dentist requires manual dexterity along with knowledge. Therefore, this book is written for both undergraduate and postgraduate dental students who find it difficult to carve and wax teeth and appreciate their features. Most students who are beginners in dentistry may not be skilled, and psychomotor and cognitive skill levels vary from person to person. This book is designed to help these students learn the skills or acquire manual dexterity. Carving skills are helpful in dental technician courses during the initial years of their syllabus for carving on wax blocks and plaster blocks as well as for making acrylic teeth and performing wax-up procedures. Skills are useful in both preparation of tooth morphology and adjustments for casting procedures in later stages of their course.

Although there are many books on dental morphology (anatomy), there are not many that teach the skillful technique of carving (which will also be useful in restorative procedures) and waxing. Cognitive and psychomotor skills strengthen students' ability to effectively achieve the learning outcome.

This book will help students to systematically learn the specific steps of the procedures. For all undergraduate students, postgraduate dental students, and dental lab assistant course students, the book will be very useful for preclinical/lab procedures.

The line diagrams in the book show live demonstrations of the techniques of carving and waxing. They help students face the challenges they encounter in their study and improve their skills. The companion website will provide an overview of the procedural steps.

For exam preparation, this book helps students practise and quickly review the procedures/steps of carving and acquire theoretical knowledge of the morphology of each tooth.

The carving skills for clinicians will help them to provide proper morphology to each tooth, especially in aesthetic procedures and posterior restorative procedures.

This book makes it easy to learn the challenging task of carving (also in restorative procedures) and waxing teeth, using illustrative diagrams in a stepwise manner. It helps in instrumentation, wax preparation for carving, and wax building technique.

Acknowledgements

First and foremost, I thank
Dr. R. Venkata Subramanyam
Professor and Coordinator
Department of Oral & Maxillofacial Surgery and Diagnostic Sciences
College of Dentistry
King Faisal University
Al Ahsa, Saudi Arabia
who has expertise in technology, for introducing me to the software, thereby making my dream come true. I also thank him for his valuable periodic suggestions.

I thank
Dr. Ravi Gummaraju Raghunath
Assistant Professor
Pediatric Dentistry Division
Department of Preventive Dentistry
College of Dentistry
King Faisal University
Al Ahsa, Saudi Arabia
for his support and guidance.

Dr. Benoy Mathews
Assistant Professor
Department of Prosthodontics & Implantology
College of Dentistry
King Faisal University
Al Ahsa, Saudi Arabia
for his support and help with the prosthodontic part of my work.

Dr. Shailesh Lele
FAIMER Institute Fellow
Professor, Department of Oral & Maxillofacial Surgery and Diagnostic Sciences
Coordinator, Department of Dental Education
College of Dentistry, King Faisal University
Al Ahsa, Saudi Arabia
for encouragement and support.

Dr. Abdel Raouf Alotaibi
Professor & Associate Dean
College of Dentistry
King Faisal University
Al Ahsa, Saudi Arabia
for encouragement and support.

Dr. Hamed Al Wadani
Dean, College of Dentistry
King Faisal University
Al Ahsa, Saudi Arabia
for encouragement and support.

About the Companion Website

Don't forget to visit the companion website for this book:

www.wiley.com/go/bangalore/toothcarving

There you will find valuable material designed to enhance your learning, including learning outcomes for all chapters, video resources and all figures as downloadable PowerPoint slides.

Scan this QR code to visit the companion website.

1

Introduction to Dental Anatomy

LEARNING OBJECTIVE
The student should be able to know the definition of dental anatomy, types of dentition, dental formula, and various tooth numbering systems.

Definition of Dental Anatomy

Dental anatomy is defined as the study of the development, morphology, function, and identity of each of the teeth in human dentition [1].

Types of Human Dentition

There are two types of dentition throughout the life of a human being: deciduous dentition and permanent dentition [1]. Deciduous dentition is also called dentition of childhood or primary dentition. This dentition begins prenatally at about 14 weeks in utero. The complete set of teeth in this dentition is seen from years 2–6. Deciduous dentition consists of 20 teeth, 10 in the upper arch and 10 in the lower arch [1, 2]. Permanent dentition is also known as dentition of adulthood or secondary dentition or *succedaneous dentition*. Permanent dentition is composed of 32 teeth, 16 in the upper arch and 16 in the lower. Teeth seen between the deciduous and permanent dentition periods are in the *transition* or *mixed dentition period* [2]. The transition period lasts from about 6–12 years of age and ends when all the deciduous teeth are shed [1].

Arch

The arch formed by the teeth and upper jawbone is the maxillary arch. The arch formed by the teeth and lower jawbone is the mandibular arch. Both the maxillary and the mandibular arches have right and left halves known as quadrants [2].

Quadrants

Each dentition is divided into four quadrants named clockwise as upper right, upper left, lower left, and lower right. The left and right quadrants on both jaws are divided by the midsagittal plane so that the upper right quadrant mirrors the upper left quadrant and the lower right quadrant mirrors the lower left quadrant. Within each quadrant there are four classes of teeth: incisors (central and lateral), canines, premolars (first and second), and molars (first, second, and third) [3].

Dental Formula

For Primary Dentition

This formula (Figure 1.1) should be read as two incisors in the maxilla and two incisors in the mandible, one maxillary canine and one mandibular canine; two maxillary and two mandibular molars, altogether 10 on one side, either right or left side [2].

For Permanent Dentition

The dental formula for permanent dentition (Figure 1.2) is read as two incisors in the maxilla and two incisors in the

An Illustrated Atlas of Tooth Carving and Wax-Up Techniques, First Edition. Anil Bangalore Shivappa.

Companion website: www.wiley.com/go/bangalore/toothcarving

$$I\frac{2}{2}\,C\frac{1}{1}\,M\frac{2}{2}=\frac{\text{5 Teeth in upper quadrant}}{\text{5 Teeth in upper quadrant}}=\text{Total 10 teeth on one side}$$

Figure 1.1 Dental formula for deciduous dentition.

$$I\frac{2}{2}\,C\frac{1}{1}\,PM\frac{2}{2}\,M\frac{3}{3}=\frac{\text{8 Teeth in upper quadrant}}{\text{8 Teeth in upper quadrant}}=\text{Total 16 teeth on one side}$$

Figure 1.2 Dental formula for permanent dentition.

mandible, one maxillary canine and one mandibular canine, two maxillary and two mandibular premolars, three maxillary and three mandibular molars [2].

Tooth Notation

Universal System

In the *universal* system for primary dentition (Figure 1.3) uppercase letters are used starting from A through J (starting from the right maxillary second molar to the left maxillary second molar) for maxillary teeth and from letters K through T (beginning from the left mandibular second molar ending at the right mandibular second molar) for mandibular teeth [2].

In the universal notation system for permanent dentition (Figure 1.4), numbers from 1 through 32 are used for the full set of teeth. The maxillary teeth are numbered from 1 through 16 (beginning from the right maxillary third molar as tooth no. 1 ending at the left maxillary third molar as tooth no. 16). Mandibular teeth are numbered from 17 through 32 (beginning from the left mandibular third molar as tooth no. 17, ending at the right mandibular third molar as tooth no. 32) [2].

Zsigmondy Palmer Notation

In this system both the maxillary and mandibular arches are divided into two quadrants, so that there are a total of four quadrants in the oral cavity, each quadrant with a set of teeth as follows [2, 3]:

For Primary Teeth

In each quadrant capital letters are used to denote teeth, from A (for central incisor) to E (for second molar); see Figure 1.5 [2].

For Permanent Teeth

In each quadrant, numbers are used to denote teeth from 1 (for central incisor) to 8 (for third molar); see Figure 1.6 [2, 3].

Right	A	B	C	D	E	F	G	H	I	J	**Left**
	T	S	R	Q	P	O	N	M	L	K	

Figure 1.3 Universal system for primary dentition.

Right	1	2	3	4	5	6	7	8	9	10	11	12	13	14	15	16
	32	31	30	29	28	27	26	25	24	23	22	21	20	19	18	17

Left

Figure 1.4 Universal system for permanent dentition.

Upper Right	Upper Left
EDCBA	ABCDE
EDCBA	ABCDE
Lower Right	Lower Left

Figure 1.5 Zsigmondy Palmer notation for primary dentition.

Upper Right	Upper Left
87654321	12345678
87654321	12345678
Lower Right	Lower Left

Figure 1.6 Zsigmondy Palmer notation for permanent dentition.

FDI System

A two-digit system proposed by Fédération Dentaire Internationale (FDI): In this system, the first number indicates the quadrant and the second number indicates a particular tooth (Figures 1.7 and 1.8) [2, 3].

For the Primary Teeth

Upper Right					Upper Left				
55	54	53	52	51	61	62	63	64	65
85	84	83	82	81	71	72	73	74	75
Lower Right					Lower Left				

Figure 1.7 FDI system for primary dentition.

For the Permanent Teeth

Upper Right								Upper Left							
18	17	16	15	14	13	12	11	21	22	23	24	25	26	27	28
48	47	46	45	44	43	42	41	31	32	33	34	35	36	37	38
Lower Right								Lower Left							

Figure 1.8 FDI system for permanent dentition.

References

1 Stanley, J.N. and Major, M.A. C. (2010). *Wheeler's Dental Anatomy and Occlusion*, 9e. St. Louis, MO: Saunders Elsevier.

2 Rickne, C.S. and Weiss, G. (2012). *Woelfel's Dental Anatomy*, 8e. Philadelphia: Lippincott Williams & Wilkins.

3 Hillson, S. (2012). *Dental Anthropology*. Cambridge University Press. Kindle Edition.

2

Armamentarium

LEARNING OBJECTIVE

At the end of the chapter, the student should have knowledge of the various applications of the armamentarium used for tooth carving and wax-up technique.

Wax Block

Carving wax (Figure 2.1) is used in dentistry to study and simulate dental anatomy.

Content of carving wax includes

i) Paraffin wax (55–60%)
Solid hydrocarbon mixture obtained from petroleum products. The straight-chain hydrocarbon has 26 carbon atoms.
ii) Beeswax (5%)
Obtained from honeycombs. Composition includes ester complex mixture, saturated and unsaturated hydrocarbons, and high molecular weight organic acid. Two types of beeswax are used: yellow beeswax and bleached beeswax.
iii) Carnauba wax (25%)
An exudate obtained from the pores of the leaves of the Brazilian wax palm tree (*Copernicia prunifera*). It is used to increase melting point and hardness of the paraffin.
iv) Inorganic filler (10–15%)
Most commonly used filler particles are silica and calcium bentonite. Increases hardness, linear thermal expansion, and melting point of carving wax. Filler materials are also added to increase toughness, improve accuracy, obtain smoother carving, avoid bubbles and flaking, and free models and instruments from tackiness [1, 2].

Inlay Wax

Inlay wax is used in waxing or building the anatomy of the tooth for crowns and bridge units that are formed by a casting process using lost-wax pattern technique. It may contain 60% paraffin, 25% carnauba, 10% ceresin, and 5% beeswax. Based on their flow, inlay waxes are classified as hard, regular (medium), or soft. The flow of the inlay wax can be reduced by increasing the percentage of composition of carnauba wax or by adding a paraffin wax with a higher melting point or small amount of resin. Inlay waxes are available in various colours such as deep blue, green, or purple and in various forms such as small pellets or cones or in jars [3].

Lecron Carver

The Lecron carver is a stainless-steel instrument used for carving tooth morphology on carving wax. It is also used for carving on inlay wax [4].

It has the following parts (Figure 2.2):

i) The knife end
ii) The spoon end/excavating end
iii) The handle
iv) The shank

The Knife End

Cutting Edge

The knife end has a cutting edge or blade which has a curved anterior part (Figure 2.3a). This edge is used for carving bulk wax. This part of the cutting edge also helps in creating concavities (Figure 2.3b) on the wax surface (eg, in creating the concave lingual or palatal outline of the anterior teeth) [5].

An Illustrated Atlas of Tooth Carving and Wax-Up Techniques, First Edition. Anil Bangalore Shivappa.

Companion website: www.wiley.com/go/bangalore/toothcarving

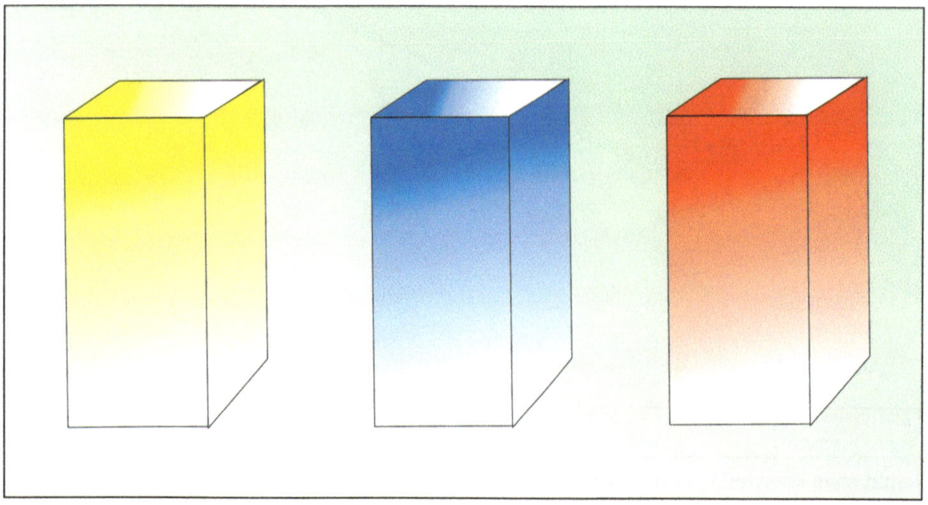

Figure 2.1 Rectangular wax block used for carving human dentition.

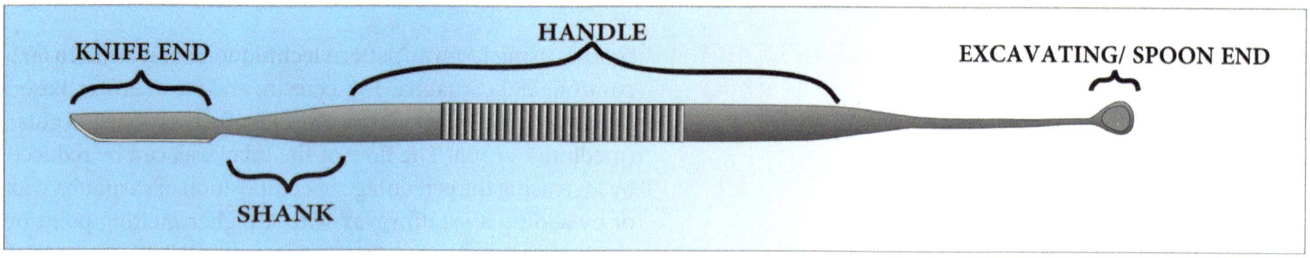

Figure 2.2 Parts of the Lecron carver.

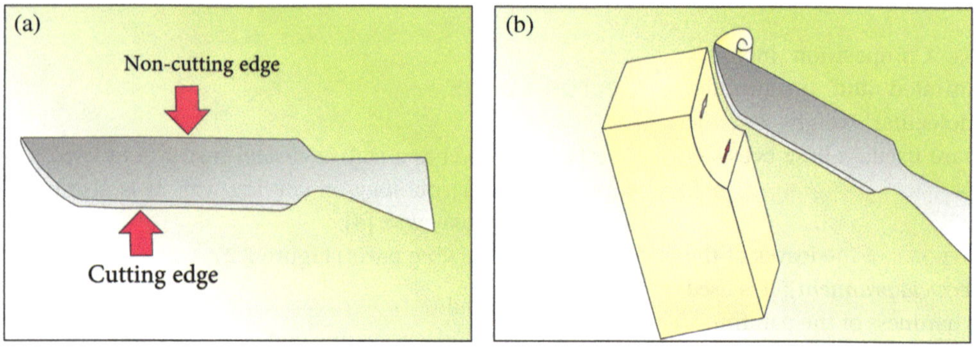

Figure 2.3 Edges of the knife end of the Lecron carver.

Non-cutting Edge/Side

The non-cutting edge/side is used for smoothing wax and creating the slopes of the triangular ridge. Figure 2.4 shows the carving of the mesial slope (2.4a) and distal slope (2.4b) of the mandibular first molar mesiobuccal cusp.

The Spoon End/Excavating End

This end is used in carving lingual or palatal fossae on the crown of anterior teeth and developmental depression on the roots of all teeth (Figure 2.5a–d), by excavating wax [6].

The Handle

This part of the instrument is used to hold the carver (Figure 2.2) [7].

The Shank

The shank connects handle to knife (Figure 2.2). It may be either straight or angled. In carvers the shank is straight [8].

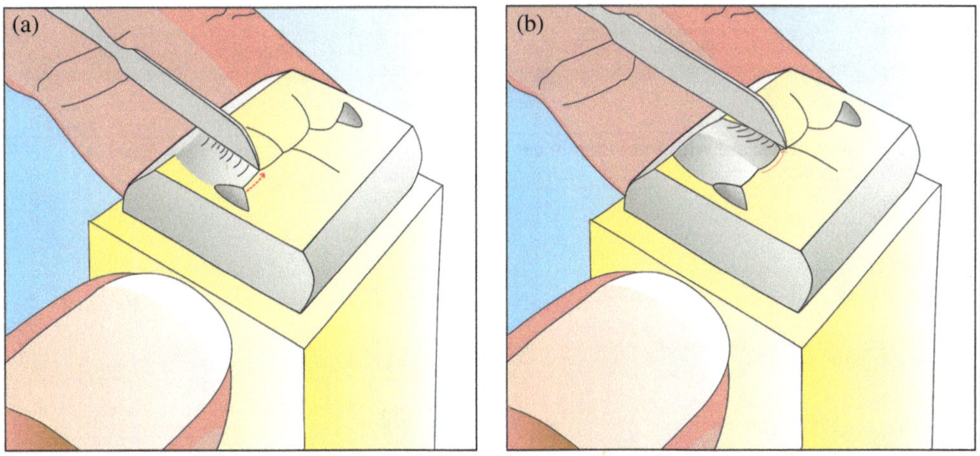

Figure 2.4 Carving the slopes of the triangular ridge using the non-cutting side of the carver.

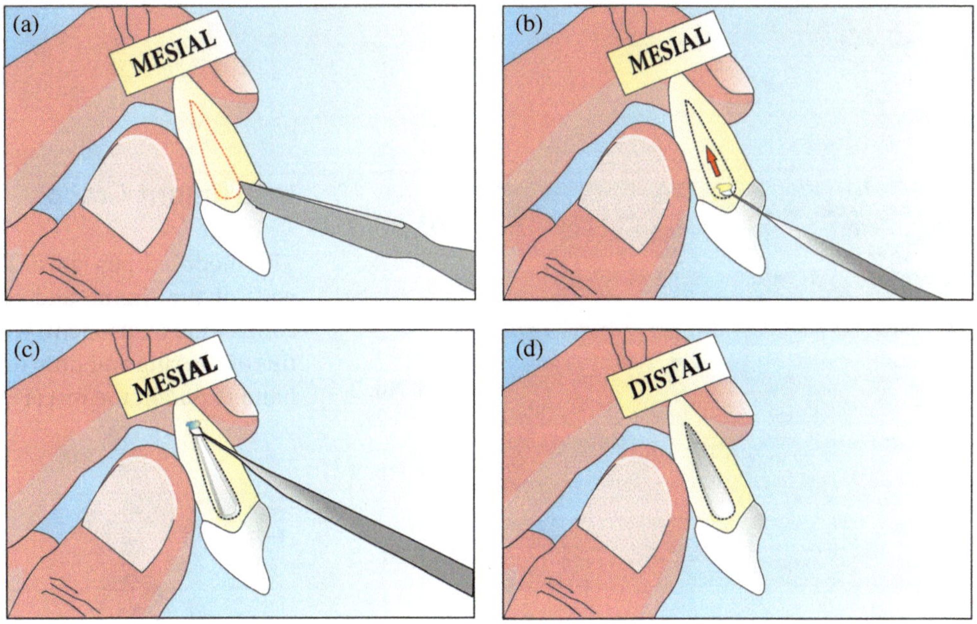

Figure 2.5 (a–d) Carving the developmental depression on the root portion using the spoon end of the carver.

Metallic Scale or Ruler

The metallic scale (Figure 2.6) is used to measure the dimension of the carving before and after the carving procedure.

Vernier Caliper

The Vernier caliper (Figure 2.7) is an aid used to measure

i) Diameter of a small spherical/cylindrical body
ii) The dimensions of a given regular body of known mass and hence to determine its density

It has a main scale and a sliding Vernier scale and four jaws [8].

Waxing Instruments

Based on their use waxing instruments are classified as wax addition, carving, or burnishing. PKT instruments (Figure 2.8) used for waxing technique were designed by

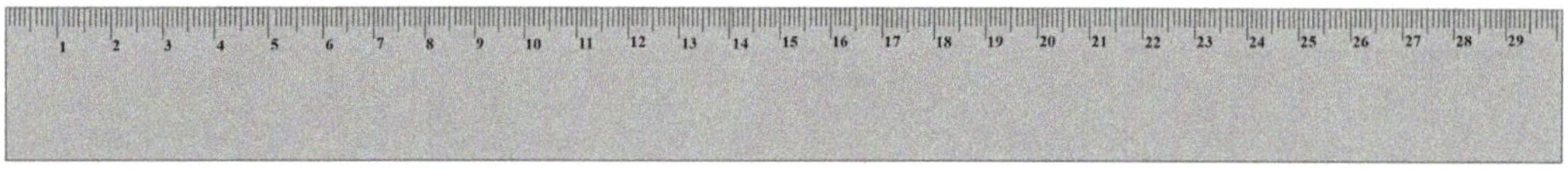

Figure 2.6 Metallic scale with markings in centimetres.

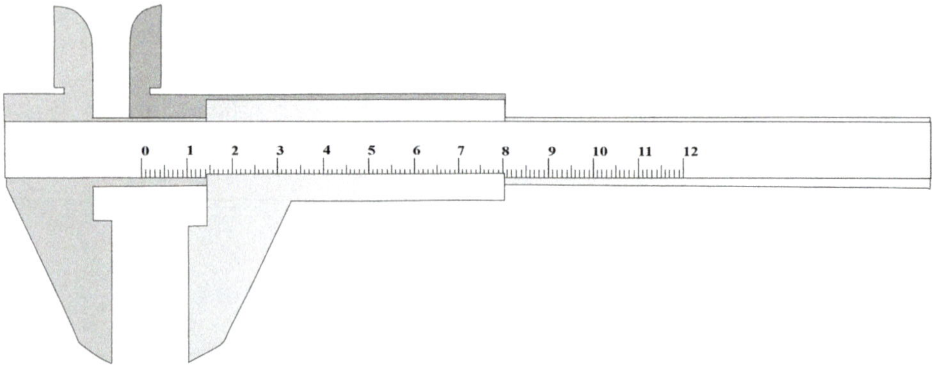

Figure 2.7 Vernier caliper.

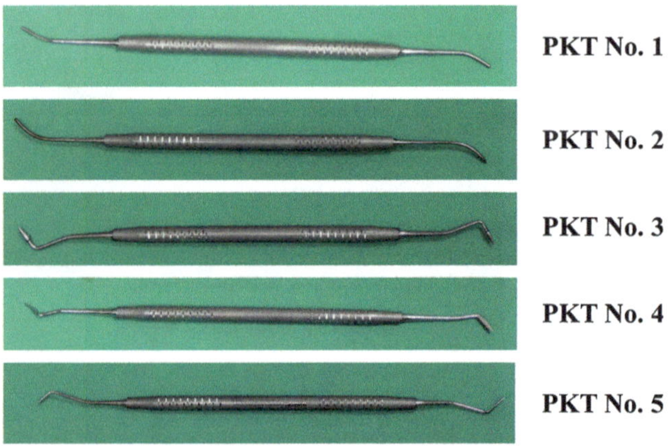

Figure 2.8 PKT instruments set.

Dr. Peter K. Thomas. PKT no. 1 and no. 2 are used for adding wax. (They can also be used for burnishing.) PKT no. 3 is a burnisher for refining the occlusal anatomy, and PKT nos. 4 and 5 instruments are wax carvers. For larger increments of wax, PKT no. 1 is used; for smaller increments, PKT no. 2 is used. A no. 7 waxing spatula is used for adding large increments of wax, especially for the initial coating. Wax is melted by heating the instrument first near its shank, then touching the wax and quickly reheating the shank [9].

Instrument Grasps

The modified pen grasp improves the tactile sense. The pads of the thumb and of the index and middle fingers contact the instrument, while the tip of the ring finger (or tips of the ring and little fingers) is placed on the opposing hand to obtain the rest (Figure 2.10a and b) [7].

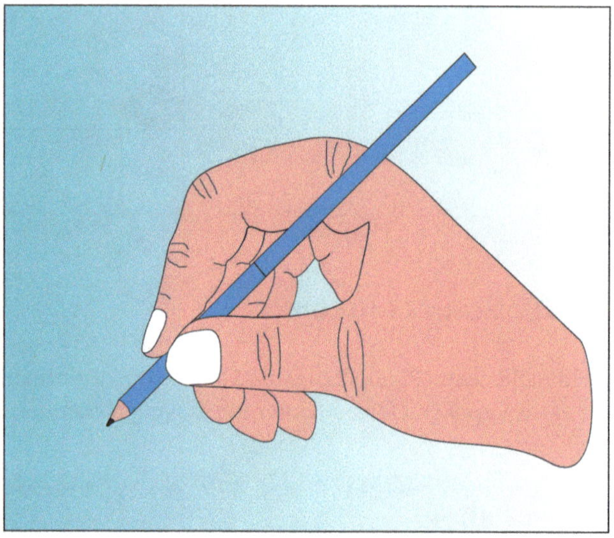

Figure 2.9 Pen grasp.

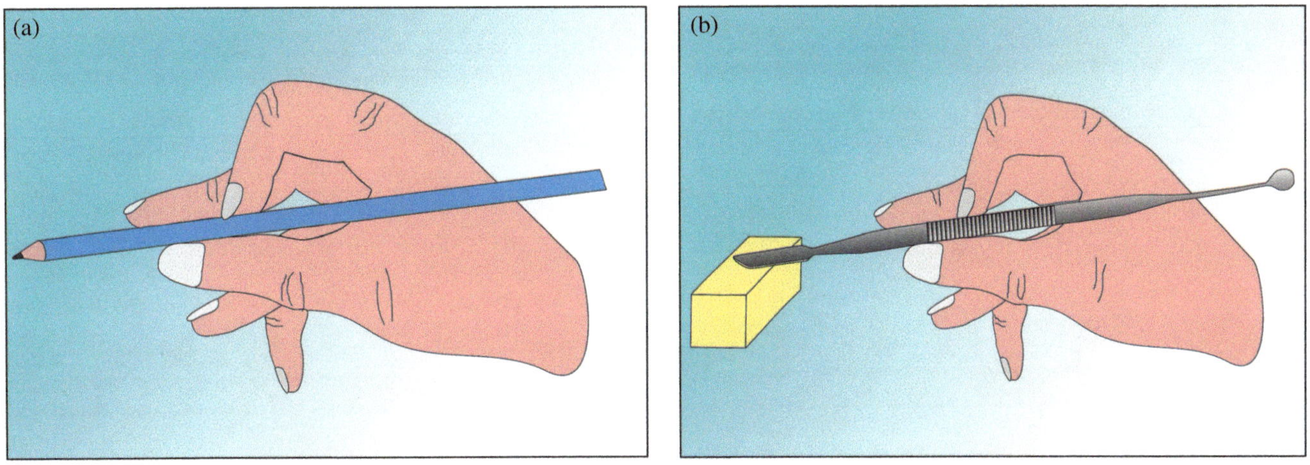

Figure 2.10 Modified pen grasp used for holding the instruments.

References

1 Widjijono Widjijono, Purwanto A, Dyah I. (2009).Mechanical properties of carving wax with various Ca-bentolite filter composition. *Dental Journal* 42. (3): 114–117

2 Widjijono (2009). Correlation between calcium bentonite concentration and paraffin wax to the hardness of carving wax. *Dental Journal* 14 (1): 20–23

3 Craig, R.G. and Powers, J.M. (2012). *Restorative Dental Materials*, 11e. St. Louis, MO: Mosby.

4 Tony, J., David, G.P., Christopher, W.S., and David, G.W. (2016). *Basics of Dental Technology: A Step by Step Approach*, 2e. West Sussex: Wiley Blackwell.

5 Veecarestores (2019). Lecron carver: Use in dentistry. https://veecaredentalinstruments.tumblr.com/post/189770090499/lecron-carver-use-in-dentistry (accessed 19 March 2020).

6 Medical Tools (2020). Lecron wax carver. https://medical-tools.com/shop/lecron-wax-carver.html (accessed 19 March 2020).

7 Harald, O.H., Edward, J.S., and Andre, V.R. (2013). *Sturdevant's Art and Science of Operative Dentistry*, 6e. St. Louis, MO: Elsevier.

8 National Council of Educational Research and Training (n.d.). Experiments. http://ncert.nic.in/ncerts/l/kelm102.pdf (accessed 19 March 2020).

9 Stephen, F.R., Martin, F.L., and Junhei, F. (2016). *Contemporary Fixed Prosthodontics*, 5e. St. Louis, MO: Elsevier.

Part I

Carving

3

Pre-carving Preparation of Wax Blocks

LEARNING OBJECTIVE
The student will be able to assess the condition of the wax block and perform preparation steps before the actual carving steps.

Smoothing the Wax Surface

Wax block obtained from the manufacturers will have irregularities, air spaces, or voids (Figure 3.1). These are created due to low filler content or entrapment of air during pouring into and hardening of the wax in the mould [1]. The wax surface should be smoothed before carving [2, 3]. Use the non-cutting edge of the carver in a single direction (Figure 3.2) to smooth surfaces (Figures 3.3 and 3.4)

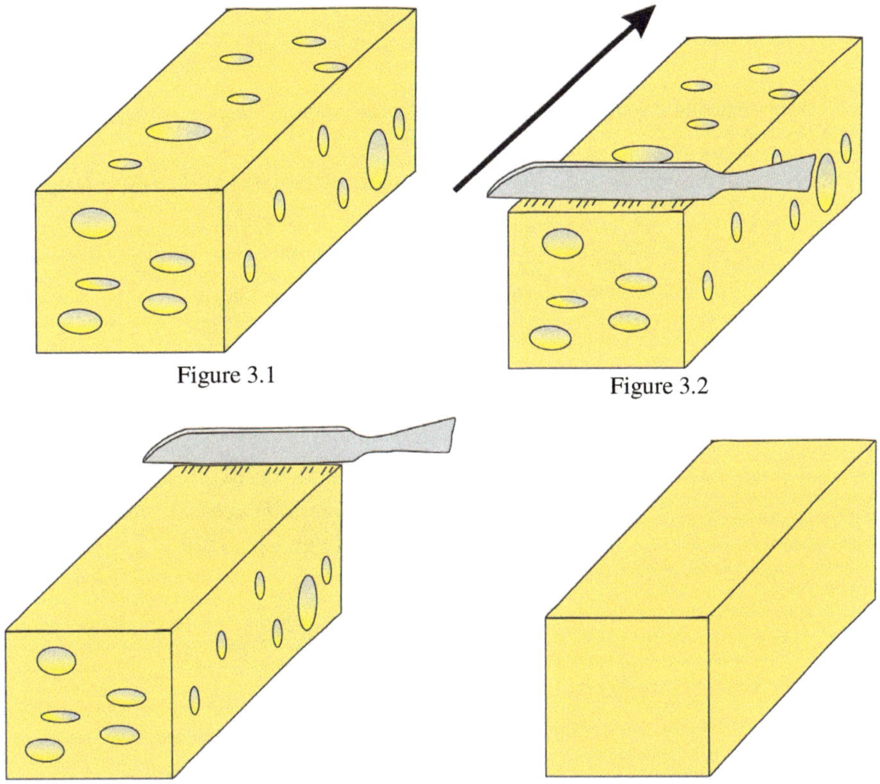

Figure 3.1

Figure 3.2

Figure 3.3

Figure 3.4

Figures 3.1–3.4 Technique to smooth wax block surface before the carving step sequence.

An Illustrated Atlas of Tooth Carving and Wax-Up Techniques, First Edition. Anil Bangalore Shivappa.

Companion website: www.wiley.com/go/bangalore/toothcarving

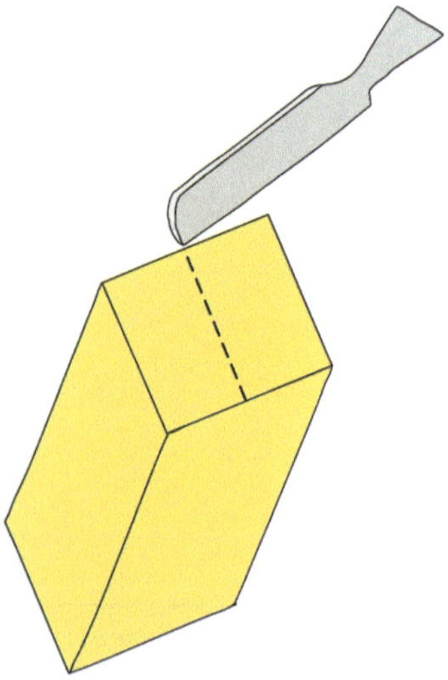

Figure 3.5

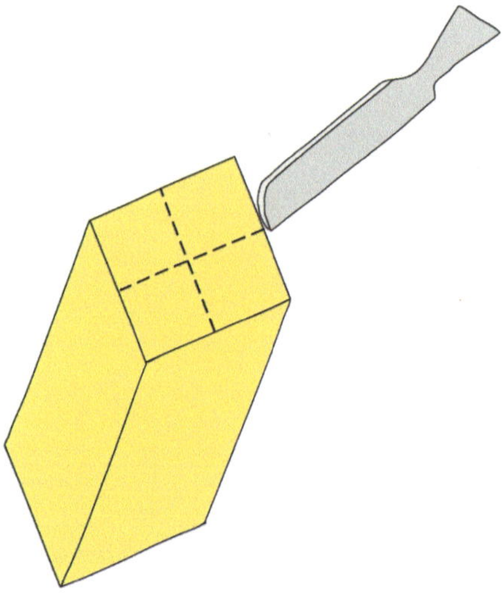

Figure 3.6

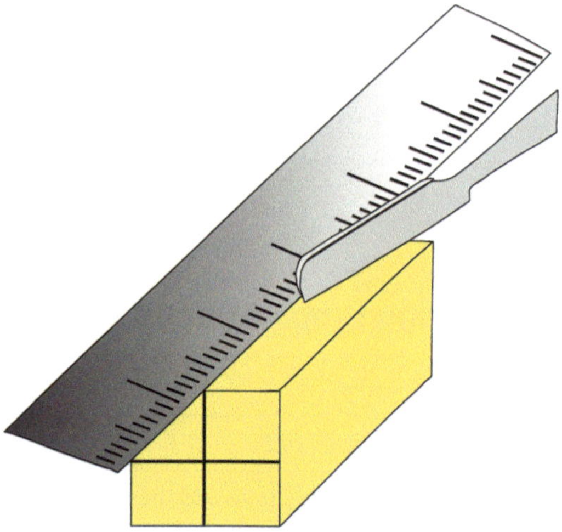

Figure 3.7

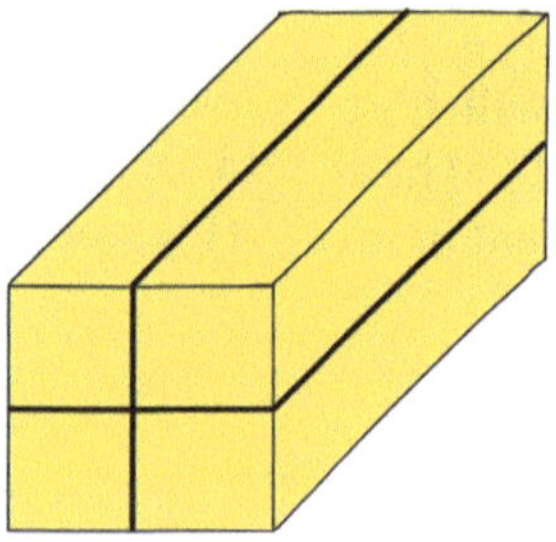

Figure 3.8

Figures 3.5–3.8 Sequence of steps to divide the wax blocks before the actual carving steps.

Division of Wax Block

Divide each end of the wax block into four equal parts. Taking the guidance of the cross lines at the ends divide each side of the wax block into two equal parts. The midline drawn on the wax block would help in placing the incisal edge of a tooth either buccally or lingually or in the centre to the long axis (the midline drawn), depending on the tooth (Figures 3.5–3.8).

References

1 Widjijono, Purwanto, A., and Dyah, I. (2009). Mechanical properties of carving wax with various Ca-bentolite filter composition. *Dental Journal* 42 (3): 114–117.

2 Linek, H.A. (1949). *Tooth Carving Manual*, 1e. Long Island City, NY: Columbia Dentoform Corporation.

3 Rashmi, G.S. (2014). *Textbook of Dental Anatomy, Physiology and Occlusion*, 1e. New Delhi: Jaypee Brothers Medical Publishers Ltd.

4

Anatomical Landmarks

LEARNING OBJECTIVE
At the end of the chapter, the student should have knowledge of various anatomical landmarks of anterior and posterior teeth that enhances the psychomotor skills for carving and waxing techniques.

Crown

Anatomic crown: Part of the tooth covered by enamel (Figure 4.1a) [1, 2].

Clinical crown: Part of the crown, visible in the oral cavity (Figure 4.1a) [1].

Root/Radicular Part

Anatomic root: Part of a tooth covered by cementum (Figure 4.1b) [1].

Clinical root: Part of a tooth covered with gingiva (Figure 4.1b) [1].

Median Line

The imaginary line that runs through the centre of the face, between the central incisors at their point of contact both in the maxilla and the mandible (Figure 4.1c) [1, 3].

Aspect

Labial Aspect

Features of the labial surface bordered by mesial, distal cervical, and incisal outlines (Figure 4.1d).

Lingual/Palatal Aspect

Features of the lingual surface bordered by mesial, distal cervical, and incisal outlines (Figure 4.1d).

Mesial Aspect

Features of the mesial surface bordered by labial, lingual/palatal, cervical, and incisal outlines (Figure 4.1e).

Distal Aspect

Features of the distal surface bordered by labial, lingual/palatal, cervical, and incisal outlines (Figure 4.1e).

Incisal Aspect

Features seen from a view bordered by labial, lingual/palatal, mesial, and distal outlines (Figure 4.1f).

Surfaces

'Facial surfaces' is a collective term for the surfaces of teeth facing towards lips or buccal surfaces. Individually, the surfaces of the anterior teeth (incisors and canine) facing towards the lips are called labial surfaces. Those surfaces of posterior teeth facing towards the cheek are known as buccal surfaces. Those surfaces of mandibular teeth facing towards the tongue are called lingual surfaces. Lingual surfaces on

An Illustrated Atlas of Tooth Carving and Wax-Up Techniques, First Edition. Anil Bangalore Shivappa.

Companion website: www.wiley.com/go/bangalore/toothcarving

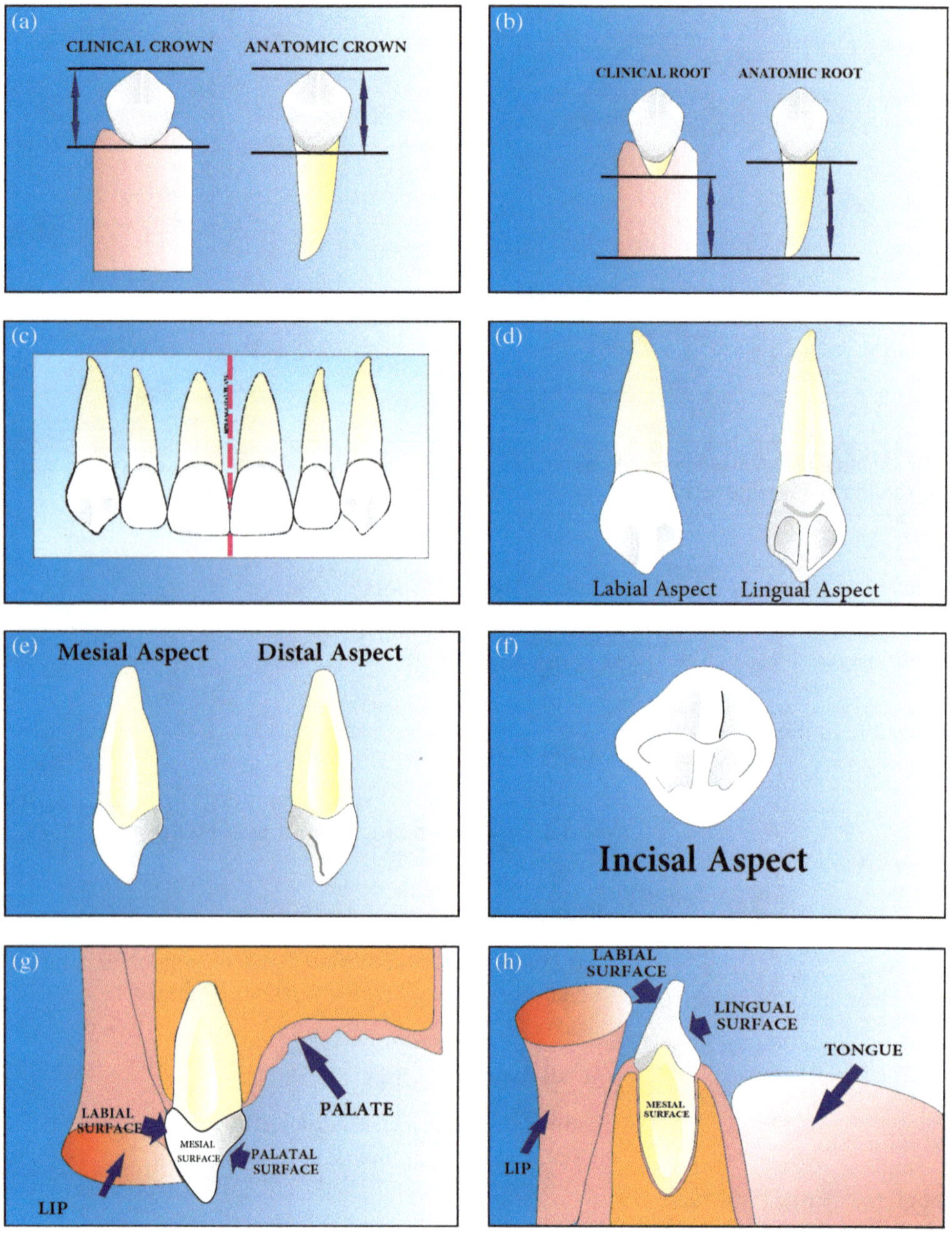

Figure 4.1 (a–h) Anatomical landmarks of human permanent dentition.

maxillary teeth are also known as palatal surfaces. Surfaces of a tooth contacting adjacent teeth in the same dental arch are called proximal surfaces. The proximal surfaces of teeth facing towards the median line are called mesial surfaces (Greek *mesos*; middle). The proximal surfaces facing away from the median line or midline of an arch are known as distal surfaces. The point at which the teeth contact each other is the contact area, which can be mesial or distal (Figure 4.1g and h) [1–3].

Surfaces of posterior teeth (premolars and molars) that contacts teeth of the opposing jaw during occlusion are called occlusal surfaces. These surfaces become incisal edges in case of incisors and cusp tips with respect to canines [1–3].

Mamelons

Rounded elevations or tubercles or protuberances at the incisal portions of incisors, seen on the newly erupted teeth formed from the facial developmental lobes (Figure 4.2a) [1, 2]. They are usually three in number and the mesial mamelon is usually the tallest [3].

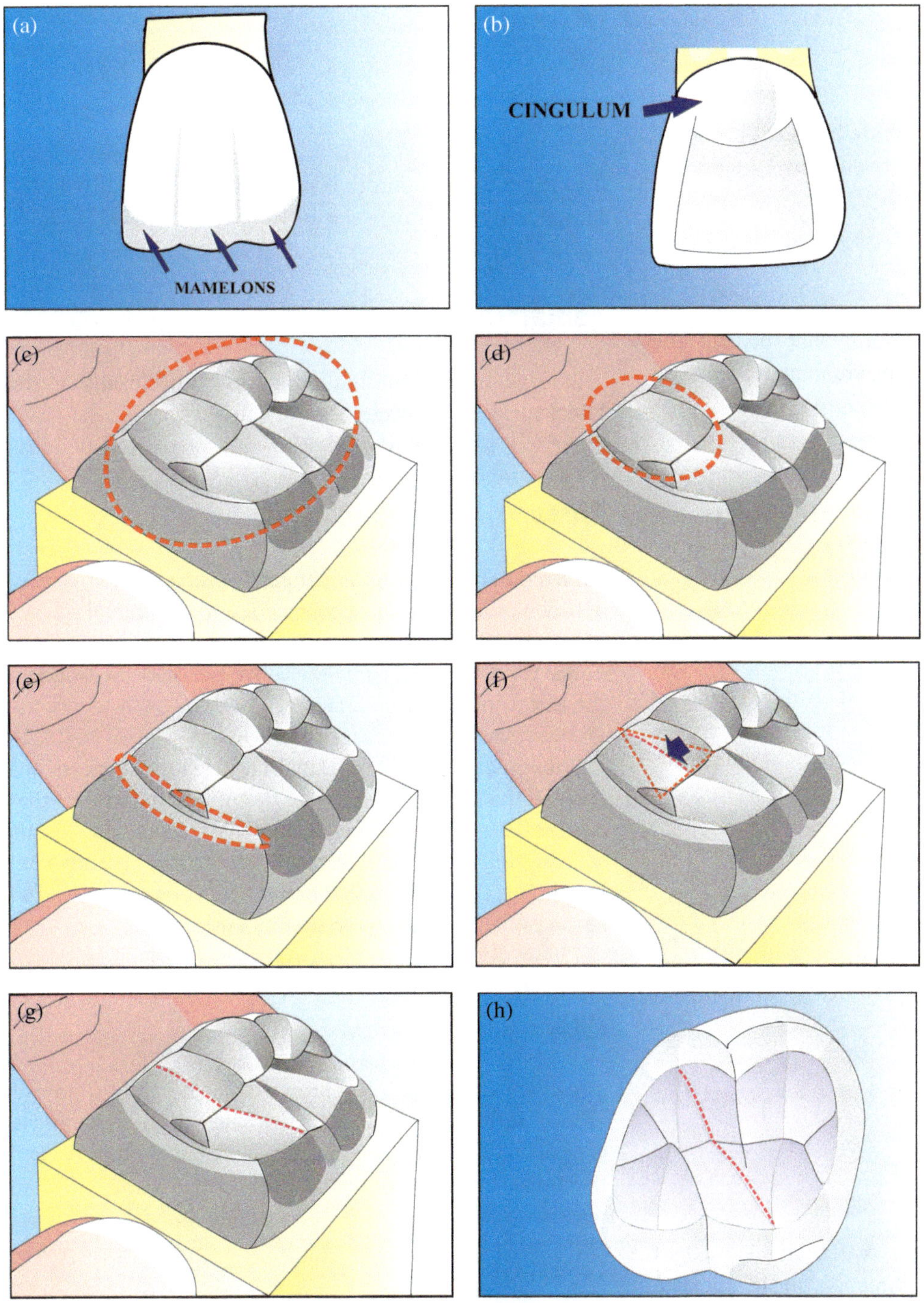

Figure 4.2 (a–h) Anatomical landmarks of human permanent dentition.

Cingulum

In Latin cingulum means girdle [3]. It is the lingual lobe among four developmental lobes of anterior teeth that makes up the bulk of the cervical third of the lingual surface (Figure 4.2b) [2].

Occlusal Table

The occlusal surface of posterior teeth, bounded by cuspal ridges buccally and lingually, and proximally by marginal ridges (Figure 4.2c) [1].

Cusp

A triangular or pyramidal elevation that divides the occlusal surface of the crown. Cusps are named according to their location (Figure 4.2d) [2].

Ridge

The linear elevation on tooth surface [2].

Marginal Ridges

The rounded borders of the enamel that forms margin of a tooth (Figure 4.2e).

Ex: Mesial and distal marginal ridges on the occlusal surface of a posterior teeth [1, 2].

Triangular Ridge

A linear elevation with slopes on either side, starting from the tip of the cusp descending towards the centre of the occlusal surface of posterior teeth. Named according to the cusp involved (Figure 4.2f) [1, 2]:

i) Buccal triangular ridge
ii) Lingual triangular ridge

Transverse Ridge

A ridge formed by the union of two triangular ridges transversely in the buccolingual direction on the occlusal surfaces of the posterior teeth (Figure 4.2g).

Ex: buccal and lingual triangular ridges join to form a transverse ridge [1, 2].

Oblique Ridge

A ridge crossing the occlusal surface of the maxillary molar teeth obliquely (Figure 4.2h).

Formed by the union of the distal cuspal ridge of the mesiopalatal cusp and the triangular ridge of the distobuccal cusp [1–3].

Buccal Ridge

The ridge or elevation that runs cervico-occlusally on the buccal surface of the posterior teeth (Figure 4.3a) [1, 2].

Labial Ridge

The ridge or elevation that runs cervico-occlusally on the labial surface of canines (Figure 4.3b) [1].

Fossa

An irregular depression or concavity seen on the surface.

Irregular depressions or concavities on the lingual surface of incisors – lingual fossae (Figure 4.3c).

The concavity formed by the convergence of the ridges at the centre of occlusal surface of posterior teeth where the groove terminal unites is the central fossa (Figure 4.3d) [1, 2].

Triangular fossae are triangular irregular depressions seen on the occlusal surfaces of premolars and molars that are mesial or distal to marginal ridges. They can also be seen on lingual surfaces of maxillary incisors (Figure 4.3e) [1, 2]. The canine fossa is a broad concavity on the mesial surface of the maxillary first premolar [3].

Pits

These are the pinpoint depressions seen at the union of groove terminals. Pits are enclosed within the fossae (Figure 4.3f). Mesial and distal pits are enclosed in respective fossae on posterior teeth [1, 2].

Central Pit

Anatomical landmark seen as pinpoint depression at the junction where developmental grooves unite in the central fossa of molars (Figure 4.3f) [1].

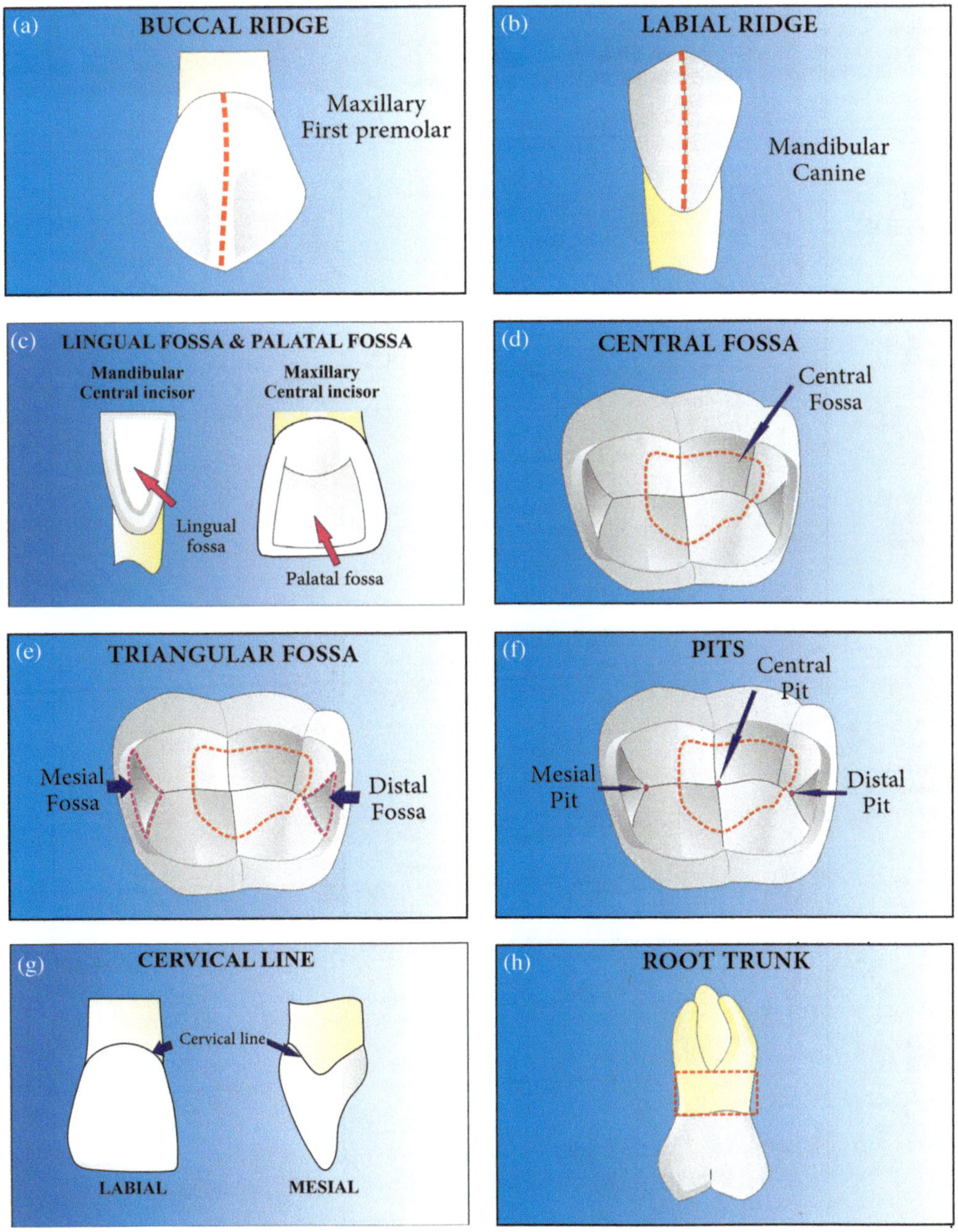

Figure 4.3 (a–h) Anatomical landmarks of human permanent dentition.

Cervical Line

Junction formed by the union of crown and root (Figure 4.3g). It represents the junction where the portion of the tooth covered with enamel meets the portion covered by cementum [4]. Proximally it curves towards the incisal edge in anterior teeth and towards the occlusal surface in posterior teeth. In general, curvature of the cervical line is more on the mesial side compared to the distal and greatest on the anterior teeth, diminishing on posterior teeth [1, 2].

Root Trunk

Part of the root on the posterior teeth between the cervical line and furcal area. Also called a trunk base (Figure 4.3h) [1].

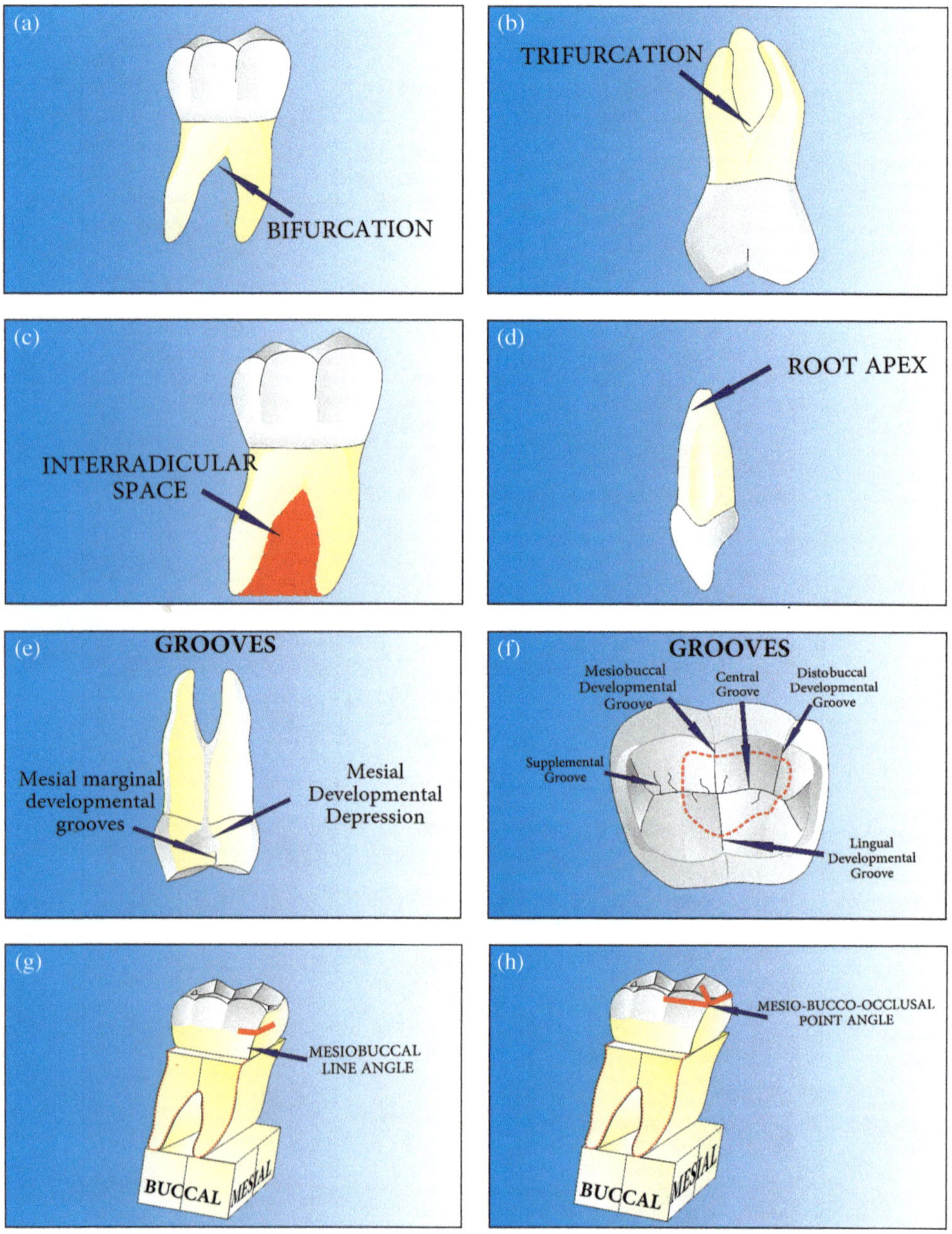

Figure 4.4 (a–h) Anatomical landmarks of human permanent dentition.

Root Furcation

It is the division of roots [1, 3].

Bifurcation

Seen on two-rooted teeth (Figure 4.4a) [1, 3].

Trifurcation

Seen on three-rooted teeth (Figure 4.4b) [1, 3].

Furcal Region or Interradicular Space

The space apical to root furcation and between the roots (Figure 4.4c) [1].

Root Apex

The tip of the root at its end (Figure 4.4d) [2, 4]

Developmental Groove

Shallow linear depression or fissure or furrow between the primary parts of the crown or root (Figure 4.4e) [2–4].

Central Groove

Groove located centrally on the occlusal surface, within the sulcus of the posterior teeth and running in a mesiodistal direction (Figure 4.4f) [1, 2].

Buccal Groove

Buccal extension from the central groove on the occlusal surface of the posterior teeth (Figure 4.4f) [1].

Lingual Grooves

Lingual extension from the central groove on the occlusal surface of the posterior teeth (Figure 4.4f) [1].

Supplemental Groove

Shallow linear depressions supplemental to a developmental groove (Figure 4.4f).

Line Angle

Angle formed by the union of two surfaces (Figure 4.4g) [1].

Point Angle

Angle formed by the union of three surfaces (Figure 4.4h) [1].

Crest of Contour

Also called crest of curvature, height of contour. It is the maximum height on a convex outline of the tooth structure [1].

References

1 Rickne, C.S. and Weiss, G. (2012). *Woelfel's Dental Anatomy*, 8e. Philadelphia: Lippincott Williams & Wilkins.
2 Stanley, J.N. and Major, M.A.C. (2010). *Wheeler's Dental Anatomy and Occlusion*, 9e. St. Louis, MO: Saunders Elsevier.
3 Hillson, S. (2012). *Dental Anthropology*. Cambridge University Press. Kindle Edition.
4 Edgar, H.J.H. (2017). *Dental Morphology for Anthropology*, (p. iii). Taylor and Francis. Kindle Edition.

5

Permanent Maxillary Central Incisor

LEARNING OBJECTIVE
At the end of the chapter, the student should be able to have knowledge of maxillary central incisor and develop the psychomotor skills for waxing and carving the same.

Permanent Maxillary Right Central Incisor

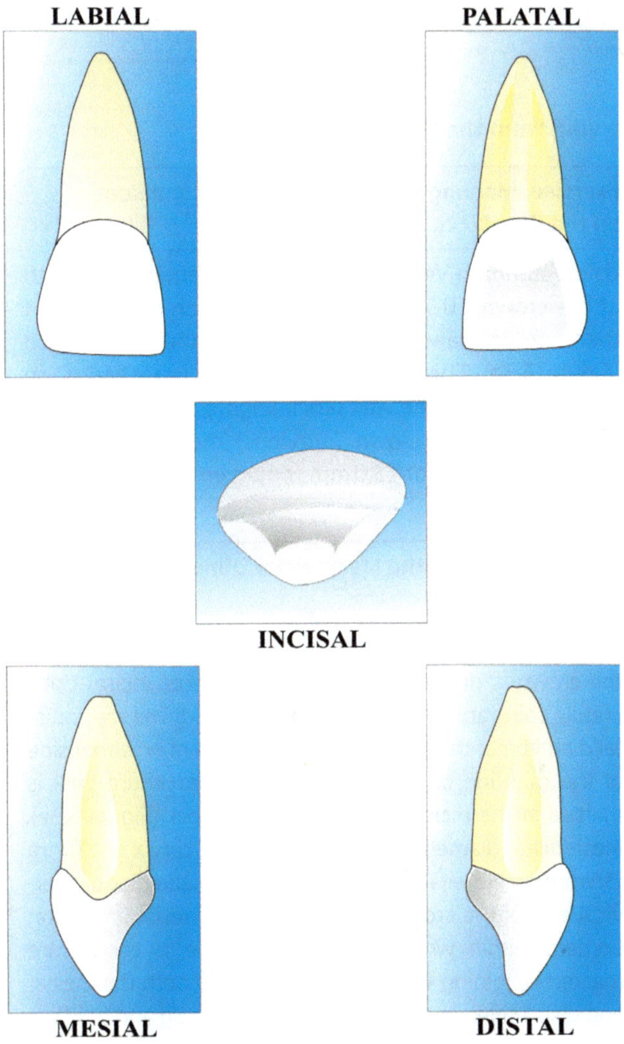

Labial Aspect

Crown

The maxillary central incisor is the first tooth from the midline (Figure 5.1). From this aspect, the crown is trapezoidal in shape, with parallel unequal sides represented by incisal and cervical outline. There are four outlines for the crown: mesial, distal, cervical, and incisal (Figure 5.2a) [1]. For the sake of describing the surface and crest of contour, the labial surface of the crown is divided into three equal parts inciso-cervically: the incisal third, middle third, and cervical third

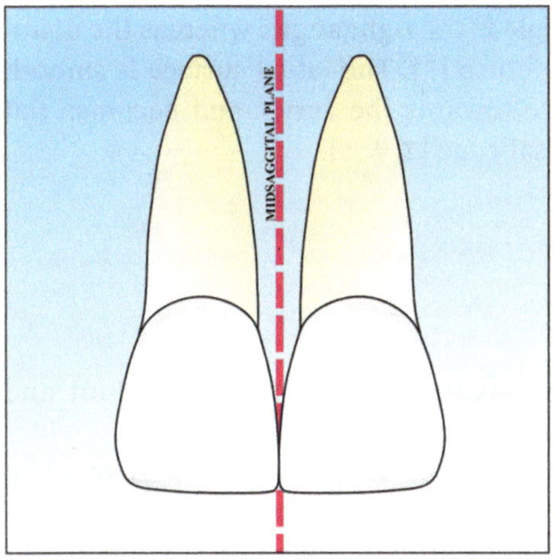

Figure 5.1 Position of the maxillary central incisor in relation to the midsagittal plane.

An Illustrated Atlas of Tooth Carving and Wax-Up Techniques, First Edition. Anil Bangalore Shivappa.

Companion website: www.wiley.com/go/bangalore/toothcarving

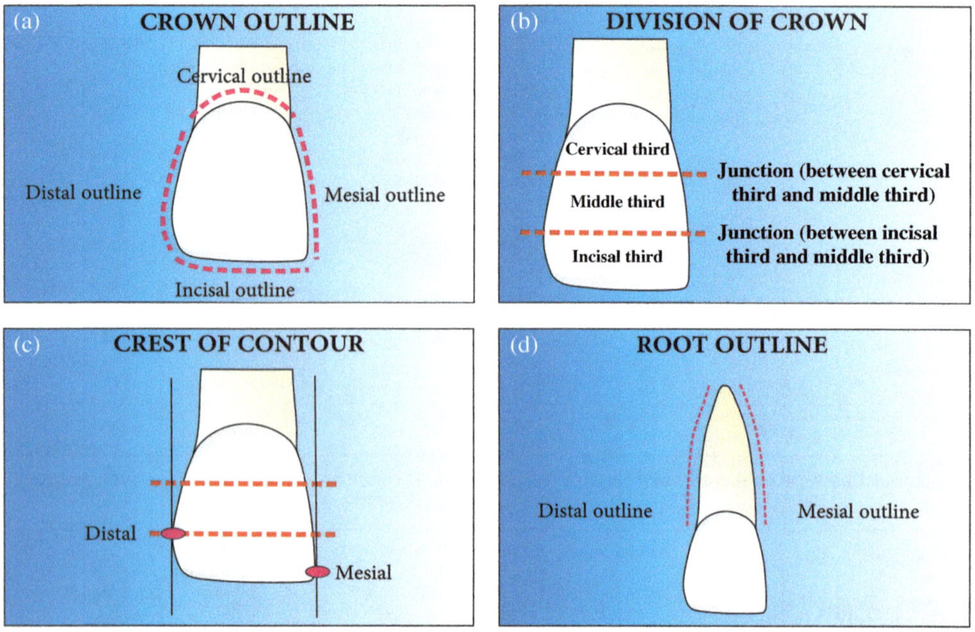

Figure 5.2 (a-d) Characteristic features of the crown and root of the maxillary right central incisor from the labial aspect.

(Figure 5.2b) [2]. The mesial and distal outline of the crown has crest of contour. The crest of curvature or crest of contour is the maximum bulge of the convex outline. It is the point at which the tooth contacts the neighbouring tooth [2, 3]. The mesial outline has crest of curvature near the mesio-incisal angle, which makes it to appear less convex. The distal outline is more convex with crest of curvature at the junction of the middle third and the incisal third (Figure 5.2b and c) [1–3]. The cervical outline is semicircular with convexity facing towards the root. The incisal edge is nearly horizontal [1, 2]. With the crest of curvatures at different levels, the mesio-incisal angle is the right angle; whereas the disto-incisal angle is obtuse [3]. The labial surface is smooth and convex more towards the cervix and becomes flat towards the incisal edge [2, 4, 5].

Root

The root of the maxillary central incisor is blunt and cone shaped with regular outlines. The root is wider mesiodistally than labiopalatally. Mesiodistally the root is thicker at the cervical third and then tapers apically in the middle and apical third of the root [2]. Long axis of the tooth parallels the mesial outline of both crown and root (Figure 5.2d) [1].

Carving from the Labial Aspect

Exercise: Marking the Length of Crown and Root on the Wax Block

Using standard Vernier caliper, measurement of length of the crown, 10.5 mm (distance between two beaks of the external jaws) is marked from the incisal end (Figure 5.3a). The same measurement is extended on other surfaces of the wax block (Figure 5.3b). At the cervical end of the crown (previous) measurement, the length of the root of 13.0 mm is marked (Figure 5.3c) [2].

Exercise: Marking the Mesiodistal Dimension of the crown

Once the crown and root length is measured and marked, the crown is divided into three equal parts: incisal third, middle third, and cervical third (Figure 5.3d). The mesiodistal diameter of the crown of 8.5 mm (4.25 mm on either side of the mid-line of wax) indicating the maximum bulk is marked at the incisal edge of the wax block (Figure 5.3e). Mesiodistal diameter of the crown at the cervix of 7.0 mm (3.5 mm on either side of the midline) is marked at the cervical end of the crown (Figure 5.3f). The mesial and distal borders within which the crown outline is carved are marked by joining the reference points on both the mesial and distal sides on the wax block (Figure 5.3g and h) [2].

Exercise: Technique to Carve Excess Wax from Mesial and Distal side

Excess unwanted wax (indicated in blue colour) mesial and distal to the crown dimension should be carved (Figure 5.3i–k). With the cutting edge of the carver facing the unwanted wax at the middle and incisal thirds on mesial side, the carver is run labiopalatally from the surface of the wax, until the mesial border is reached (Figure 5.3l and m). Remaining excess wax in the cervical third is carved using the front part of non-cutting side of the carver facing wax and tip towards the cervix, as shown (Figure 5.3n). Then the carver is run in the labiopalatal direction. The same technique is applied on the distal side (Figure 5.3o and p)

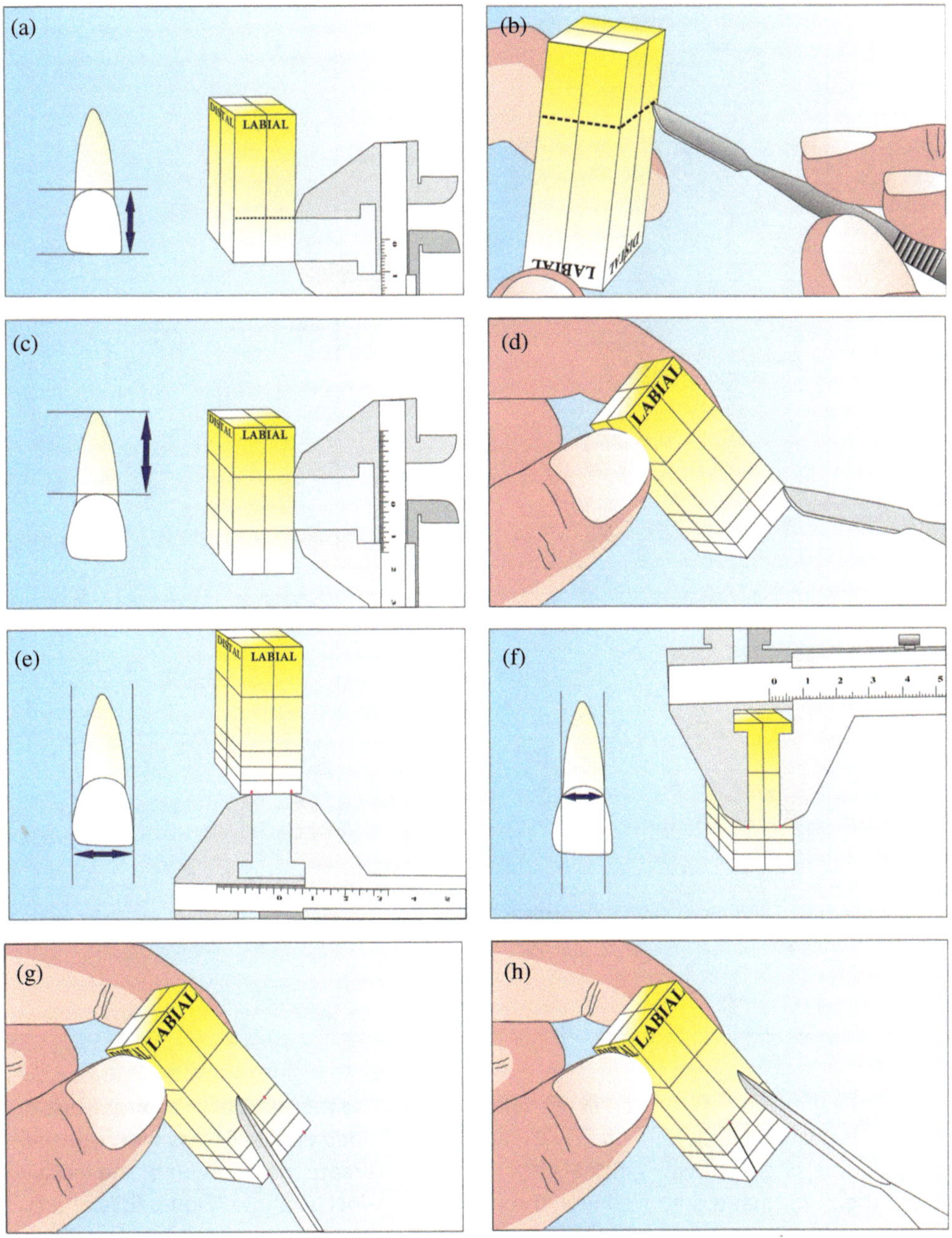

Figure 5.3 (a–h) Measuring and marking the crown dimension and root length on the labial surface.

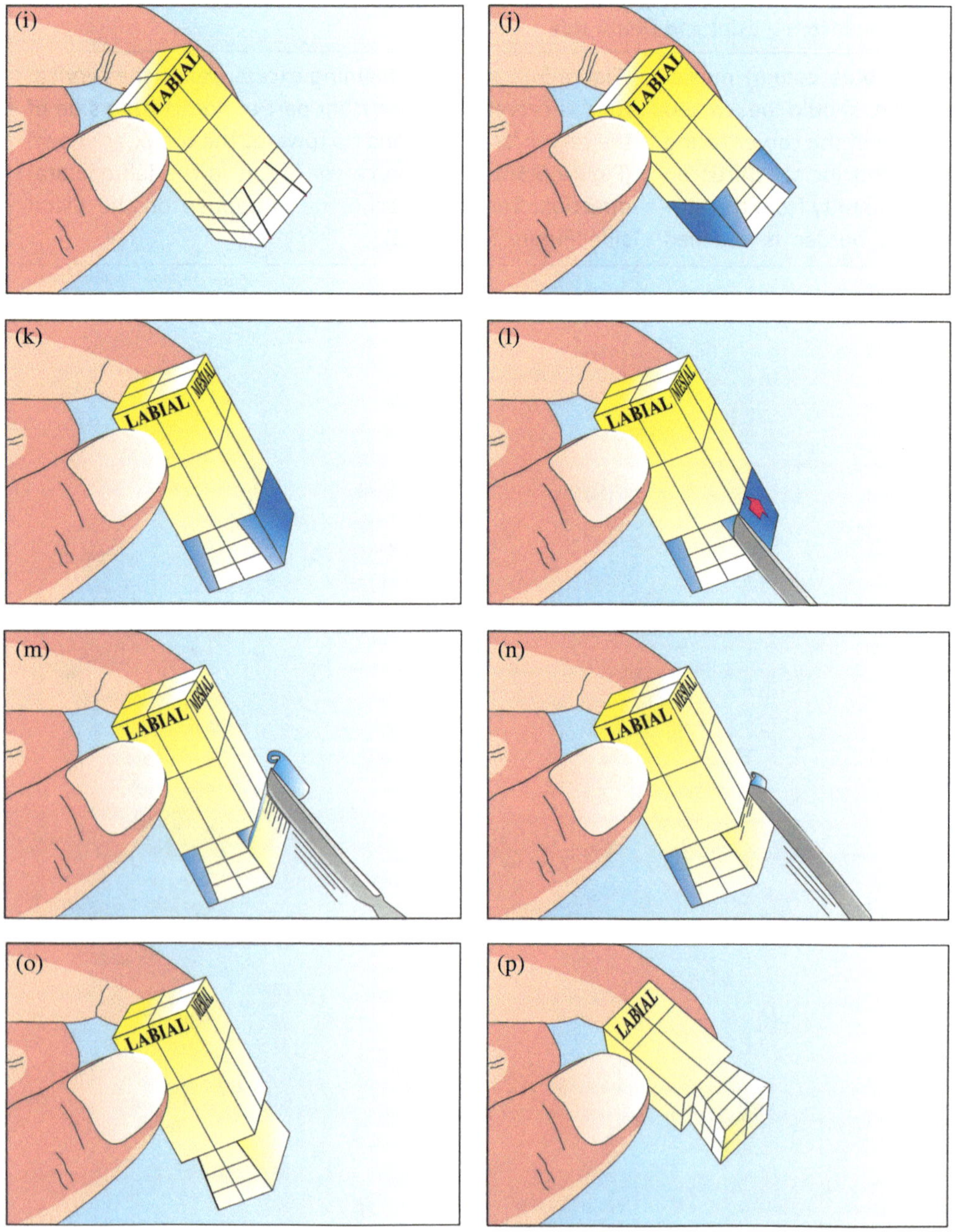

Figure 5.3 (i–p) Carving excess wax from the mesial and distal side of the crown border.

Exercise: Marking and Carving the Outline of the Crown

The crest of contour is marked mesially near mesio-incisal angle, distally at the junction between incisal and middle third (Figure 5.3q and r). Then the outline of the crown drawn (Figure 5.3r) beginning from the point marked at the cervical line (on the mesial side) to the mesial crest of contour then to the incisal edge, continuing to the distal crest of contour and back to the cervical line (on the distal side), with features described earlier. Excess wax near the incisal edge is carved to create the distal lift of the incisal edge and rounded disto-incisal angle (Figure 5.3s and t). In the same way, the excess wax is carved in other areas to get a proper outline.

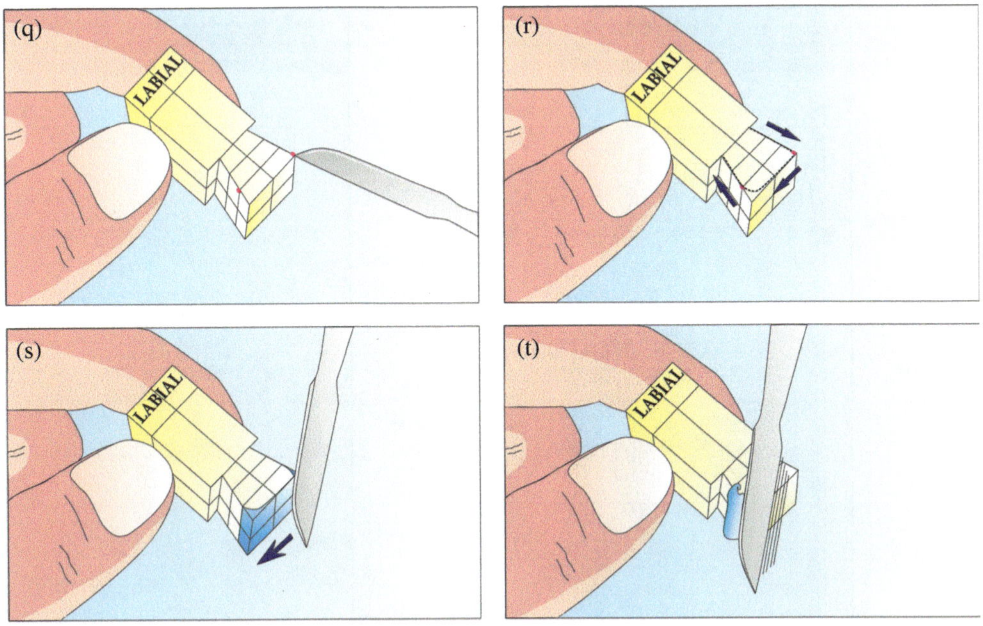

Figure 5.3 (q–t) Marking and carving the outline of the crown on labial surface.

Mesial Aspect

From this aspect, the crown appears wedge or triangular shaped, with the base at the cervix and the apex near the incisal edge (Figure 5.4a) [1, 2]. The incisal edge is slightly labial or in line with the long axis of the tooth [2, 3]. From this aspect, the crown exhibits three outlines – labial, palatal, and cervical – and an incisal edge [2]. The labial outline starts from the cervical line to the crest of contour, which is in the cervical third just coronal to the cervical line (Figure 5.4b and c). From the crest of contour, the outline becomes less convex uniformly, up to the incisal ridge or edge (Figure 5.4d). The palatal outline forms an 'S' shape. It starts from the cervical line with crest of contour at the cervical third just coronal to the cervical line (Figure 5.4e). The outline in this cervical third represents the cingulum with convex outline (Figure 5.4f). Below the cingulum the outline becomes concave until the incisal edge, where it becomes convex (Figure 5.4g and h) [1–4]. The cervical line in this aspect curves more incisally than that seen from the distal aspect [3].The root from this aspect appears blunt and cone shaped, wider in the labiopalatal direction [1]. The labial outline is nearly straight whereas the palatal outline is straight at the cervical third and tapers labially towards the tip at the middle and apical third [3].

Carving from Proximal (Mesial or Distal) Aspect

Exercise: Marking the Labiopalatal Dimension of the crown

The labiopalatal dimension of the crown at the cervix of 7.0 mm (3.5 mm on either side of the midline) is marked at the cervix (Figure 5.5a and b). The labiopalatal dimension of the crown which is the bulkiest dimension of the crown measuring 8.0 mm (4.0 mm on either side of the midline) is marked at the occlusal edge of the wax (Figure 5.5c and d) [2].

Exercise: Marking the Outline of the Crown on Mesial / Distal Surface

Within the dimension obtained in the previous exercise, the outline of the crown is drawn starting from the reference point on the labial side of the cervical line to the labial crest of contour, from here to the incisal edge. Then the palatal outline is drawn, starting from the palatal reference point at the cervical line to the crest of contour palatally, completing the convexity in the cervical third representing the cingulum. Then the concave outline is drawn in the middle third and incisal third. Near the incisal edge, once again the convexity is drawn connecting the labial outline (Figure 5.5e).

The wax outside the crown outline is excess wax (blue coloured part on the wax), which should be carved from labial and palatal surface of the wax until the respective outline (Figure 5.5f).

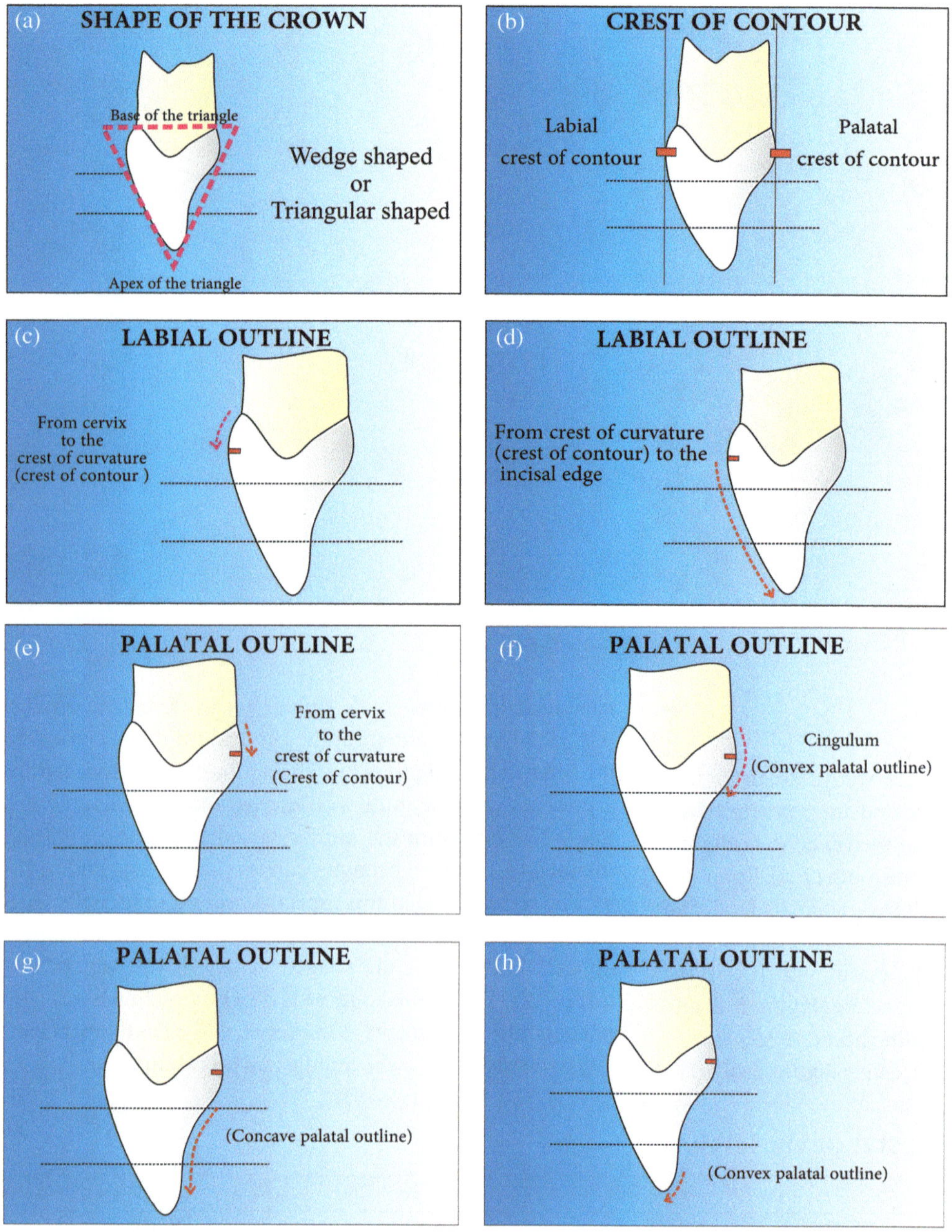

Figure 5.4 (a–h) Description of the right maxillary central incisor crown from the mesial aspect.

Exercise: Steps to Carve Excess Wax on Labial Side

While the cutting edge of the carver is facing the excess wax (in blue) on the lower half of the labial surface, it is moved in mesiodistal direction until the labial outline is reached (Figure 5.5g and h). Above the crest of the contour, the carver should be held in the reverse way with non-cutting edge facing the wax and the carver is moved in a mesiodistal direction until the outline is reached (Figure 5.5i and j).The triangular excess wax near the crest of contour is smoothed out to get the smooth labial surface (Figure 5.5k and l).

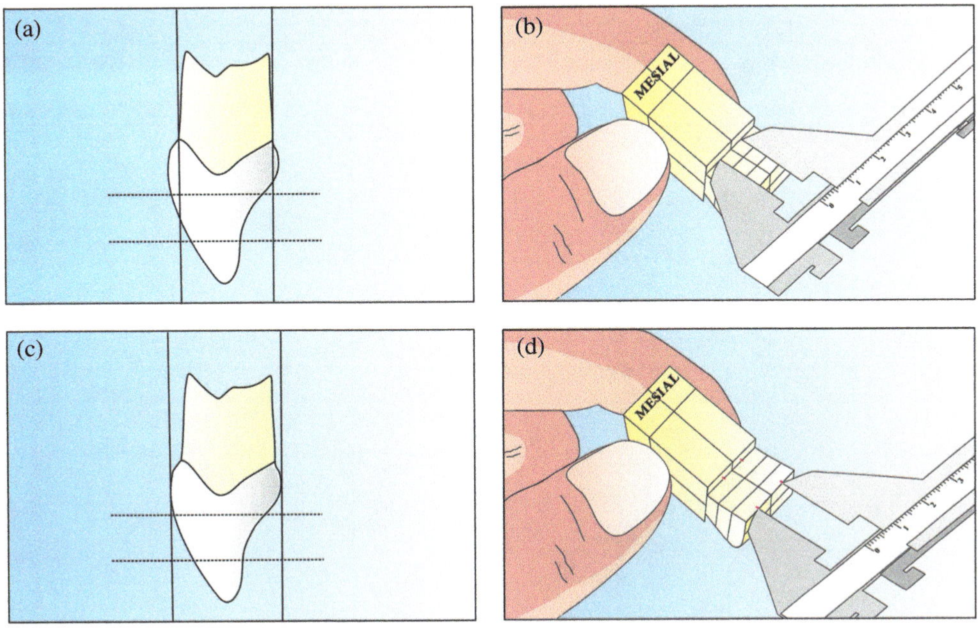

Figure 5.5 (a–d) Measuring and marking the crown dimension on the mesial aspect of the wax.

Exercise: Steps to Carve Excess Wax from the Palatal Side

The palatal side excess wax is carved in two steps. The convex or the curved part of the cutting edge of the carver should be used to carve the concave palatal outline. The excess wax (blue) is carved by moving the carver mesiodistally from the surface of the wax until the palatal concave outline is reached (Figure 5.5m and n). At the cervical third, above the crest of contour, the carver should be held in the reverse way with the non-cutting edge towards the wax and the tip of the carver facing the cervical line; the carver is then moved mesiodistally until the outline is reached (Figure 5.5o and p). The wedge of the wax near the crest of contour is carved to get the smooth labial surface (Figure 5.5q and r).

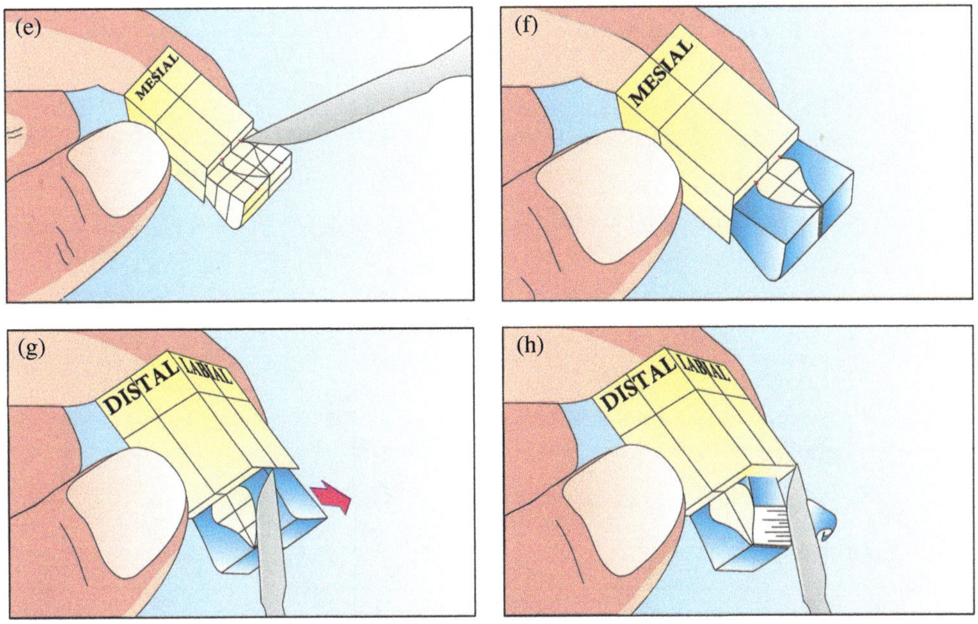

Figure 5.5 (e–l) Drawing the crown outline and carving excess wax from the labial surface.

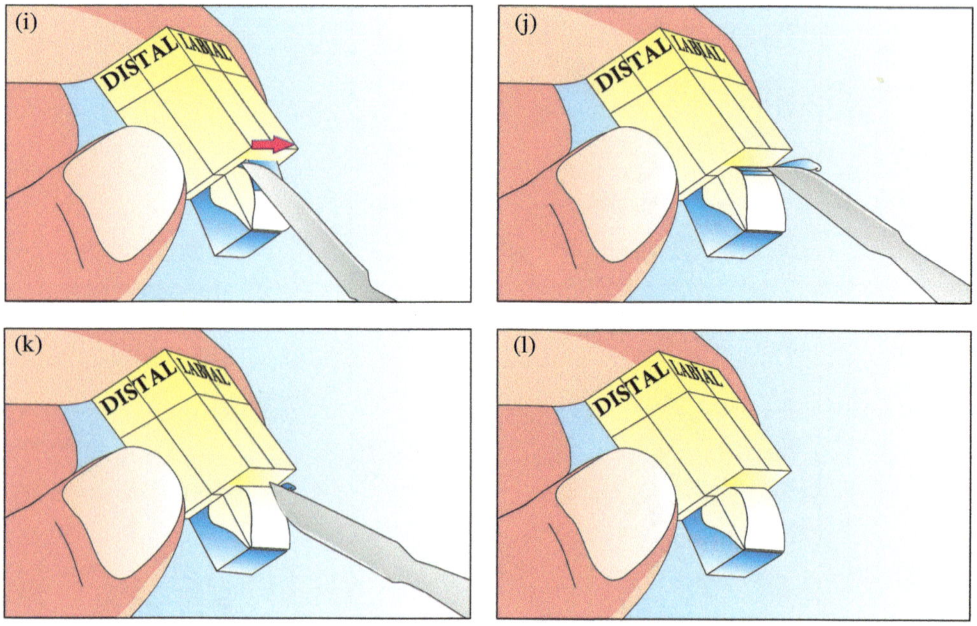

Figure 5.5 (Cont'd) (e–l)

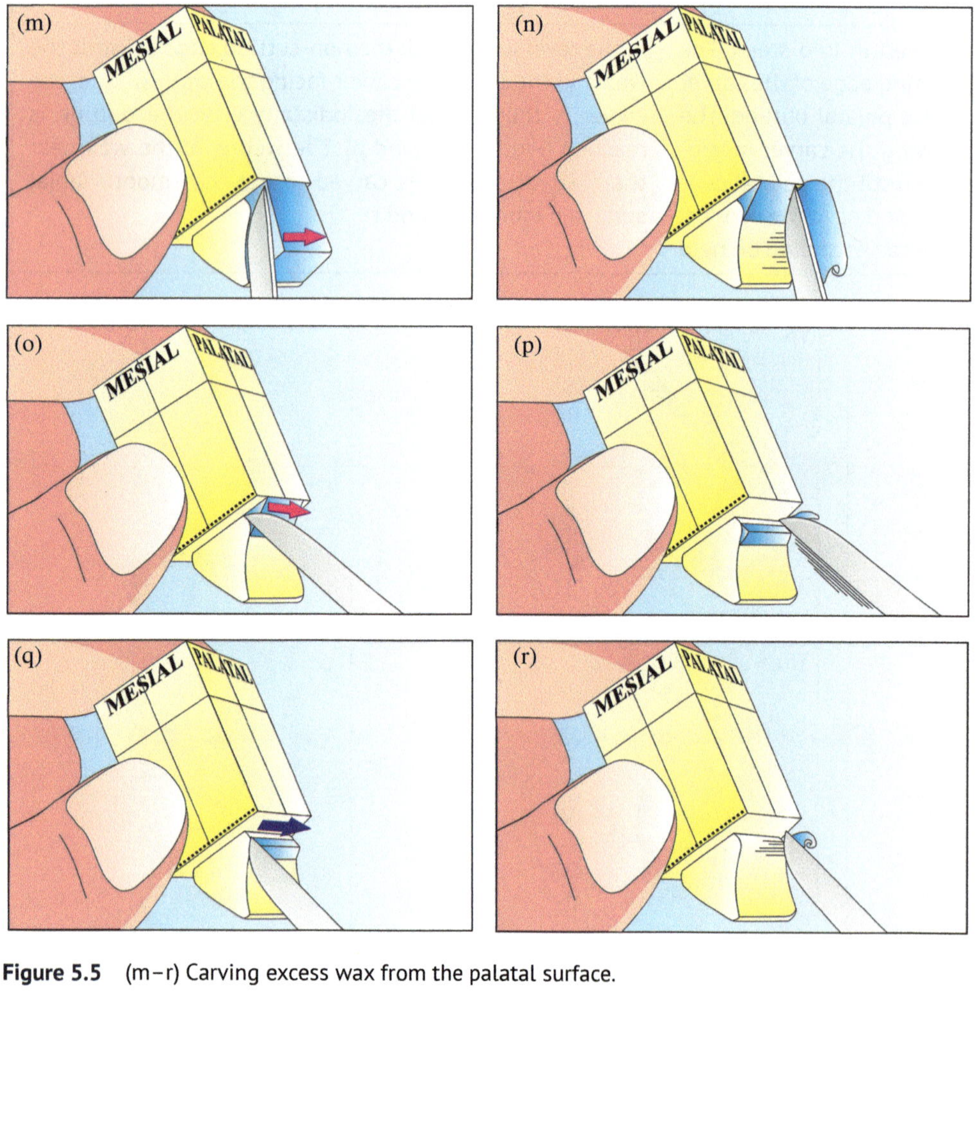

Figure 5.5 (m–r) Carving excess wax from the palatal surface.

Palatal Aspect

The outline of the crown from the palatal aspect is the mirror image of the labial aspect but shows convergence that makes the palatal surface appear narrower [1, 2]. The palatal surface has convexities and a concavity. Convexity immediately below the cervical line represents the cingulum. Concavity at the middle and incisal third is bordered by the cingulum cervically, mesially by the mesial marginal ridge, distal marginal ridge distally, and incisal ridge incisally. This concavity is the palatal fossa. The mesial marginal ridge is slightly longer than the distal marginal ridge, because of the tilt of the incisal edge cervically near distal side [1, 3]. Small accessory palatal ridge can be seen sometimes, extending from the lower portion of cingulum that runs within the fossa for a short distance towards the incisal ridge. The cingulum is placed distal to the long axis of the tooth, so that more of the mesial surface can be seen compared to the distal [3]. In some cases, the palatal pit can be seen at the junction where the cingulum unites with marginal ridges (Figure 5.6a) [6]. Cervical line is asymmetrical with more curvature offset to distal side [1].

The root from this aspect is blunt and conical shaped cervico-apically, with the convergence of mesial and distal surfaces. Cross-section of the root at the cervix shows a scalene triangle with unequal sides. The biggest side is labial, followed by mesial, and the last one is distal (Figure 5.6b) [3].

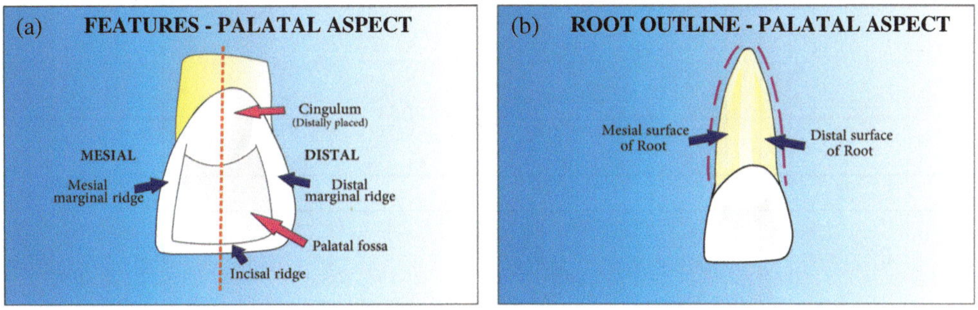

Figure 5.6 (a–b) Description of the maxillary right central incisor from the palatal aspect.

Carving from the Palatal Aspect

Exercise: Creating the Palatal Convergence of the Crown

The mesial and distal surface of the crown should be narrowed palatally to create convergence. More convergence is created on the mesial side than the distal side. This is done by drawing lines on either side of the midline on the palatal surface as shown (Figure 5.7b). The mesial line is closer to midline than the distal one. The mesial convergence is created by carving excess wax on the mesial side using the anterior part of the cutting edge of the carver, moved palatolabially form the line drawn till the mesiolabial line angle (Figure 5.7c to e). (NOTE: Care should be taken not to touch the mesiolabial line angle (to prevent damage to the mesial outline of the labial aspect). The same carving step is repeated on the distal side (Figure 5.6f and g).

Exercise: Carving the Palatal Fossa

Outline for the maxillary central incisor fossa is roughly 'M' shaped. This outline is drawn on the palatal surface (Figure 5.8a). Using the excavating end of the carver, the excess wax is carved out within the border drawn as shown (Figure 5.7b–g). The fossa is carved in such a way that it is deep near the cingulum and shallow as it approaches the incisal edge. At the incisal edge, the incisal ridge is created by halting the excavation at a distance from the incisal edge (Figure 5.8d, e, and g) and smoothing the ridge (Figure 5.8h).

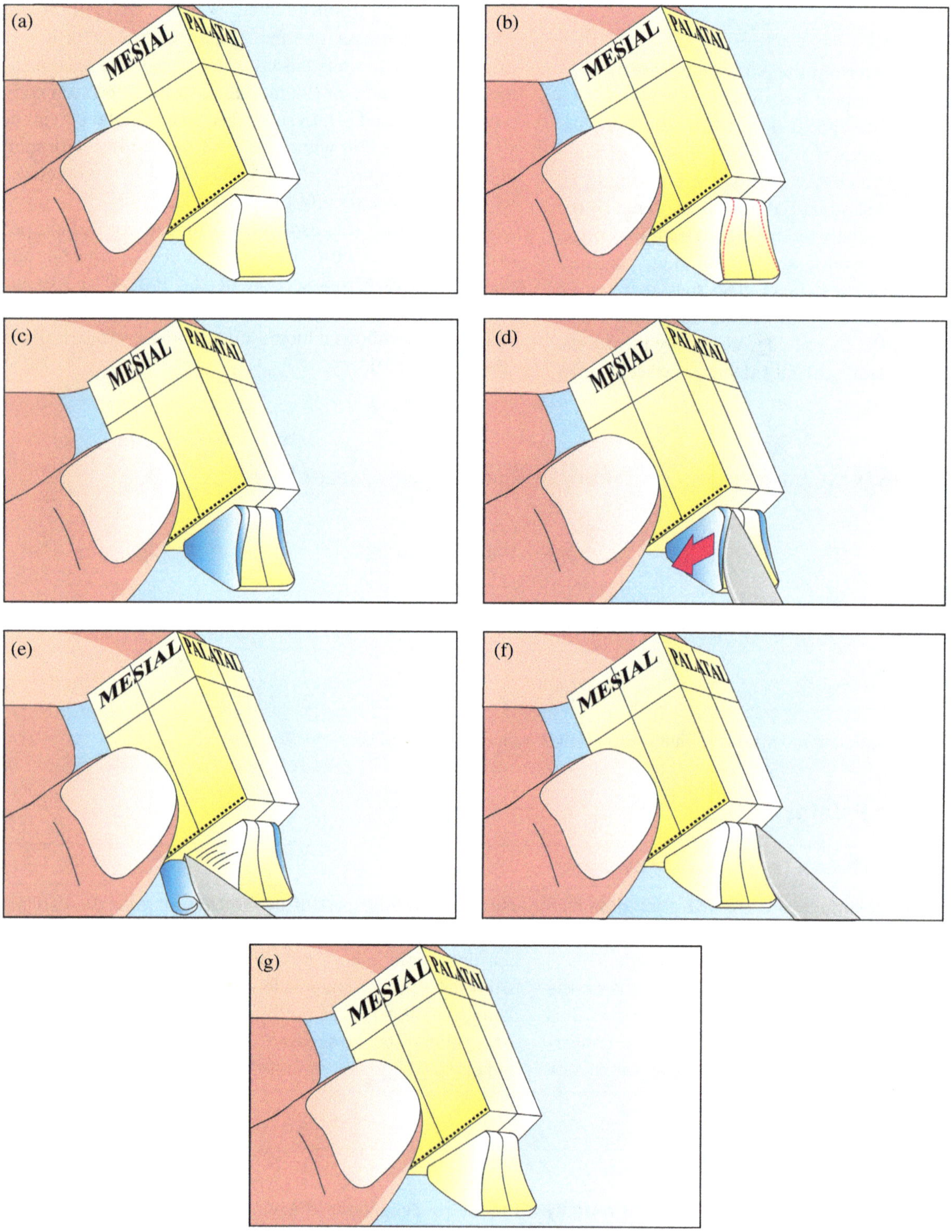

Figure 5.7 (a–g) Creating the palatal convergence.

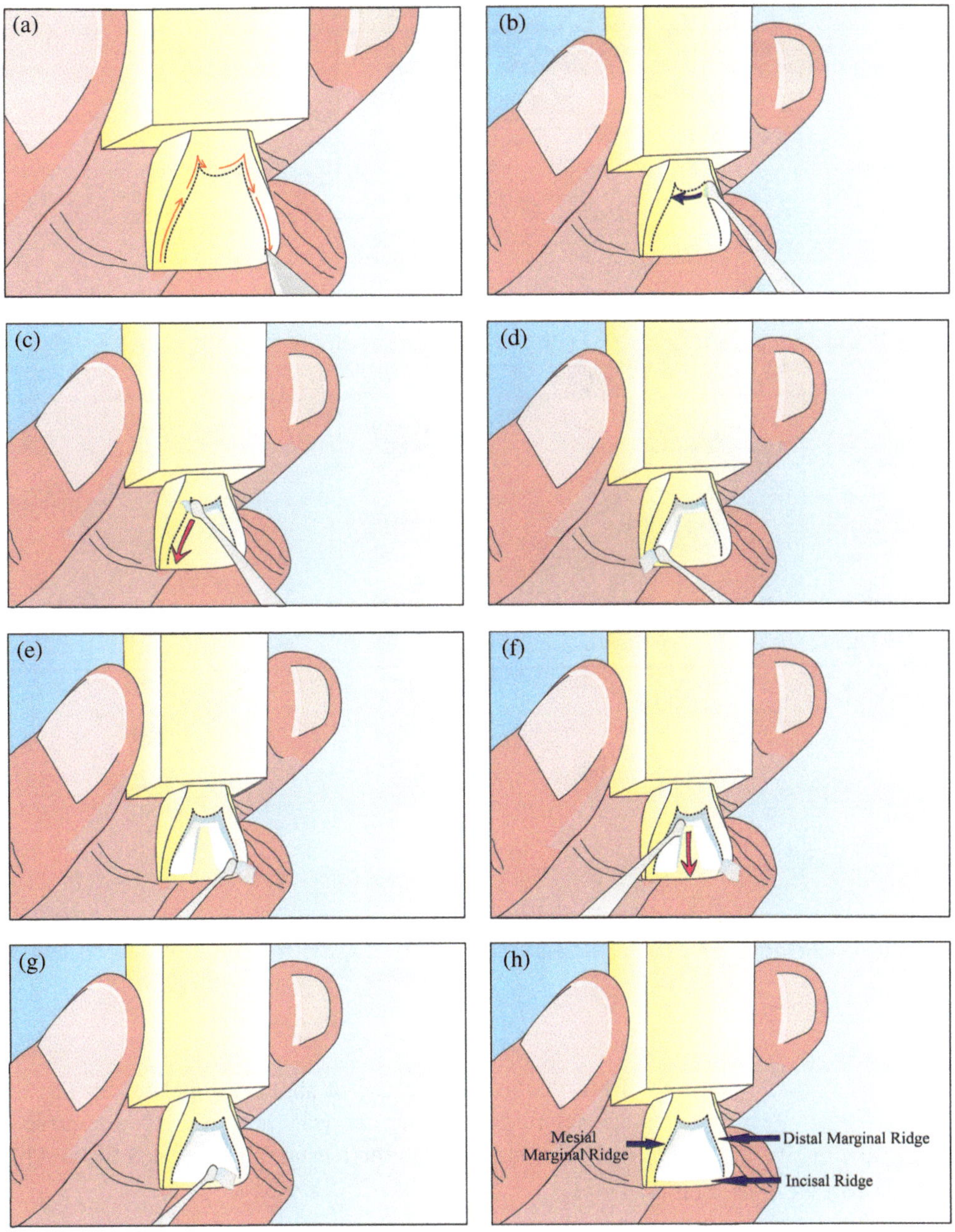

Figure 5.8 (a–h) Marking and carving the palatal fossa.

Incisal Aspect

The crown from this aspect appears roughly triangular shaped with rounded borders (Figure 5.9a–b) [1, 3]. The crown appears to be placed in the centre of the root as the root is entirely confined within the crown. The crown is wider mesiodistally than labiopalatally. The labial surface appears wider than the palatal surface and is less convex (Figure 5.9c) [2]. The crown has well-defined mesiolabial and distolabial line angles compared to the palatal ones [1]. The distolabial line angle is placed slightly palatal to the mesiolabial line angle. This shows slight distopalatal tilt of crown. The mesial and distal surface tapers palatally towards the cingulum. The distance from the line angles to the centre of the cingulum is greater on the mesial side than the distal side (Figure 5.9d). The cingulum is located distal to the long axis of the crown (Figure 5.9e) [3].

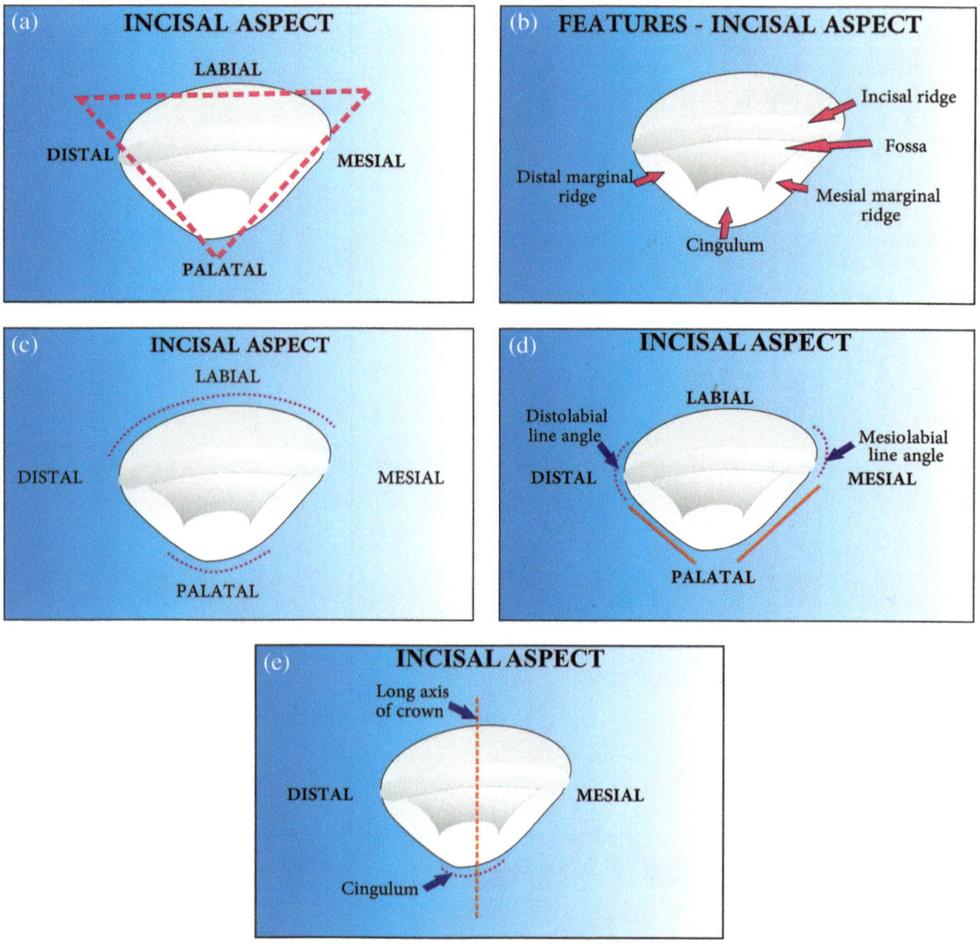

Figure 5.9 (a–e) Description of the maxillary right incisor from the incisal aspect.

Distal Aspect

The crown appears shorter and becomes thicker at the incisal portion [1, 2]. Part of the labial surface can be seen from this aspect because of slight distopalatal tilt of the incisal ridge [3]. The cervical line appears less curved incisally compared to the mesial side (Figure 5.10a and b) [1–3].

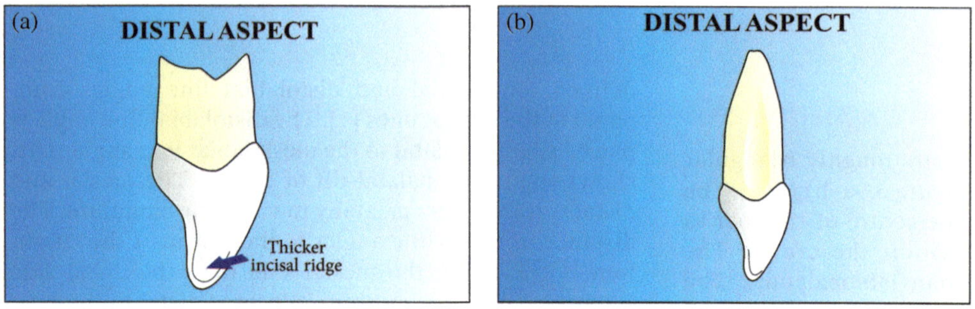

Figure 5.10 (a–b) Description of the maxillary right incisor from the distal aspect.

Root Carving

Exercise: Carving the Root from the Mesial or Distal Aspect

Outline of the root, as described earlier, is drawn on the proximal surface (distal) as shown (Figure 5.11a). The excess wax outside the root outline indicated in blue needs to be carved (Figure 5.11b). Excess wax at the cervical and middle third of labial surface is carved using the anterior part of the cutting-edge of the carver facing wax (Figure 5.11c) and moved in distal to mesial direction from the surface until the outline is reached (Figure 5.11d).The remaining wax near the apical portion of the labial surface is carved with the non-cutting edge of the carver facing the excess wax (Figure 5.11e) and excess wax is carved in the same way as previously described (Figure 5.11f).Excess wax on the palatal side is carved in the same way as on the labial side(Figure 5.11g).

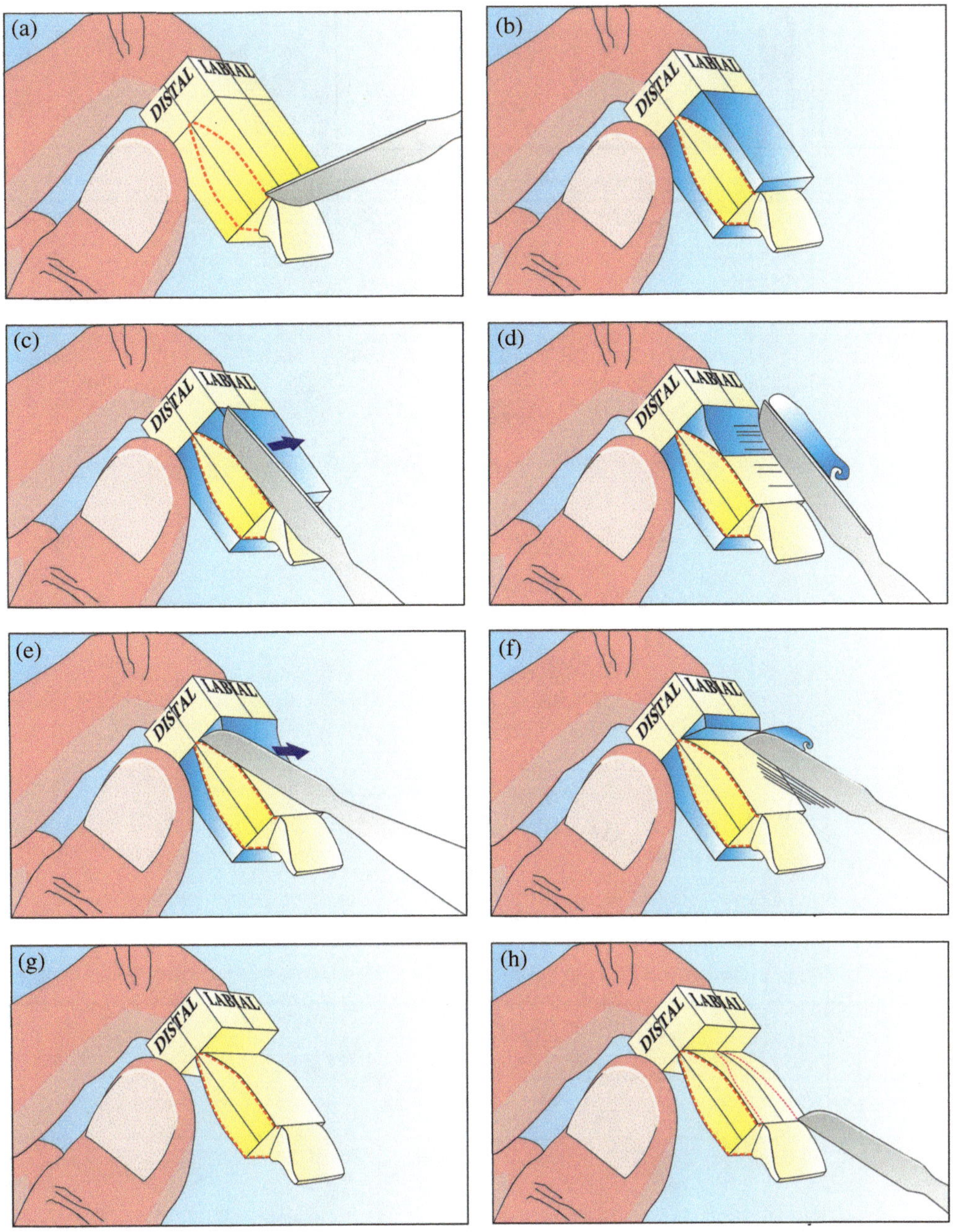

Figure 5.11 (a–r) Sequence of carving the root.

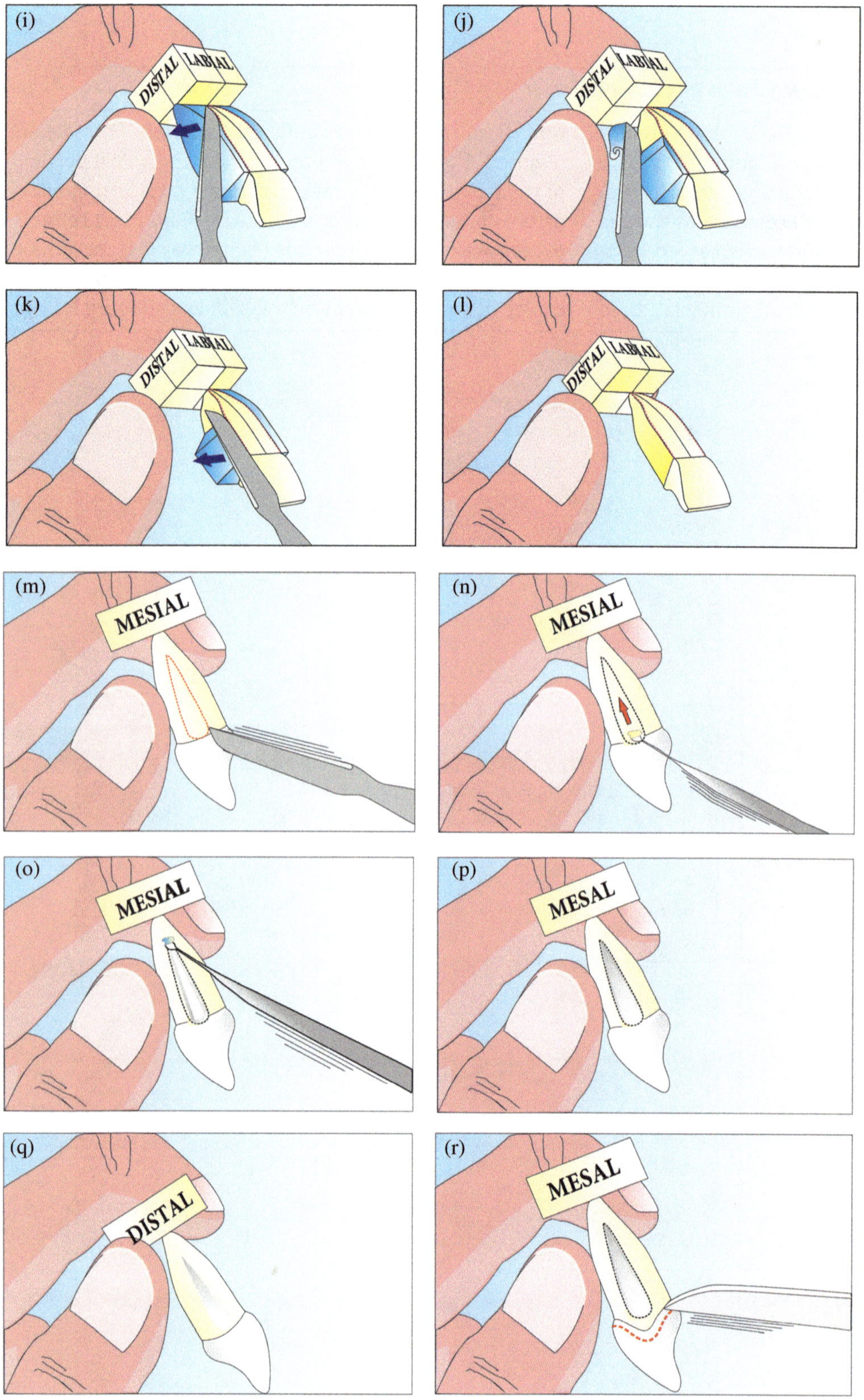

Figure 5.11 (Cont'd) (a–r)

Exercise: Carving the Root from the Labial Aspect

The mesiodistal root outline is drawn on the labial wax surface, with the mesial root outline being parallel to the long axis of the tooth (Figure 5.11h). Excess wax distal to the apical third of root is carved with the convex part of the carver facing the concave root outline (Figure 5.11i) and moved in a labiopalatal direction (Figure 5.11j) along with root convergence palatally. Remaining wax on the distal side is carved out (Figure 5.11k) along with excess wax on the mesial side (Figure 5.11l).

Exercise: Creating Developmental Depression on Root Surfaces

Outline of developmental depression is drawn on the mesial side (Figure 5.11m). Using the excavating end of the Lecron carver the wax is carved in a cervico-apical direction, deeper at the centre and shallower near the border of the outline (Figure 5.11n–p). The same step is repeated on the distal side of the root (Figure 5.11q). The curvature of the cervical line is drawn on both the mesial and distal sides of the root. The mesial cervical line curves more towards the incisal edge than the distal side (Figure 5.11r).

References

1 James, L.F., Gerald, E.D., and Thomas, M. (2001). *Concise Dental Anatomy and Morphology*, 4e. Iowa City, IA: University of Iowa College of Dentistry.
2 Stanley, J.N. and Major, M.A.C. (2010). *Wheeler's Dental Anatomy and Occlusion*, 9e. St. Louis, MO: Saunders Elsevier.
3 Rickne, C.S. and Weiss, G. (2012). *Woelfel's Dental Anatomy*, 8e. Philadelphia: Lippincott Williams & Wilkins.
4 Geoffrey, C.B. (1983). *Dental Morphology. An Illustrated Guide*, 2e. Philadelphia: Wright Elsevier.
5 Scott, G.R. (2017). *Human Tooth Crown and Root Morphology*, (p. iii). Cambridge University Press. Kindle Edition.
6 Hillson, S. (2012). *Dental Anthropology*. Cambridge University Press. Kindle Edition.

6

Permanent Maxillary Lateral Incisor

LEARNING OBJECTIVE
At the end of the chapter, the student should have knowledge of the permanent maxillary lateral incisor and develop the psychomotor skills for carving and waxing the same.

Permanent Maxillary Right Lateral Incisor

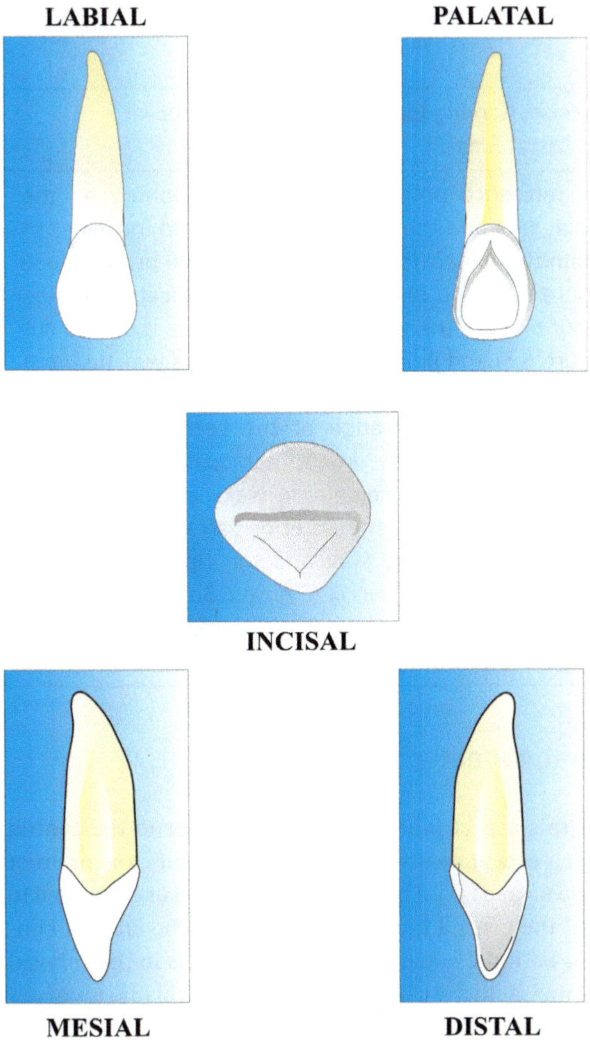

Labial Aspect

The maxillary lateral incisor is the second tooth from the midline (Figure 6.1). From this aspect, the maxillary lateral incisor appears similar to the central incisor. However, it is more curved, with rounded mesial and distal line angles [1, 2]. The crown's overall dimension is smaller compared to the central incisor [2]. The mesial outline is rounded (Figure 6.2a). The mesial crest of contour is at the junction between the incisal and middle third, making mesio-incisal line angles more rounded (Figure 6.2b). The distal outline of the crown is more rounded than the mesial, as the crest of curvature is placed at the middle of the middle third (Figure 6.2a and b) [1, 2].Sometimes the distal outline appears semicircular [1, 3]. The incisal edge slopes cervically on the distal side [1–3]. The labial surface of the crown is more convex [1, 3]. Root length is about 1.5 times the length of the crown (Figure 6.2c) [1]. The mesial and distal outline

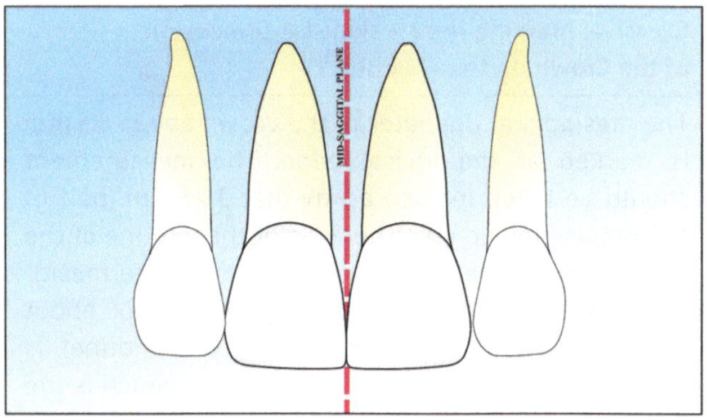

Figure 6.1 Location of the lateral incisor in relation to the midsagittal plane.

An Illustrated Atlas of Tooth Carving and Wax-Up Techniques, First Edition. Anil Bangalore Shivappa.

Companion website: www.wiley.com/go/bangalore/toothcarving

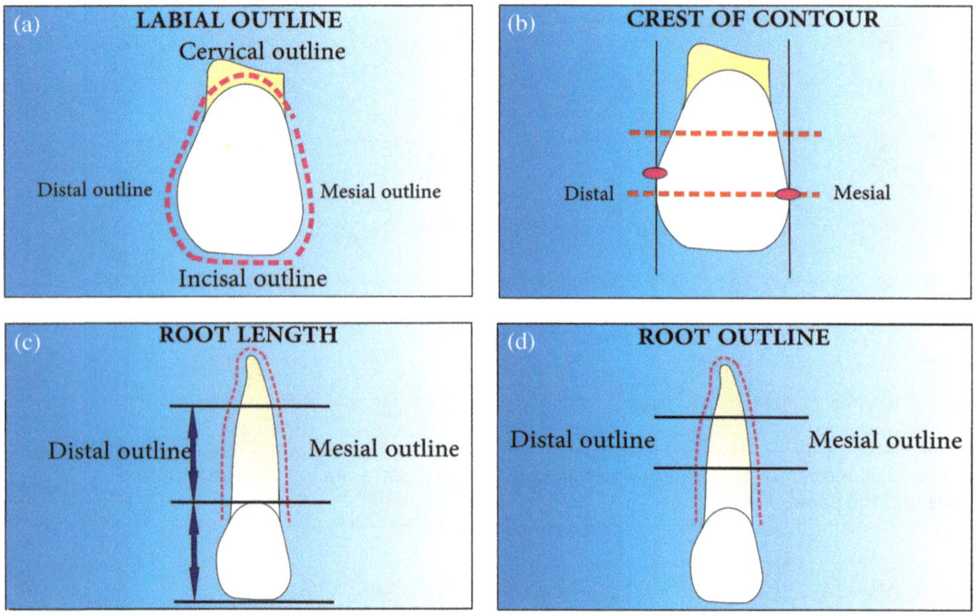

Figure 6.2 (a–d) Characteristic features of the permanent maxillary right lateral incisor from the labial aspect.

of the root tapers evenly from the cervical line to two thirds of the root length apically. The apical third of the root appears pointed, very often curving distally (Figure 6.2d) [2].

Carving from the Labial Aspect

> **Exercise: Marking the Length of Crown and Root on the Wax Block**
>
> Using standard Vernier caliper, the cervico-incisal length of the crown about 9.0 mm and the length of the root about 1.3 mm are marked on the prepared wax block (Figure 6.3a–c). After this, the crown is divided into three equal parts (Figure 6.3d) [1]

> **Exercise: Marking the Mesiodistal Dimension of the Crown on the Wax Block**
>
> The mesiodistal diameter of the crown about 6.5 mm is marked at the incisal edge. The measurement should be taken in such a way that 3.25 mm (half of 6.5 mm) is marked on either side of the midline of the wax block (Figure 6.3e). In a similar way, the mesiodistal diameter of the crown at the cervix about 5.0 mm (2.5 mm on either side of the midline) is marked at the cervical end of the crown, which is the line of demarcation between the crown and the root (Figure 6.3f) [1].

> **Exercise: Carving Excess Wax from the Mesial and Distal Side**
>
> The reference points of marking are joined on the mesial side and the distal side of the midline, so as to obtain the dimension of the crown at the proper place (Figure 6.3g and h). The excess wax indicated by blue colour on both the mesial and distal sides is carved out (Figure 6.3i and j). The bulk of the excess wax near the incisal and middle third is carved using the anterior part of the cutting edge of the Lecron carver and moving the carver in a labiopalatal direction (Figure 6.3k and l). Remaining wax near the cervical third is carved using the anterior part of the non-cutting edge facing the wax and the tip of the carver pointing toward the cervix (Figure 6.3m). The carver is then moved labiopalatally to complete the step (Figure 6.3n).

Mesial Aspect

From this aspect the tooth appears similar to the central incisor, except with shorter crown and longer root (Figure 6.4a–d) [1]. The incisal ridge is thicker compared to that of the central incisor (Figure 6.4e). The crest of contour of both the labial and palatal outline is in the cervical third, incisal to the cervical line. The cervical line is curved

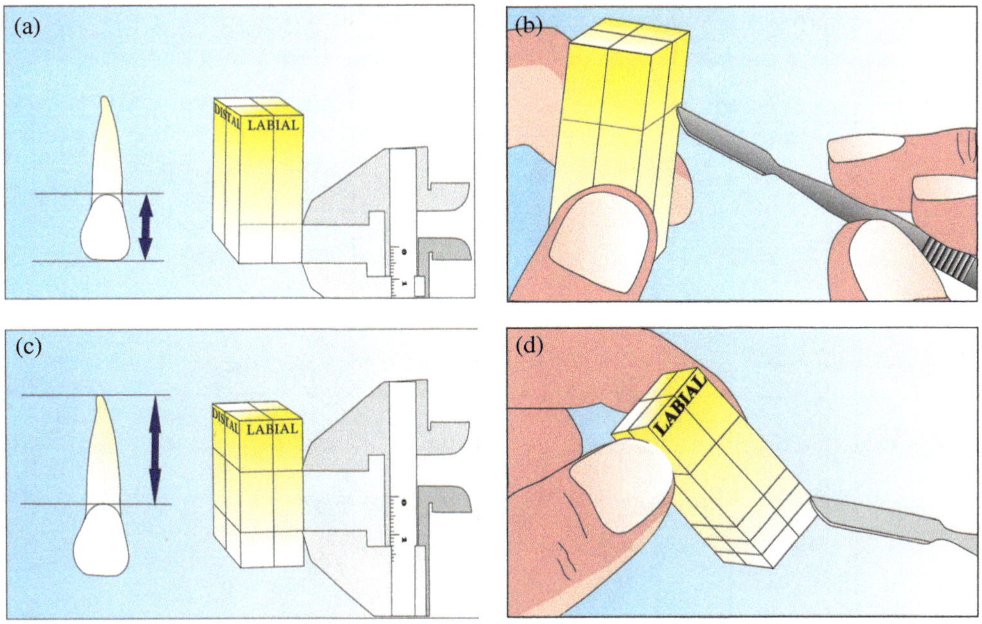

Figure 6.3 (a–d) Measuring and marking the length of the crown and root on the labial aspect.

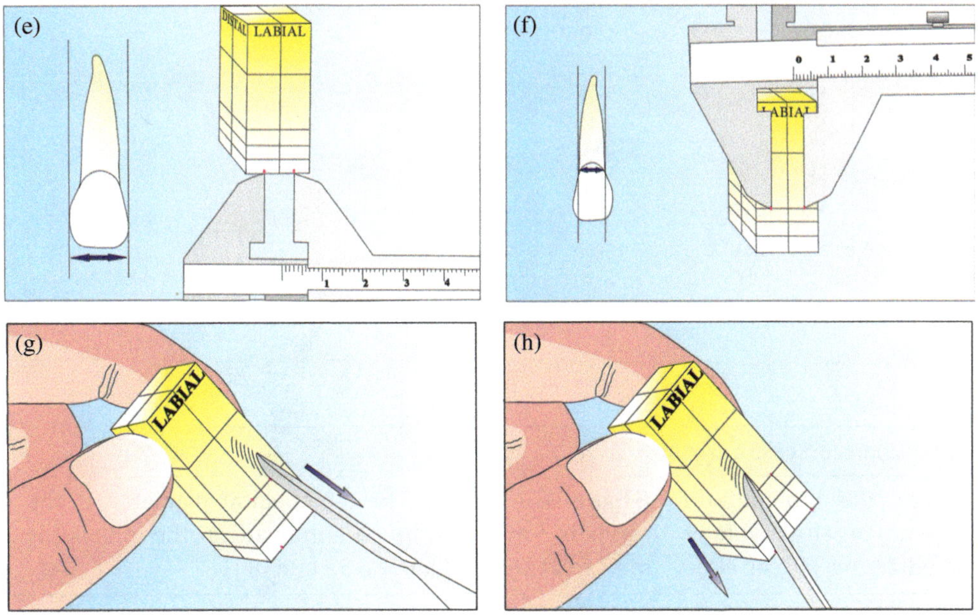

Figure 6.3 (e–h) Measuring and marking the crown dimension on the labial surface of the wax block.

in the direction of the incisal ridge for about 3 mm [2, 3]. The root is blunt and cone shaped with uniform taper. A line drawn through the centre of the root tends to bisect the incisal ridge of the crown (Figure 6.4f) [1, 2].

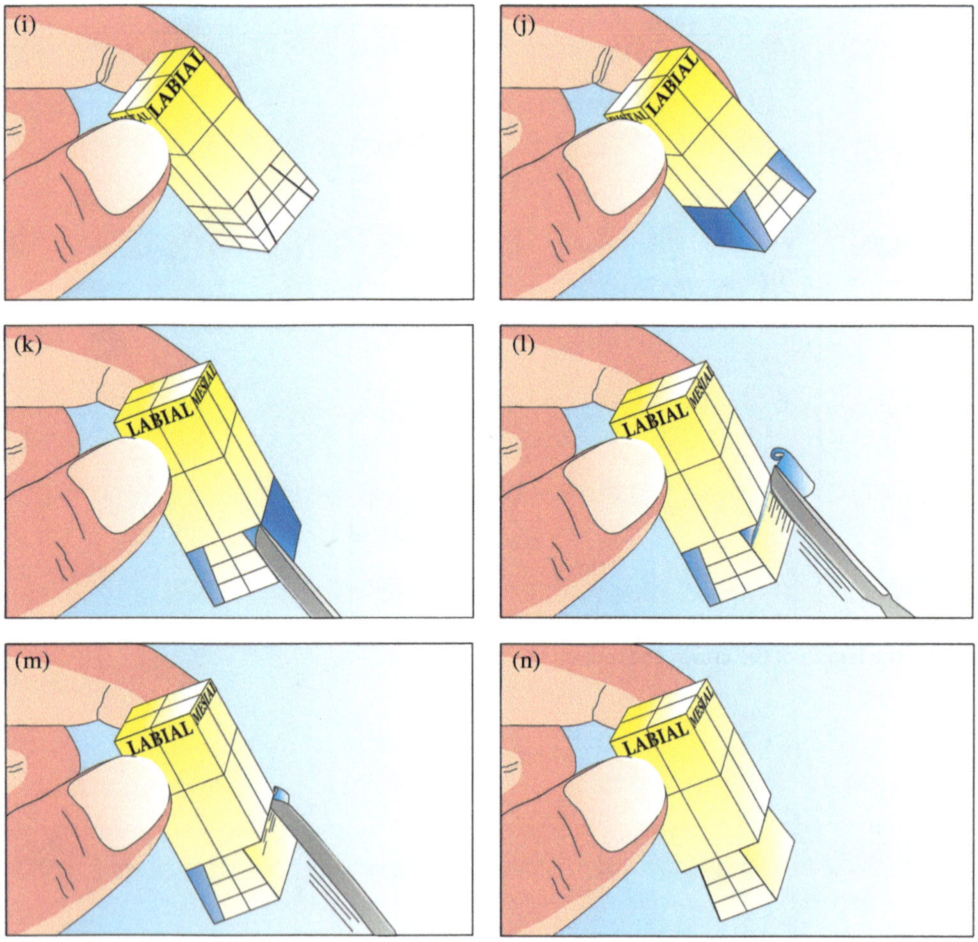

Figure 6.3 (i–n) Carving the mesial and distal excess wax of the crown from the labial aspect.

Carving from the Mesial Aspect

Exercise: Marking the Labiopalatal Dimension of the crown

On the mesial/distal of the wax, the labiopalatal diameter of the crown of 6 mm (3 mm on either side of the midline of the wax) is marked at the incisal edge (Figure 6.5c and d). The labiopalatal diameter at the cervix of 5 mm (2.5 mm on either side of the midline) is marked at cervix (Figure 6.5a and b) [1].

Exercise: Marking the Outline of Crown on the Mesial surface

The reference points of measurements taken are joined on the labial and the palatal half, so the dimension of the crown is obtained. The crown is divided into three equal parts and the crest of curvatures on labial and palatal side are marked. The crest of curvature of both the labial and palatal outlines are at the cervical third with the labial crest being more incisal than the palatal. The outline of the crown is drawn, by joining the reference points near the cervical, at the crest of contour and at the incisal edge (Figure 6.5e). The excess wax indicated in blue colour is carved out (Figure 6.5f).

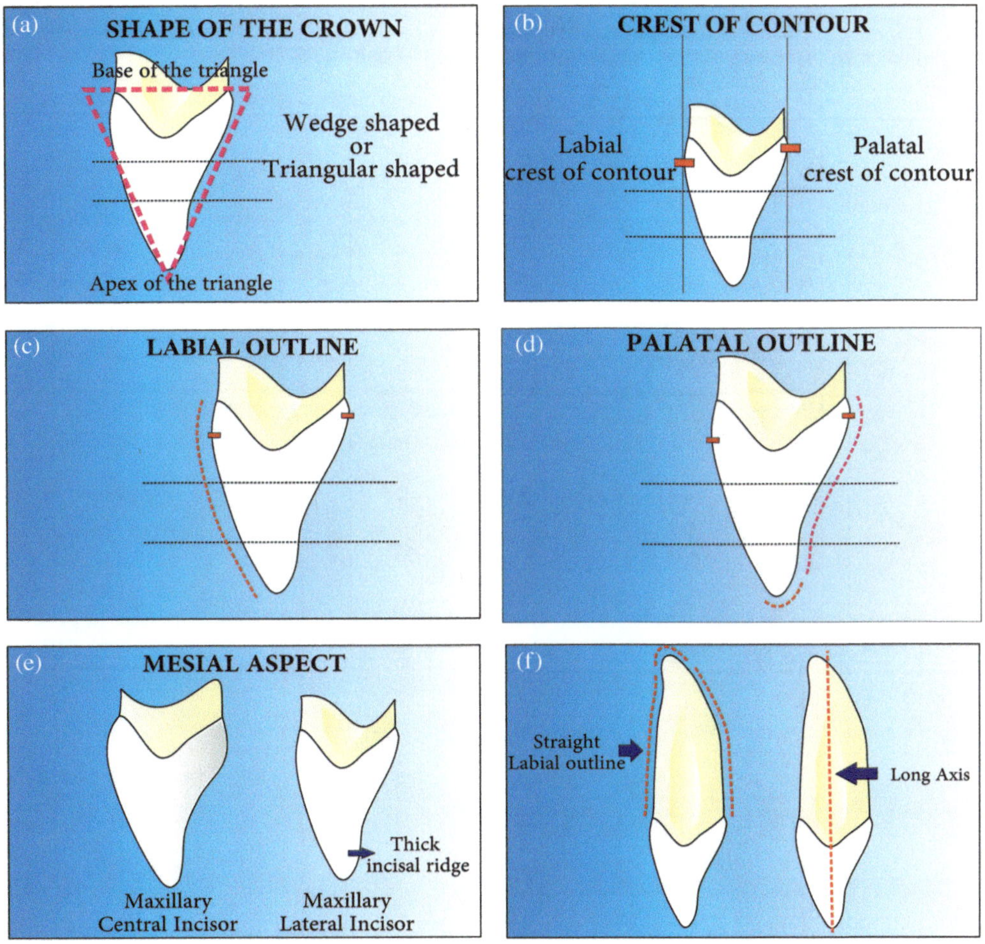

Figure 6.4 (a–f) Descriptive features of the permanent maxillary right lateral incisor from the mesial aspect.

Exercise: Carving Excess Wax on the Labial and palatal surfaces

Excess wax labially is carved in two steps. The bulk of wax on the middle and the incisal third of the labial surface is carved (Figure 6.5g) with the curved part of the cutting edge moved in a mesiodistal direction (Figure 6.5h). The cervical third on the labial surface is carved with the non-cutting (back) side of the carver facing excess wax and the tip of the carver facing the cervical line and moved in the same direction as mentioned previously (Figure 6.5i and j). The remaining part of the wax on the labial surface is carved out. Wax from the palatal surface is carved in similar way following the crown outline.

Palatal Aspect

From this aspect, the cingulum appears more prominent along with well-developed marginal ridges both mesially, distally, and incisally, making the palatal fossa more concave [1, 3]. More frequently, a pit is seen at the incisal part of the cingulum, where the mesial and distal marginal ridges unite. This is called a palatal pit [2]. Developmental grooves can be found bordering the cingulum, especially the distal side extending to the root (Figure 6.6a) [2, 3]. The tooth tapers palatally, so that most of the mesial and distal surfaces can be seen (Figure 6.6b).

Carving on the Palatal Aspect

Exercise: Creating the Palatal Convergence of the Crown

The palatal convergence is created by drawing the mesial and distal outlines, approaching the midline as they start from the incisal angle to the cervical line (Figure 6.7a). The excess wax indicated by the blue colour is carved using the curved part of the cutting edge of Lecron carver (Figure 6.7b). The carver is moved palatolabially as shown (Figure 6.7c).

NOTE: Care should be taken not to damage the outline at mesiolabial and distolabial line angle (Figure 6.7d).

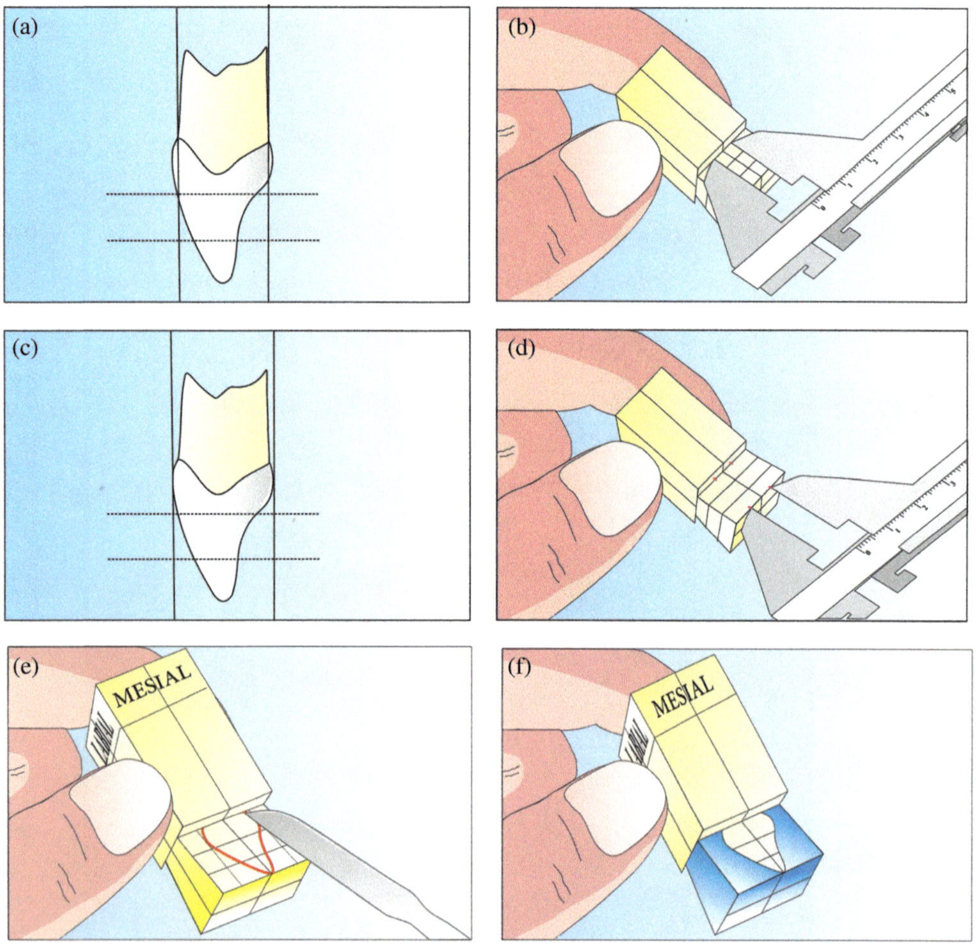

Figure 6.5 (a–f) Measuring and marking the dimension and outline of the crown on the mesial aspect of the wax.

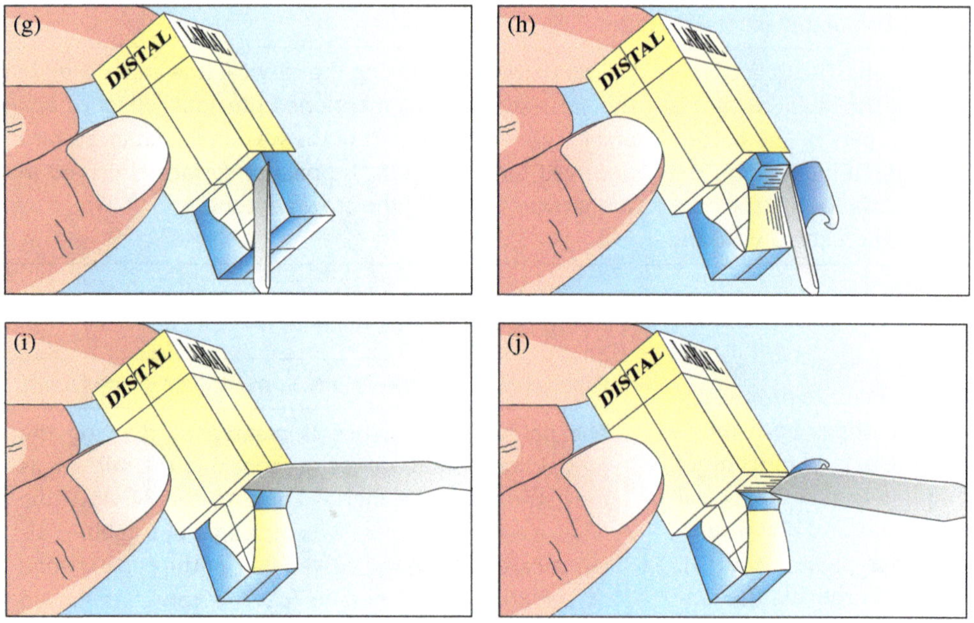

Figure 6.5 (g–j) Carving excess wax from the labial and palatal surfaces.

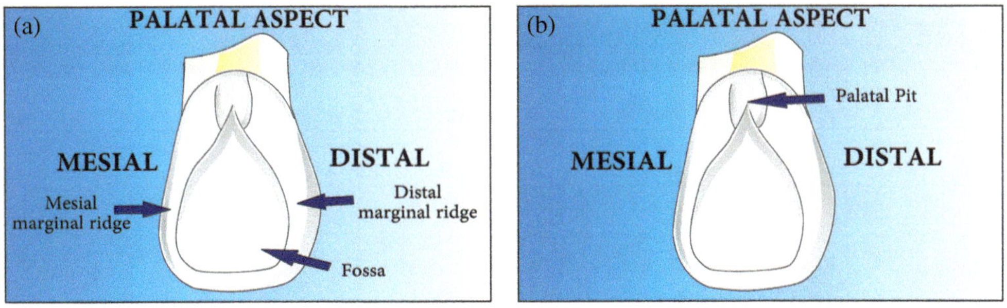

Figure 6.6 (a and b) Description of the permanent maxillary right lateral incisor from the palatal aspect.

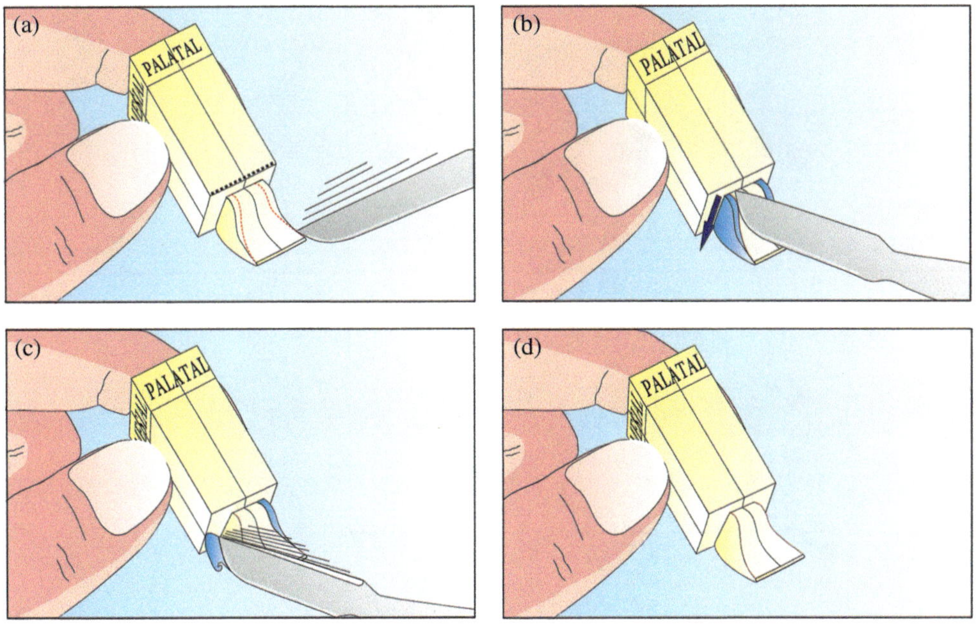

Figure 6.7 (a–d) Creating the palatal convergence of the crown.

Exercise: Carving the Palatal Fossa

The pointed dome-shaped outline of the fossa is drawn on the incisal and the middle third of the palatal surface (Figure 6.7e). Using the excavating end of the carver, the wax is removed/excavated near the marginal ridges, shallow near the incisal ridge and deep as the carver is moved towards the cingulum (Figure 6.7f–j). The centre of the fossa is carved in a similar way, so that the concave fossa is created within the outline drawn (Figure 6.7k–m).

Exercise: Carving the Outline on the Labial Aspect

Here the proper outline is drawn on the labial surface, after joining the crests of curvature with reference points at the mesial and distal of the cervix and the incisal edge. The excess wax is carved using the cutting edge of the wax to get the proper outline (Figure 6.8a and b).

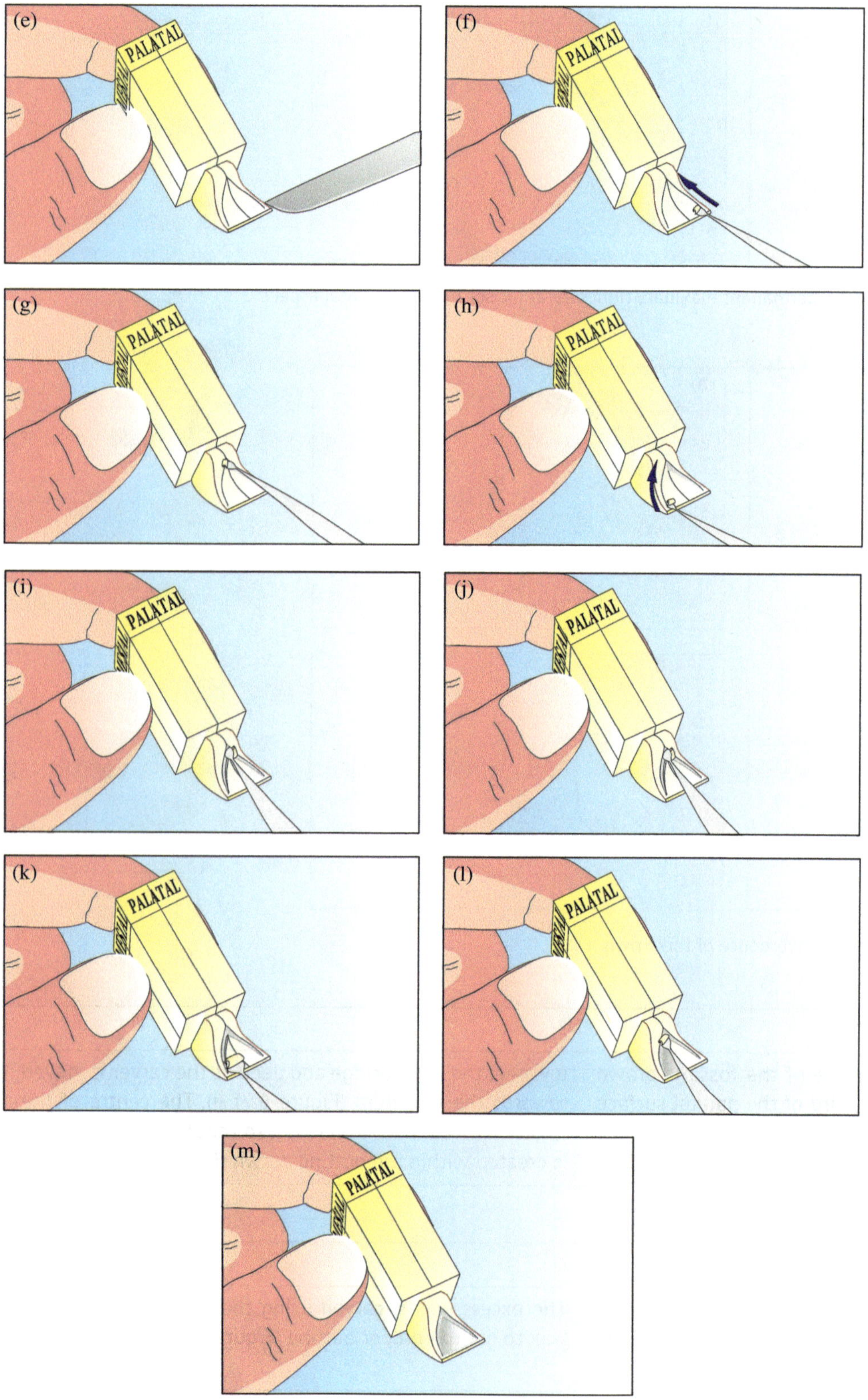

Figure 6.7 (e–m) Marking and carving the palatal fossa.

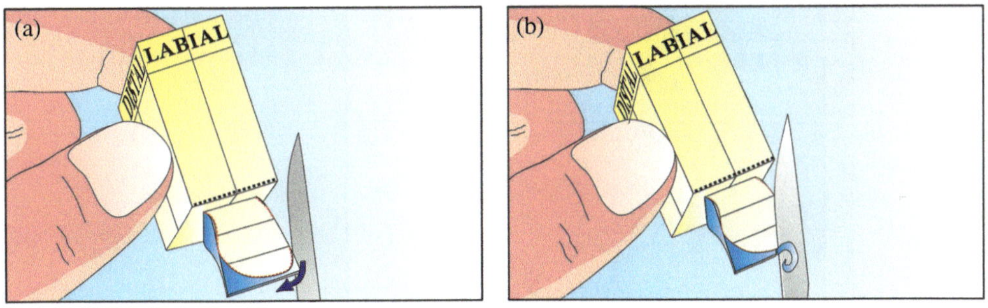

Figure 6.8 (a–b) Drawing and carving the outline of the crown (Labial aspect).

Distal Aspect

The crown appears similar to that seen from the mesial aspect, except thicker. The developmental groove can be seen from this aspect of crown, extending on to the root. The cervical line is curved in the direction of the incisal edge for about 2 mm (Figure 6.9a and b) [1, 2].

Incisal Aspect

The crown appears wider mesiodistally than labiopalatally but less wide when compared to the central incisor [3]. The outline of the crown is more rounded. The crown appears more convex labially and palatally from the incisal aspect than does the maxillary central incisor. The cingulum is centred along the axis of the crown [3, 4]. The incisal edge is straight when compared to the traits of central incisor [3] (Figure 6.10a and b).

Root Carving

Exercise: Carving the Root from the Labial Aspect

The mesial and distal outline of the root as described in Figure 6.2d is drawn on the labial surface (Figure 6.11a). The excess wax indicated in blue colour should be carved on both the mesial and distal sides (Figure 6.11b). Excess wax at the cervical third and part of the middle third on the mesial surface is carved using the anterior part of the Lecron carver running labiopalatally (Figure 6.11c and d). The wax at the apical part is carved with the tip of the carver at the apex and the non-cutting edge of the carver facing the wax (Figure 6.11e). The wedge of wax remaining should be carved using the curved part of the cutting edge, so as to get the mesial outline of the root (Figure 6.11f). The aforementioned procedures are repeated on the distal surface (Figure 6.11g).

NOTE: Palatal convergence of both mesial and distal surface is also included.

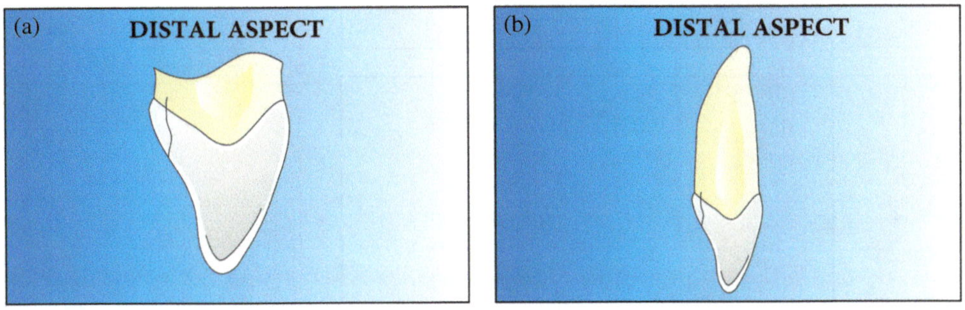

Figure 6.9 (a–b) Description of the permanent maxillary right lateral incisor from the distal aspect.

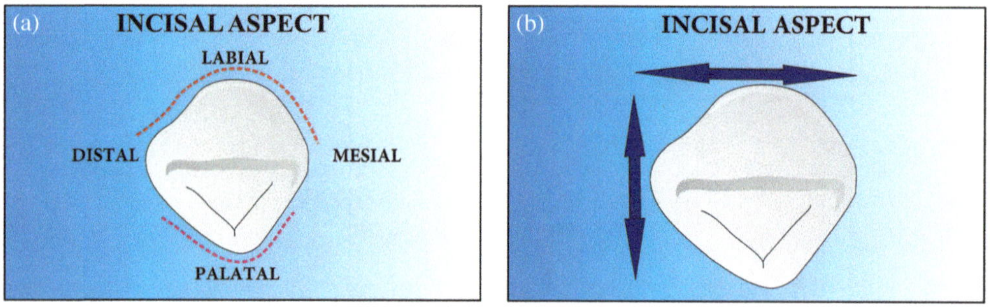

Figure 6.10 (a–b) Description of the permanent maxillary right lateral incisor from the incisal aspect.

Exercise: Carving the Root from the Distal Aspect

The labial and palatal outline on the distal surface of the root portion of wax is drawn with features as described. Excess wax on the labial and the palatal surface should be carved. To get the labial tilt of the root tip, the carver is placed at the apex in such a way that the curved part of the Lecron carver is facing the wax and the tip facing the root apex (Figure 6.11h). The carver is moved mesiodistally unidirectional until the outline of the root is reached (Figure 6.11i). The remaining bulk of the wax is carved with the curved part of the Lecron carver to get the labial outline of the root (Figure 6.11j). The carving is repeated on the palatal surface of root portion (Figure 6.11k). The developmental depression is carved by drawing the outline as shown (Figure 6.11l). The inner part of the outline is carved with the excavating end of the carver, moving it deeper near the cervical part and shallower as moved towards the apex of the root (Figure 6.11m and n). Finally, the cervical line is drawn on both mesial and distal sides.

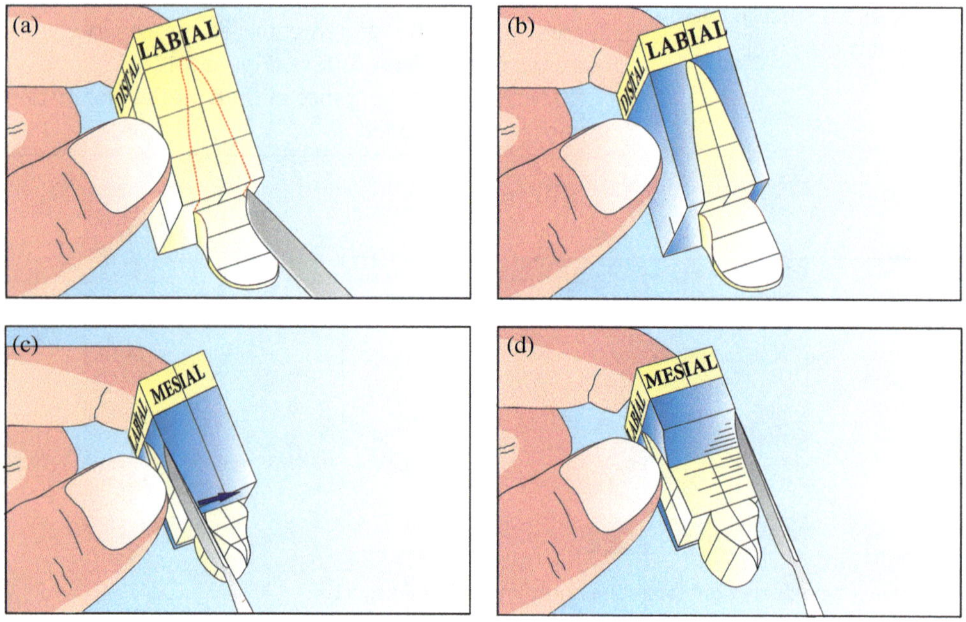

Figure 6.11 (a–d) Step sequence to carve the root.

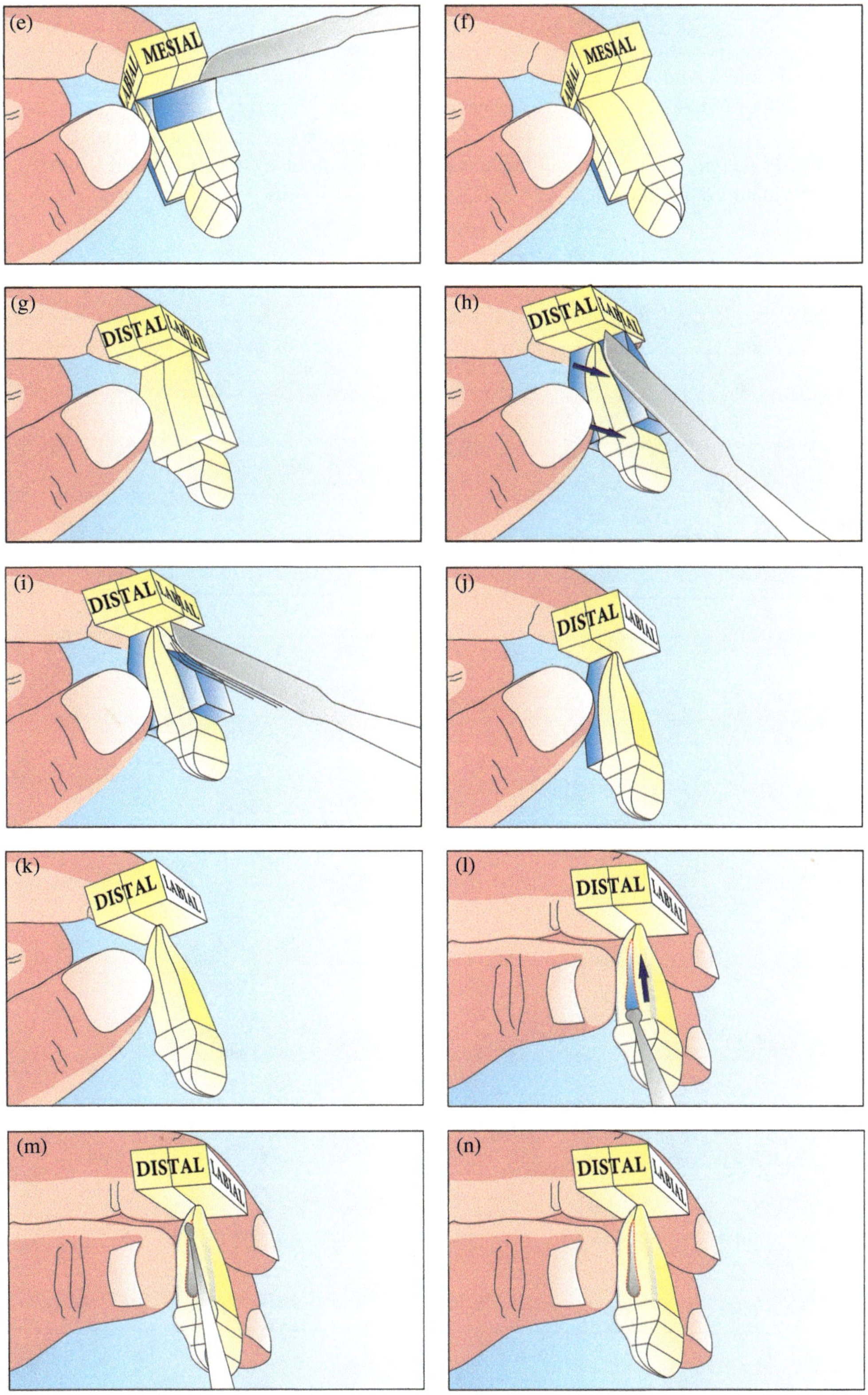

Figure 6.11 (e–n) Step sequence to carve the root.

References

1 Stanley, J.N. and Major, M.A.C. (2010). *Wheeler's Dental Anatomy and Occlusion*, 9e. St. Louis, MO: Saunders Elsevier.

2 Rickne, C.S. and Weiss, G. (2012). *Woelfel's Dental Anatomy*, 8e. Philadelphia: Lippincott Williams & Wilkins.

3 Hillson, S. (2012). *Dental Anthropology*. Cambridge University Press. Kindle Edition.

4 Scott, G.R. (2017). *Human Tooth Crown and Root Morphology* (p. iii). Cambridge University Press. Kindle Edition.

7

Permanent Mandibular Central Incisor

LEARNING OBJECTIVE
At the end of the chapter, the student should have knowledge of the permanent mandibular central incisor and develop the psychomotor skills for waxing and carving the same.

Permanent Mandibular Right Central Incisor

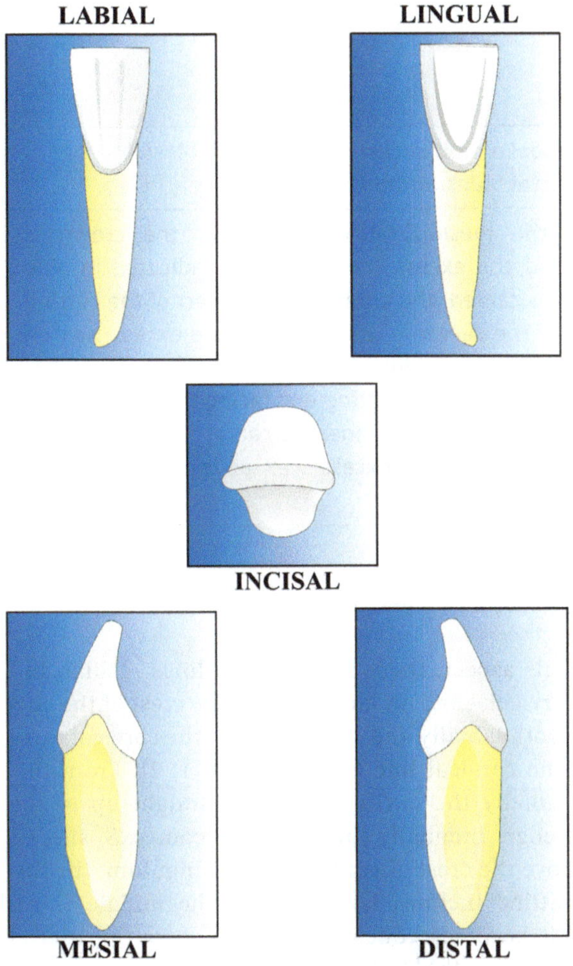

Labial Aspect

The permanent mandibular central incisor is the first tooth from the midline (Figure 7.1). The crown appears bilaterally symmetrical. The crest of contour on both the mesial and distal sides is at the incisal third, more towards the incisal edge (Figure 7.2a). From the contact areas the mesial and distal outlines converge uniformly towards the cervical line (Figure 7.2c). The incisal edge is perpendicular to the long axis of the tooth (Figure 7.2b) [1–3]. Both the mesio-incisal and disto-incisal angles are nearly at a right angle [2]. The mesio-incisal angle is sharper whereas the disto-incisal angle is slightly rounded [1]. The labial surface of the crown is flat [1, 3]. The outline of the root is uniform and tapering with the apex bent distally (Figure 7.2d) [1, 2].

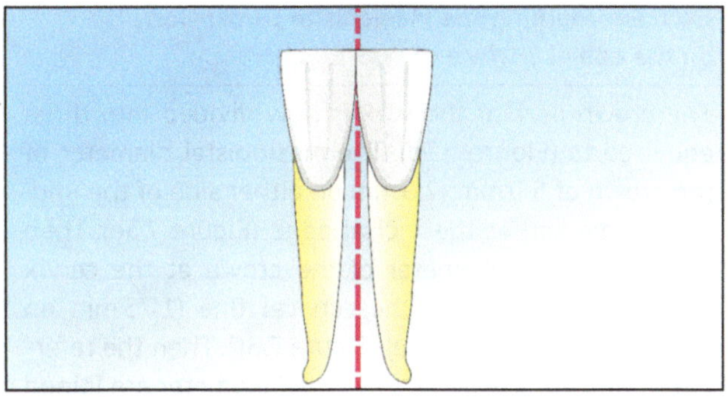

Figure 7.1 Position of the mandibular central incisor in relation to the midsagittal plane.

An Illustrated Atlas of Tooth Carving and Wax-Up Techniques, First Edition. Anil Bangalore Shivappa.

Companion website: www.wiley.com/go/bangalore/toothcarving

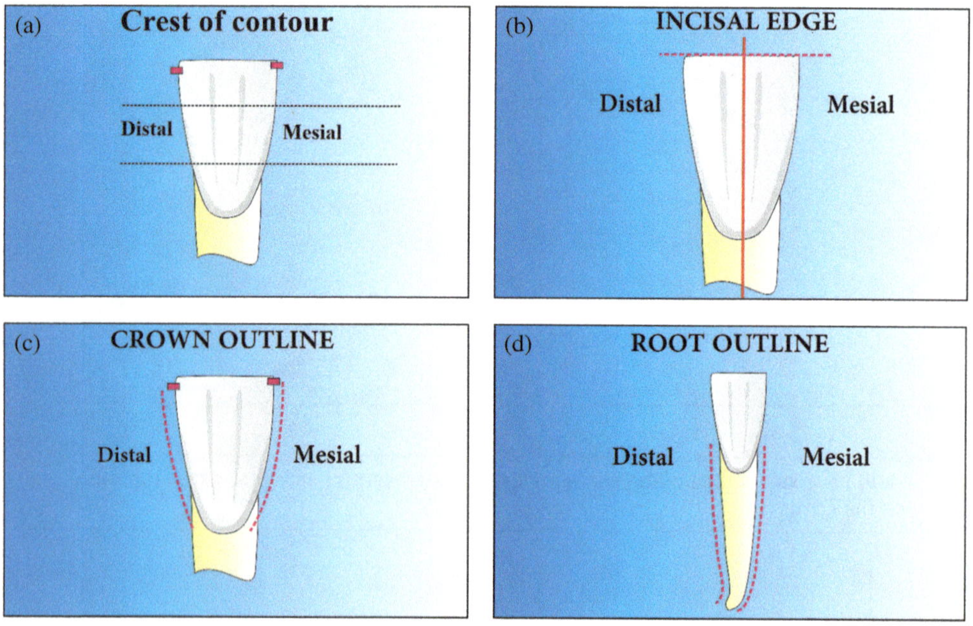

Figure 7.2 (a–d) Descriptive features of the permanent mandibular right central incisor from the labial aspect.

Carving from the Labial Aspect

Exercise: Marking the Length of Crown and Root on the Wax Block

On the prepared wax block, the length of the crown (9.5 mm) is marked from the incisal end on the labial surface (Figure 7.3a). The markings are extended on the remaining surfaces (Figure 7.3b). From the cervical end of the crown, the length of the root (12.5 mm) is marked (Figure 7.3c) [1].

Exercise: Marking the Mesiodistal Dimension on the Labial Surface of Wax Block

The crown part of the wax is now divided into three equal parts (Figure 7.3d). The mesiodistal diameter of the crown of 5.0 mm (2.5 mm on either side of the midline) is marked at the incisal edge (Figure 7.3e). Then the mesiodistal diameter of the crown at the cervix (3.5 mm) is marked at the cervical line (1.75 mm on either side of the midline) (Figure 7.3f). Then the reference points of the aforementioned diameter are joined on the mesial (Figure 7.3g) and distal sides (Figure 7.3h) to get the dimension of the crown within which the crown needs to be carved [1].

Exercise: Carving Excess Wax from the Mesial and Distal Sides of the Crown

Once the mesiodistal dimension of the crown is obtained, the excess wax outside it, indicated in blue colour, is carved. The anterior curved part of the cutting edge of the carver is used to carve the excess wax on the incisal and middle third of the crown (Figure 7.3i and j). With the non-cutting end facing the wax and the tip facing the cervical line, the carver is run buccolingually to carve the excess wax at the cervical third (Figure 7.3k–m).

Mesial Aspect

From this aspect, there are three outlines –labial, lingual, cervical – and an incisal edge. The crest of the curvature both labially and lingually is in the cervical third above the cervical line (Figure 7.4a) [1, 2]. From this crest, labially the outline becomes straight up to the incisal edge. Lingually the outline becomes 'S' shaped [2]. Above the crest of contour at the cingulum, the lingual outline inclines labially until the middle third, where it becomes concave and ends near the incisal ridge (Figure 7.4b) [1]. The cervical line curves approximately about one third to one fourth the length of the

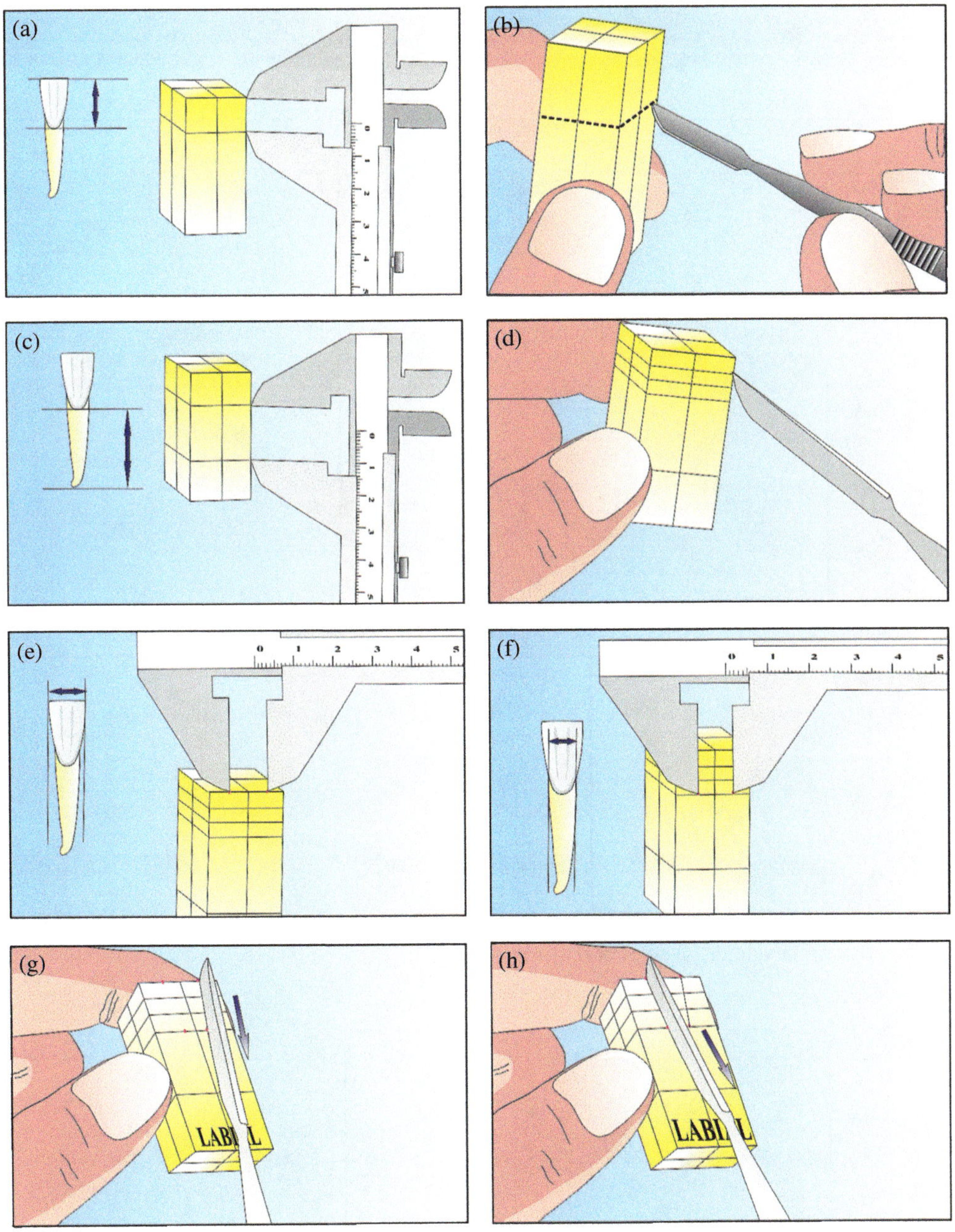

Figure 7.3 (a–h) Marking crown dimensions and root length on the labial surface of the wax block.

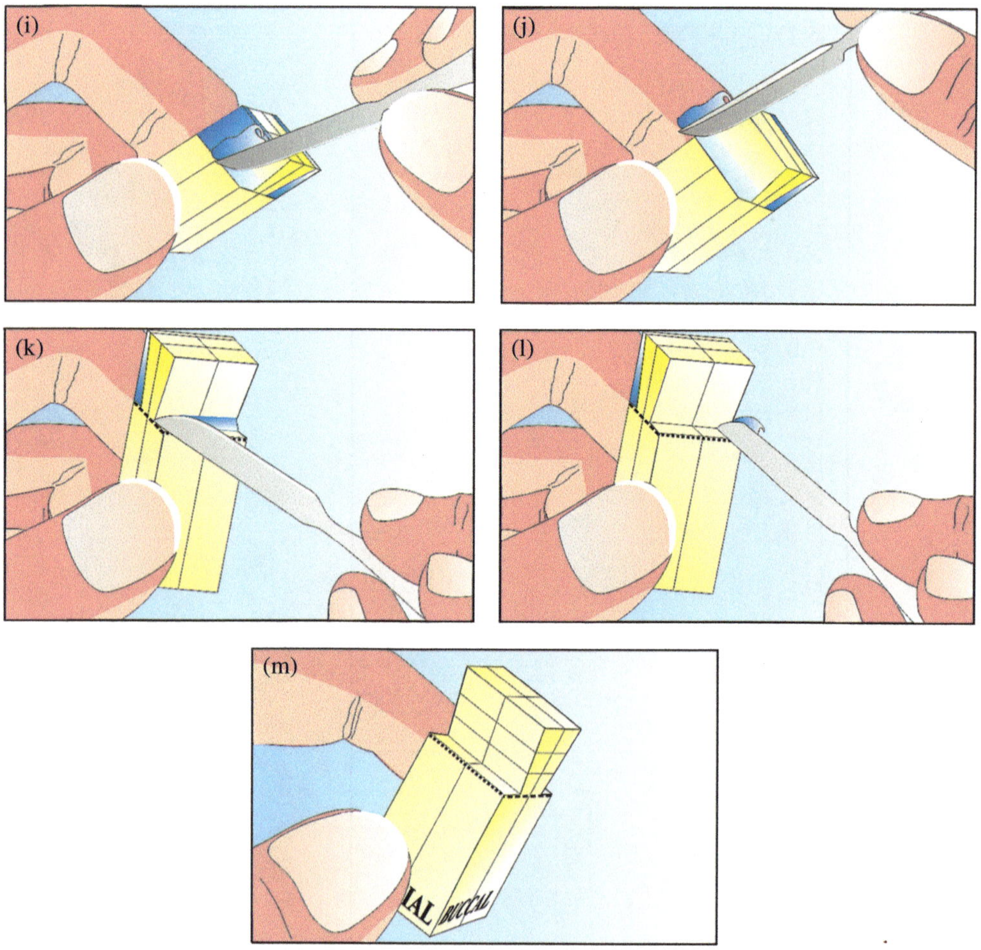

Figure 7.3 (i–m) Carving excess wax from the mesial and distal sides of the crown.

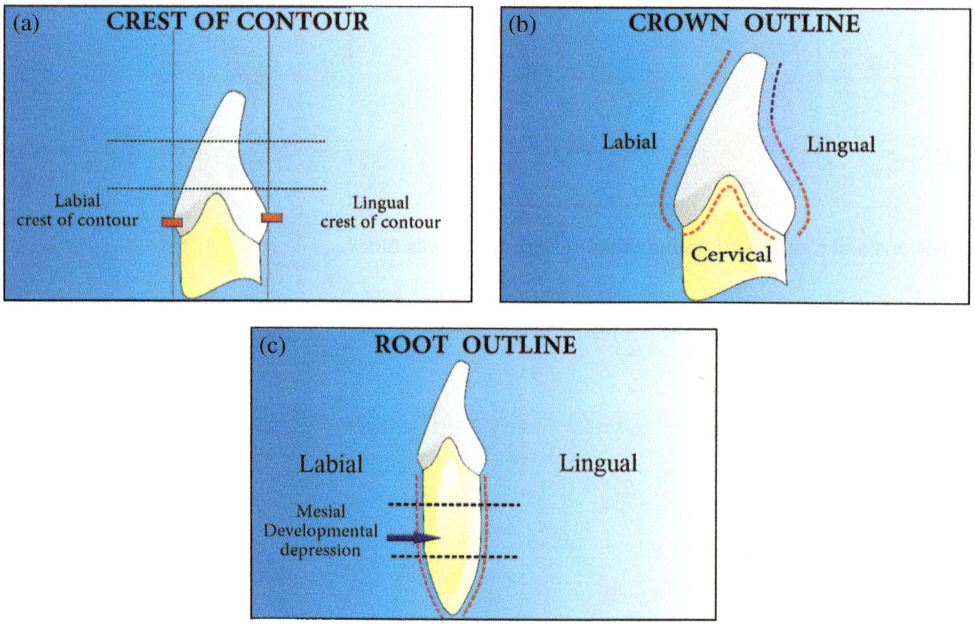

Figure 7.4 (a–c) Description of the permanent mandibular right central incisor from the mesial aspect.

crown [1, 2]. The incisal edge is lingual to the long axis of the tooth [2]. The mesial surface is smooth convex at the incisal third, concave in the middle third, and flattened at the cervical third [1].

The root outline is almost straight in the cervical third and middle third, which gradually taper at the apical third, ending in a blunted or pointed root apex [1]. The mesial surface of the root shows the developmental depression over the entire root, deeper at the middle and apical third (Figure 7.4c) [2].

Carving from the Mesial Aspect

Exercise: Marking the Labiolingual Dimension on the Wax Block

On the mesial surface, the labiolingual diameter of the crown at the cervix measuring 5.3 mm (2.65 mm on either side of the midline) is marked at the cervix (Figure 7.5a and b). The labiolingual diameter of the crown of 6 mm (3 mm on either side of the midline) is then marked near the incisal edge (Figure 7.5c and d) [1].

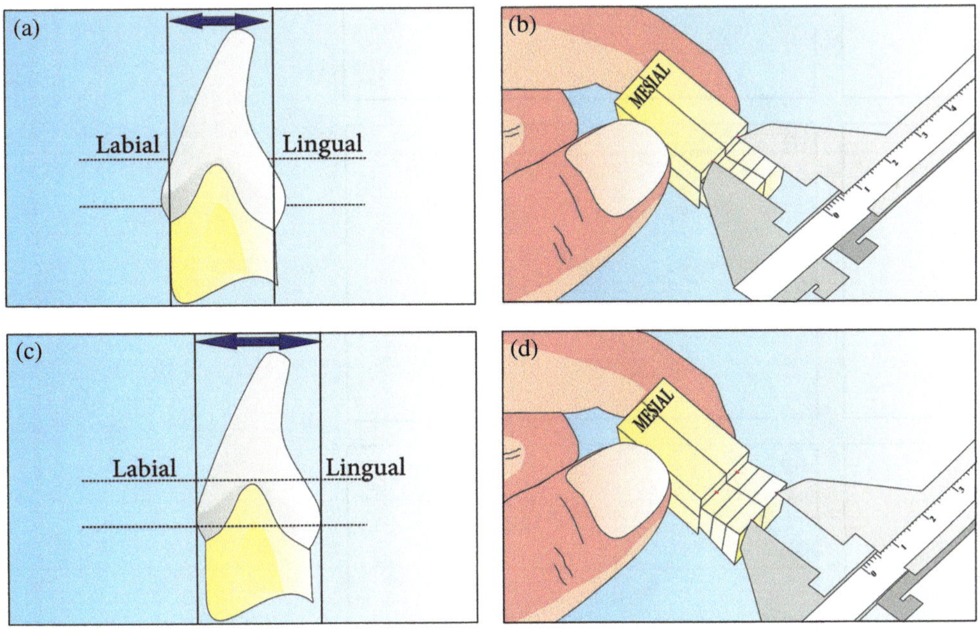

Figure 7.5 (a–d) Measuring and marking the dimension of the crown on the mesial aspect of the wax.

Exercise: Marking the Outline of the Crown on the Mesial Aspect

After obtaining the dimensions, the outline is drawn with features mentioned previously (Figure 7.6a). The excess unwanted wax marked in blue colour should be carved (Figure 7.6b).

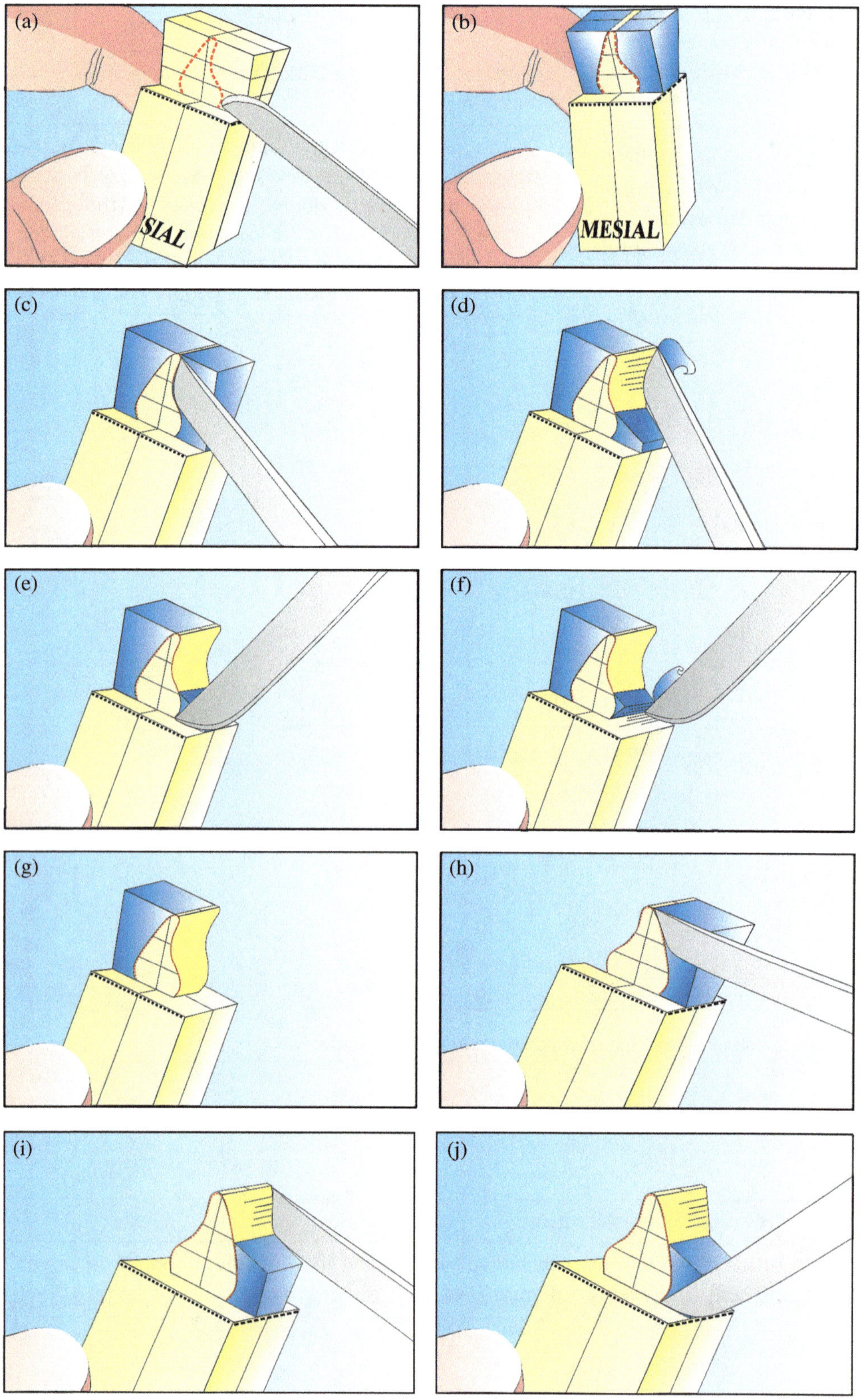

Figure 7.6 (a–l) Drawing the crown outline and carving excess wax from the labial and lingual surfaces.

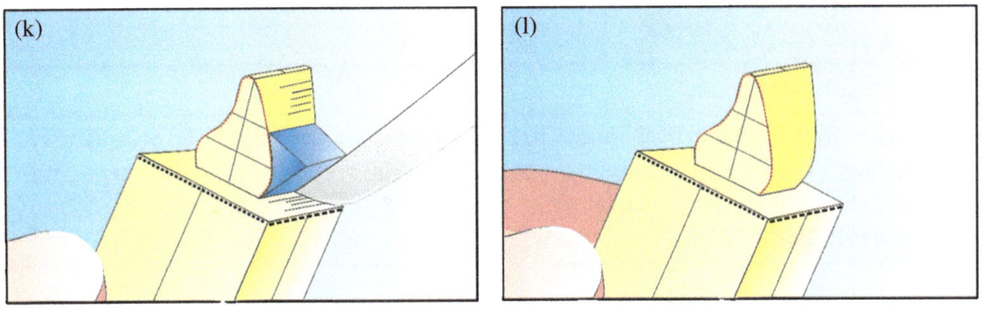

Figure 7.6 (Cont'd) (a–l)

Exercise: Carving Excess Wax on the Lingual Side
The incisal third and middle third of the lingual surface are carved using the convex part of the Lecron carver to get the concave surface (Figure 7.6c). The carver is moved in a mesiodistal direction from the surface until the outline is reached (Figure 7.6d). The cervical third of the wax below the crest of contour is carved moving the carver in a mesiodistal direction with the non-cutting edge of the carver facing the wax and the tip facing the cervix (Figure 7.6e and f). The remaining wax is then carved to get a smooth lingual surface (Figure 7.6g).

Lingual Aspect

The crown outline from this aspect is exactly the opposite of the labial aspect. The crown shows the slight lingual convergence. The lingual fossa is a smooth, shallow, and concave area at the incisal and middle third bordered on the mesial and distal sides by marginal ridges. The cingulum at the cervical third is convex, less prominent, and centred on the long axis of tooth (Figure 7.7a and b) [2].

Exercise: Carving Excess Wax on the Labial Side
Excess wax on the labial half of the crown is carved with the curved part of the cutting edge (Figure 7.6h and i). The cervical half of the wax is carved in a similar manner as was done to carve the area below the crest of contour at the cervical part of the lingual surface (Figure 7.6j and k). A smooth labial surface is obtained after removing the remaining wedge of wax (Figure 7.6l).

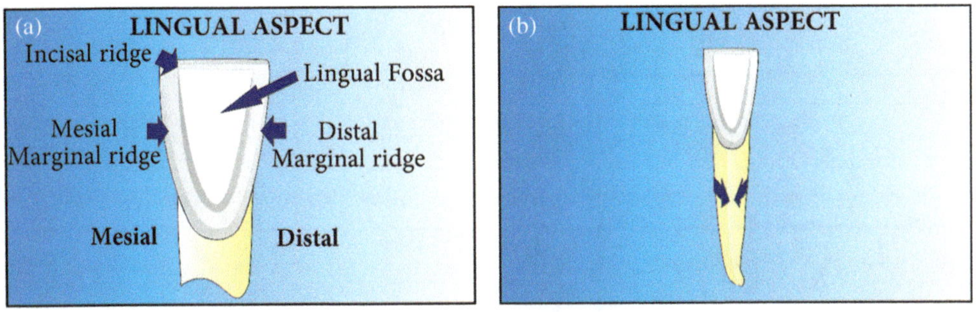

Figure 7.7 (a–b) Description of the mandibular right central incisor from the lingual aspect.

Carving from the Lingual Aspect

Exercise: Creating the Lingual Convergence of the Crown
To create the lingual convergence of the crown, the outline is marked on the both the mesial and distal part of lingual surface. The outline should be such that it follows the labial outline but is narrower towards the midline (Figure 7.8a). The excess wax indicated in blue is then carved on both the mesial and distal sides by moving the carver incisocervically (Figure 7.8b–d).

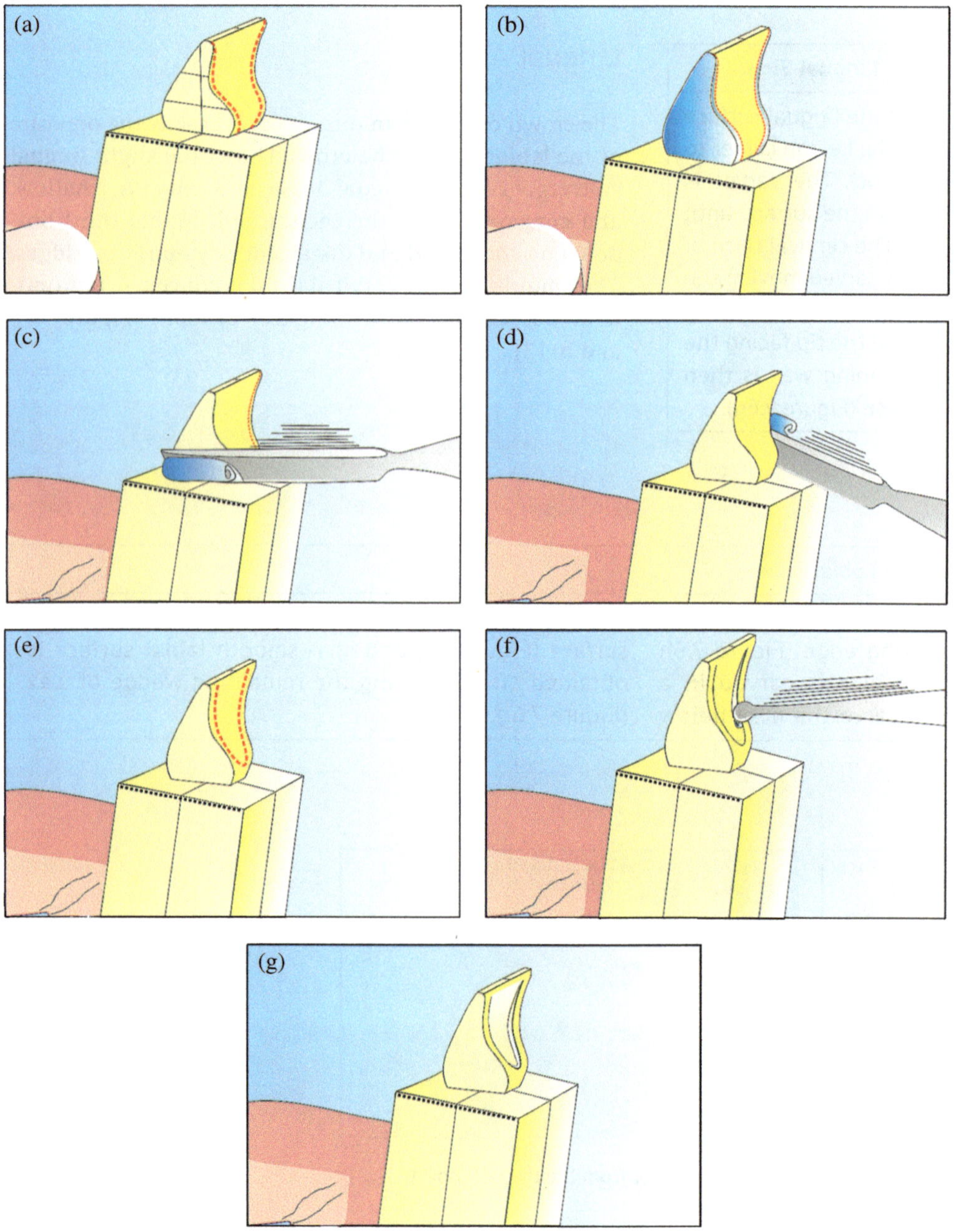

Figure 7.8 (a–g) Creating lingual convergence and carving the lingual fossa.

Exercise: Carving the Fossa on the Lingual Surface

The outline of the fossa is drawn resembling the letter 'V' (Figure 7.8e). Then the concavity is created within the boundary of the 'V' using the excavating end of the carver, deeper near the cingulum and shallower as moved towards the incisal edge (Figure 7.8f and g).

Distal Aspect

The distal aspect is similar to that of the mesial aspect. The cervical line curvature is less towards the incisal edge compared to the mesial side. The root surface shows the presence of deeper developmental depression [2].

Incisal Aspect

The crown is wider labiolingually than mesiodistally [2]. The tooth is bilaterally symmetrical with the mesial half equal to the distal half. The labial surface is wider than the lingual surface. The incisal edge is perpendicular to the long axis of the crown and is about 2 mm thick [1–3]. Most of the labial surface is seen from this aspect. The cingulum is placed in the centre of the crown (Figure 7.9a and b) [1].

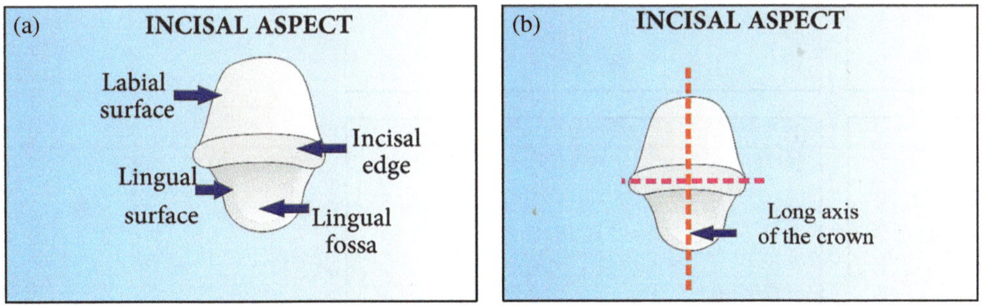

Figure 7.9 (a–b) Description of the mandibular right central incisor crown from the incisal aspect.

Carving the Root

Exercise: Carving the Root from the Labial Aspect

The labial outline is drawn on the labial surface of the root portion of the wax block with features described earlier in the chapter (Figure 7.10a). The wax outside the outline is excess wax that needs to be carved (Figure 7.10b). The wax indicated in blue is carved on the distal side in two steps. With the curved part of the cutting edge of carver facing the cervical part of the wax, the carver is moved buccolingually (Figure 7.10c and d). Then with the non-cutting edge facing the wax near the apical portion, the carver is moved in the same direction as mentioned previously (Figure 7.10e). The remaining bulk of wax is carved (Figure 7.10f). Similarly, the wax is then carved out on the mesial side to complete the outline of the root from the labial aspect (Figure 7.10g).

Exercise: Carving the Root from the Mesial or Distal surface

The buccolingual outline is drawn on the distal aspect (Figure 7.10h). The excess wax is carved labially and lingually to get the outline of the root on the distal aspect (Figure 7.10i and j).

Exercise: Creating the Lingual Convergence of the Root

The root convergence is created by carving the wax on mesial and distal side, more in the lingual portion than the labial (Figure 7.10k and l).

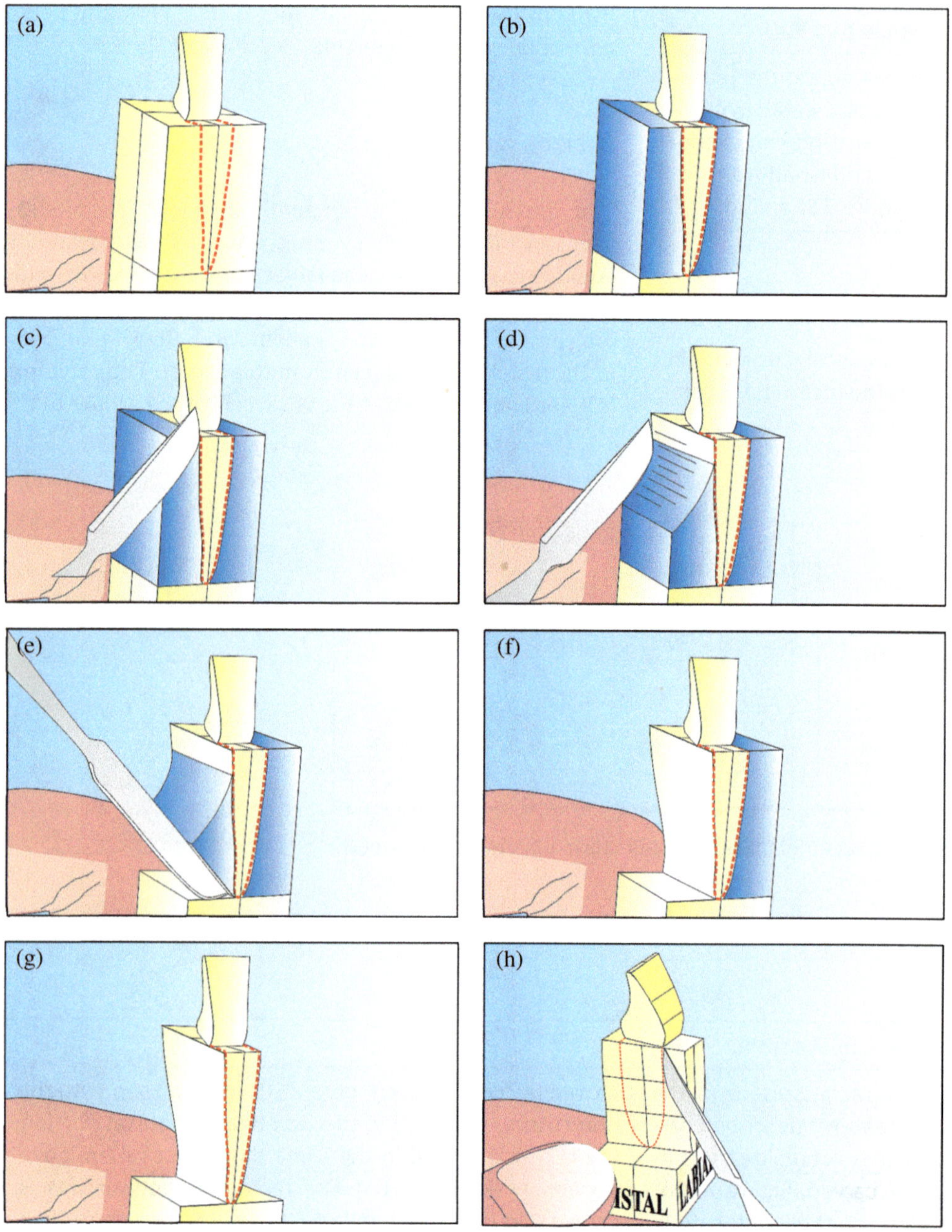

Figure 7.10 (a–p) Carving the root of the permanent mandibular right central incisor from the labial and distal aspects.

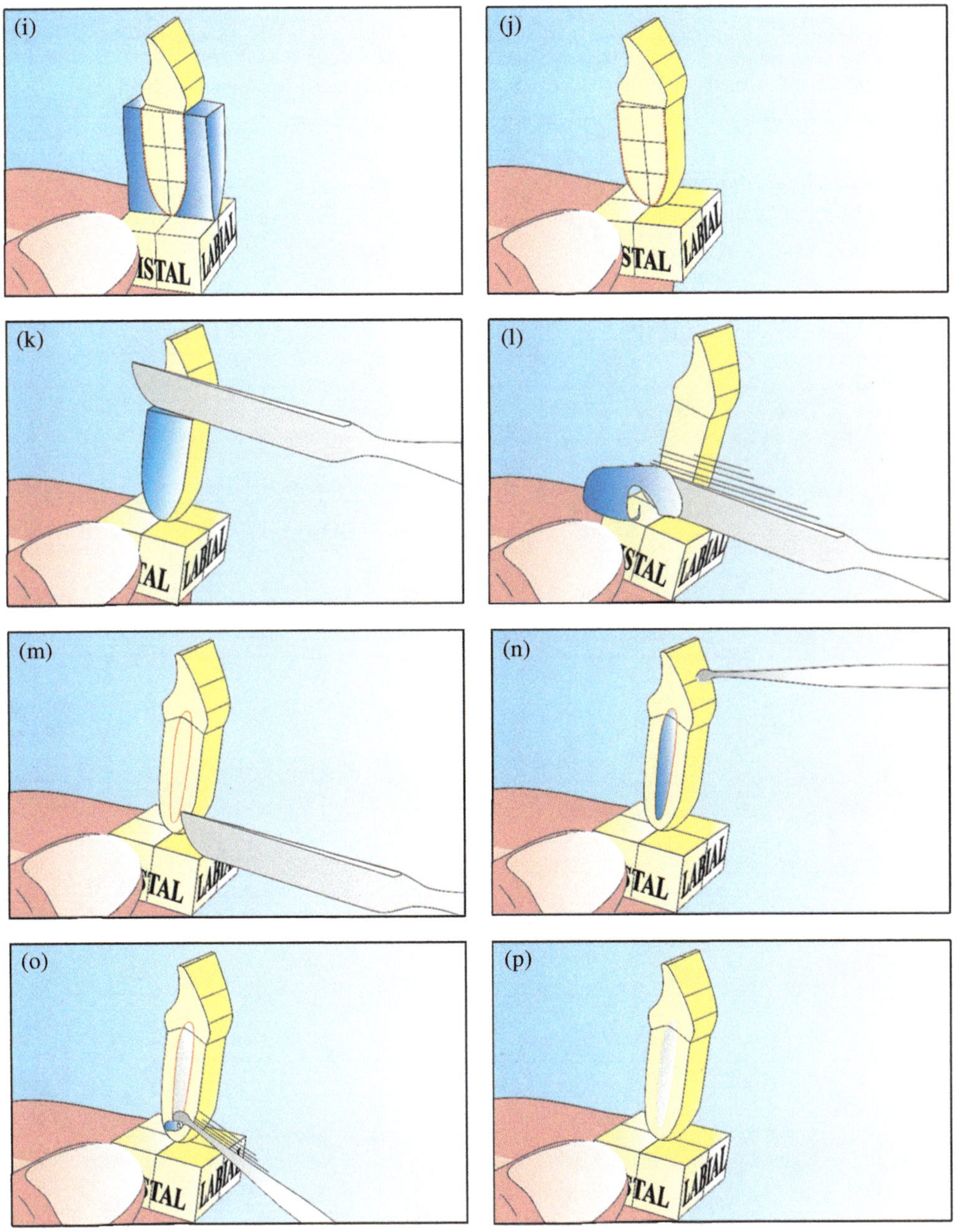

Figure 7.10 (Cont'd) (a–p)

Exercise: Creating Developmental Depression on Root Surfaces

The outline for the developmental depression on the root is drawn and the concavity of the depression is created using the excavating end of the carver moving it cervico-occlusally (Figure 7.10m–o). At the end of the carving procedure, the cervical line is drawn at the cervix of both the mesial and distal sides (Figure 7.10p).

Exercise: Drawing the Cervical Line on the Mesial and Distal Aspects

The cervical line is marked with its curvature of 3 mm, facing incisally on the mesial aspect. On the distal surface, the curvature of the cervical line is 2 mm.

References

1 Stanley, J.N. and Major, M.A.C. (2010). *Wheeler's Dental Anatomy and Occlusion*, 9e. St. Louis, MO: Saunders Elsevier.

2 Rickne, C.S. and Weiss, G. (2012). *Woelfel's Dental Anatomy*, 8e. Philadelphia: Lippincott Williams & Wilkins.

3 Hillson, S. (2012). *Dental Anthropology*. Cambridge University Press. Kindle Edition.

8

Permanent Mandibular Lateral Incisor

LEARNING OBJECTIVE
At the end of the chapter, the student should have knowledge of the permanent mandibular lateral incisor and develop the psychomotor skills for waxing and carving the same.

Permanent Mandibular Right Lateral Incisor

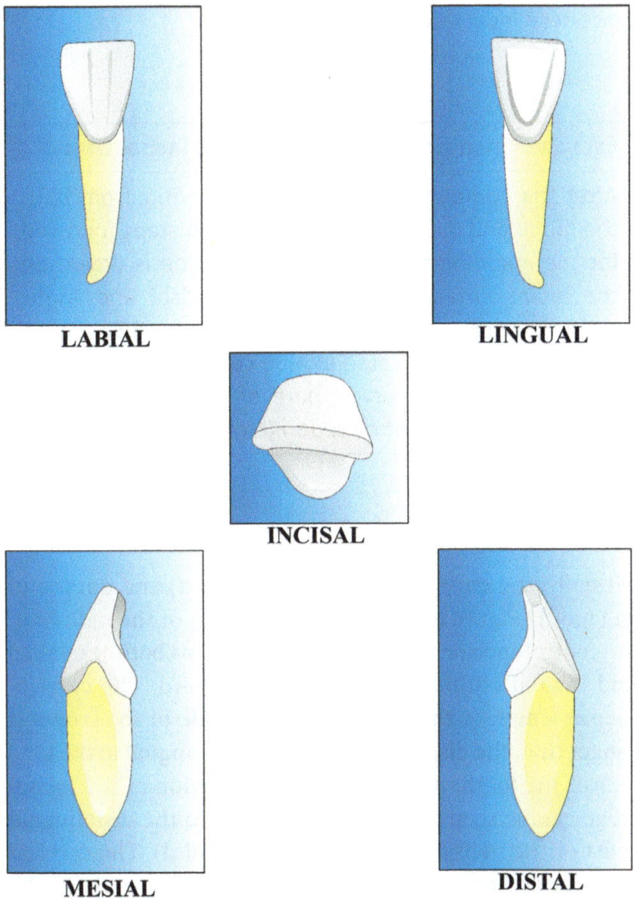

Labial Aspect

The permanent mandibular lateral incisor is the second tooth from the midline (Figure 8.1). Compared to the mandibular central incisor, this tooth is wider mesiodistally with bulk added to the distal side (Figure 8.2a) [1]. The crest of contour on both the mesial and distal sides is in the incisal third. The distal crest of curvature is more cervical than the mesial crest and the distal outline is more curved than the mesial outline (Figure 8.2c). The incisal edge is tilted cervically towards the distal portion (Figure 8.2b). The root has a uniform outline from the cervix to the root apex, which tilts distally in most cases. The length of the root is longer compared to that of the mandibular central incisor. In some cases, bifurcation of the root can be seen (Figure 8.2d) [2].

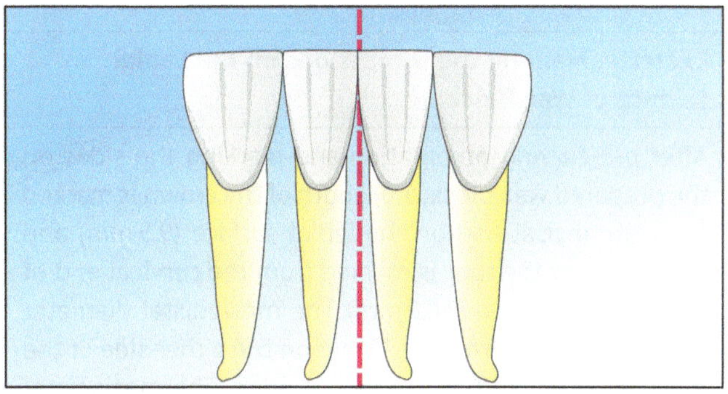

Figure 8.1 Position of the mandibular lateral incisor in relation to the midsagittal plane.

An Illustrated Atlas of Tooth Carving and Wax-Up Techniques, First Edition. Anil Bangalore Shivappa.

Companion website: www.wiley.com/go/bangalore/toothcarving

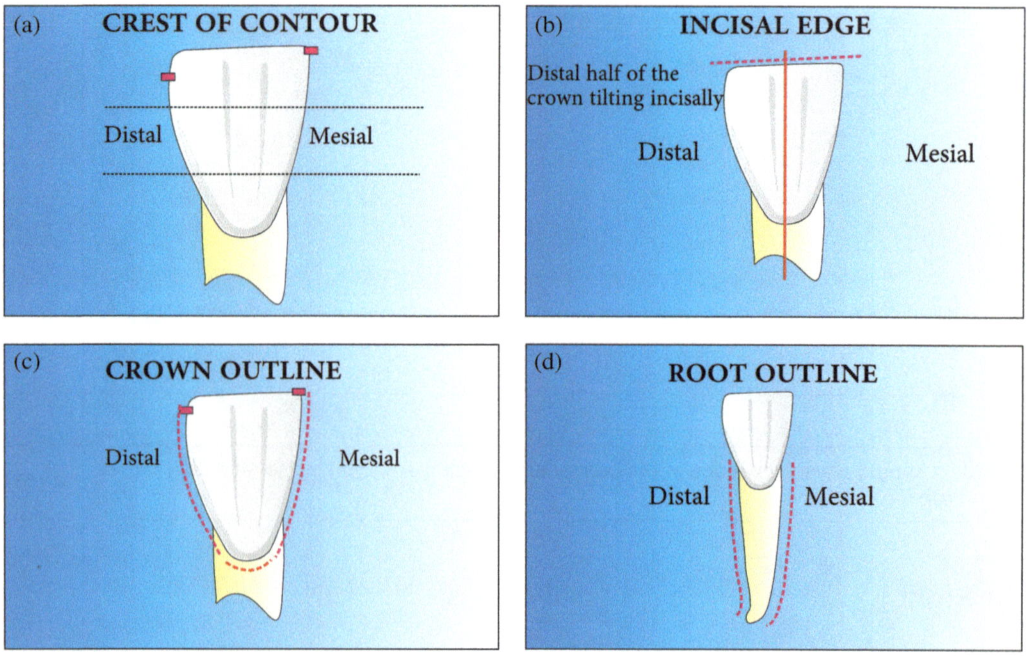

Figure 8.2 (a–d) Descriptive features of the permanent mandibular right lateral incisor from the labial aspect.

Carving from the Labial Aspect

Carving from this aspect is similar to the steps followed for the mandibular central incisor, with slight variations in the steps as follows:

- The distal bulk is added to the outline to increase the mesiodistal dimension of the tooth.
- The root length is increased by 1.5 mm.
- The cervico-incisal length of the crown is reduced distally than mesial, so the crown appears to tilt distally.

Exercise: Marking the Dimensions on the Labial Surface of Wax Block

After pre-carving preparation and marking the sides on the prepared wax block,the length of the crown is marked from the incisal end on the labial surface (9.5 mm) and the length of the root is marked from the cervical end of the crown marking (14.0 mm). The mesiodistal diameter of the crown of 5.5 mm (2.75 mm on the either side of the midline) is marked at the incisal edge. The mesiodistal diameter of the crown at the cervix is marked at the cervix, about 4.0 mm (2.0 mm on either side of the midline). Then the points are joined on both mesial and distal sides to get the dimension of the crown [1].

Exercise: Creating the Distal Tilt of the Incisal Edge

After the completion of the crown carving, from both the labial and mesial aspects (similar to steps followed for the mandibular central incisor), a line is drawn on the labial surface, from the mesio-incisal line angle, tilting cervically towards the distal (Figure 8.3a and b). The excess wax indicated in blue colour (Figure 8.3c) is carved using the curved part of the Lecron carver moved in mesiodistal direction (Figure 8.3d–f).

Mesial Aspect

Mesially, the crest of contour (Figure 8.4a) and outline of the tooth (Figure 8.4b) are similar to that of the mandibular central incisor. The crest of contour on both the labial and lingual outlines is at the cervical third. The cervico-incisal length of the crown on mesial side of the crown is longer than the distal. The incisal edge is lingual to the long axis of the tooth. A part of the distal portion of the incisal ridge can be seen from this aspect, due to the distolingual twist of the incisal ridge (Figure 8.4c and d). The cervical line curves incisally about one fourth the length of the crown. The root appears similar to the central incisor (Figure 8.4e), except the length is greater. In some instances, bifurcation of the root can be seen [1, 2].

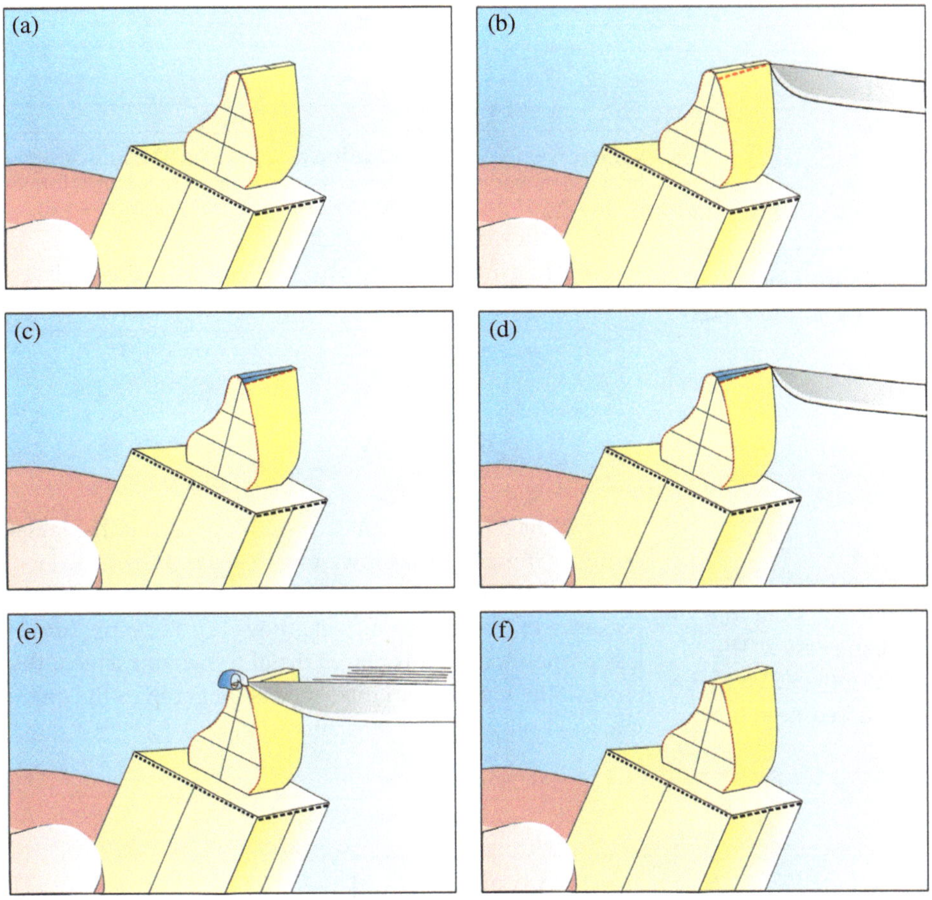

Figure 8.3 (a–f) Creating the distal tilt of the incisal edge of the crown.

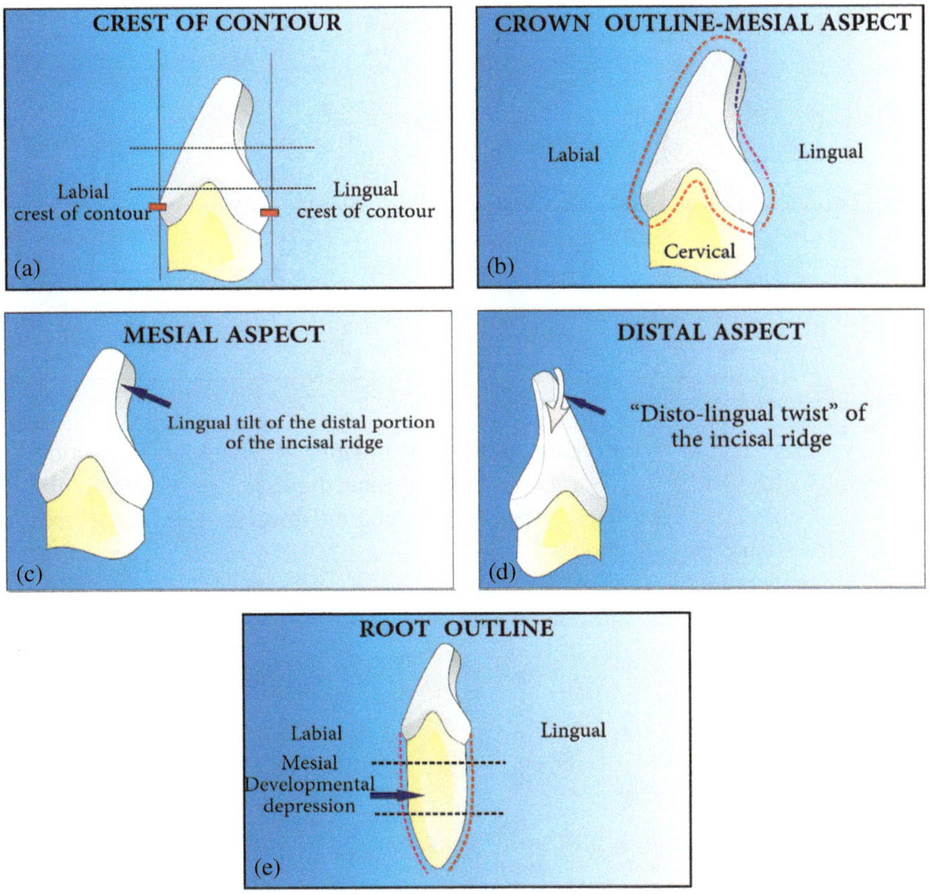

Figure 8.4 (a–e) Description of the permanent mandibular right lateral incisor from mesial and distal aspect.

Distal Aspect

From this aspect, the tooth outline appears similar to that of the mesial side. The incisal edge appears slanting towards the distal, because of the reduced distal marginal ridge height. Because of the distolingual twist, the distal part of the labial surface can be seen [2].

Carving from the Mesial Aspect

Exercise: Marking the Dimensions on the Mesial Surface of Wax Block
On the mesial surface, the labiolingual diameter of the crown at the cervix measuring 5.8 mm (2.9 mm on either side of the midline) is marked at the cervix. The labiolingual diameter of the crown of 6.5 mm (3.25 mm on either side of the midline) is then marked near the incisal edge [1].

Exercise: Carving the Outline of Crown on Mesial Aspect
Carving steps from the mesial aspect are similar to the steps followed for the mandibular central incisor. **NOTE:** While drawing the outline, keep the incisal edge thicker than the central incisor.

Lingual Aspect

The outline from the lingual aspect is opposite of the labial outline. The crown narrows towards the lingual surface. The lingual surface is smooth and sometimes shows the presence of the cervico-incisal groove [1]. The cingulum is less pronounced and is placed distal to the long axis of the crown. The mesial marginal ridge is longer than the distal marginal ridge (Figure 8.5a and b) [2].

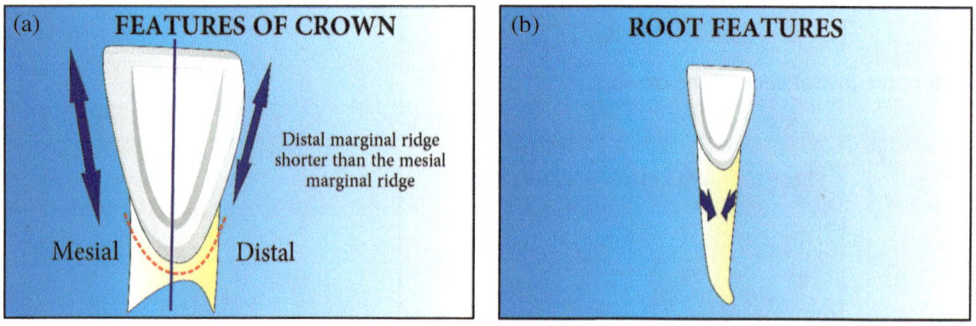

Figure 8.5 (a–b) Description of the permanent mandibular right lateral incisor from the lingual aspect.

Carving from the Lingual Aspect

Exercise: Carving step sequence from the Lingual Aspect
Carving steps from the lingual aspect are similar to the steps followed for the mandibular central incisor with significant modification. • Lingual convergence of the mesial surface should be more than that of the distal surface. This convergence is created by marking the mesial convergence line more towards the midline than the distal convergence line. This shifts the cingulum towards the distal side (Figure 8.6a–d).

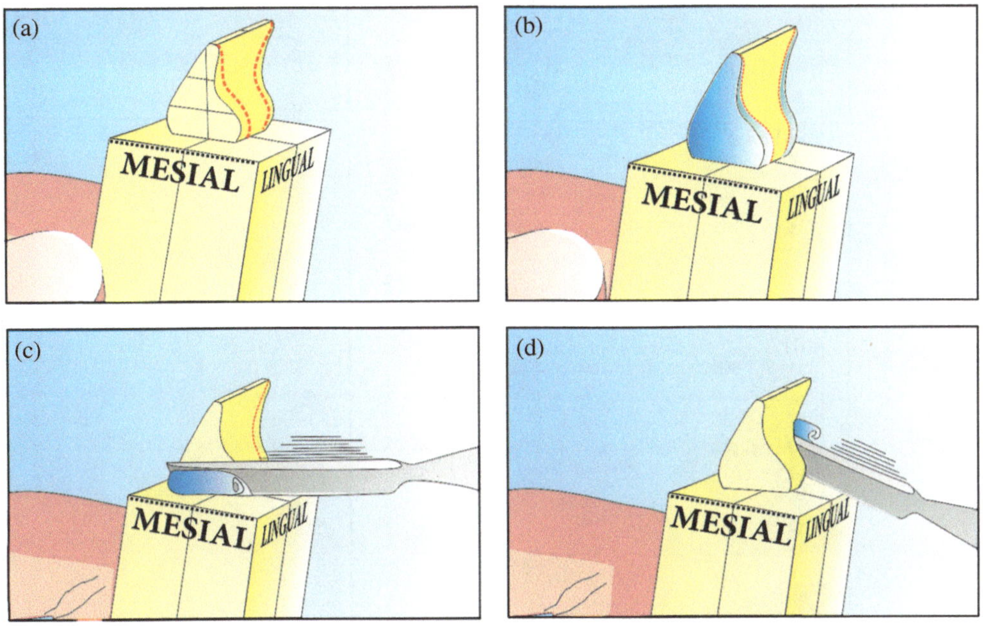

Figure 8.6 (a–d) Creating lingual convergence and distal placement of the cingulum.

Incisal Aspect

Labiolingual dimension of the crown is greater than the mesiodistal dimension. Disto-incisal twist of the incisal ridge to the long axis of crown is seen, which follows the curvature of the mandibular arch (Figure 8.7a). The cingulum is also positioned distal to the long axis of the crown (Figure 8.7b) [2].

Carving from the Incisal Aspect

The incisal edge, which was kept thicker while carving the mesial aspect, is utilized for creating the lingual twist of the distal half of the incisal edge (Figure 8.8a). The outline on the thick incisal edge is drawn, such that the distal half of the edge tilts lingually. Excess wax (in blue colour) is carved from the lingual surface in such a way that more from the mesial half is carved (Figure 8.8b and c). In a similar way, more wax is carved from the distal half of the labial surface (Figure 8.8d and e).

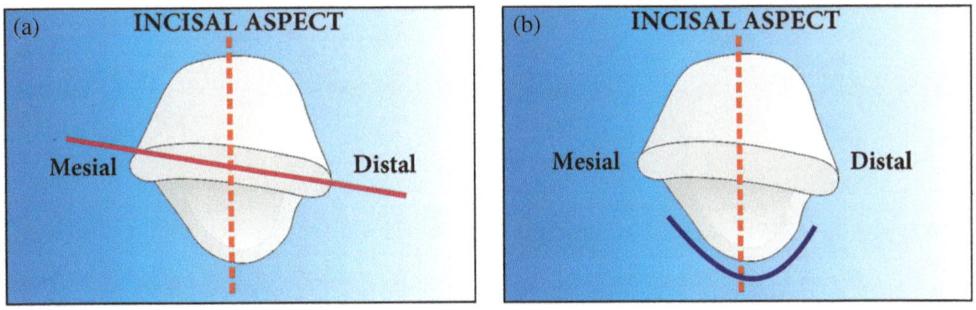

Figure 8.7 (a–b) Description of the mandibular right lateral incisor crown from the incisal aspect.

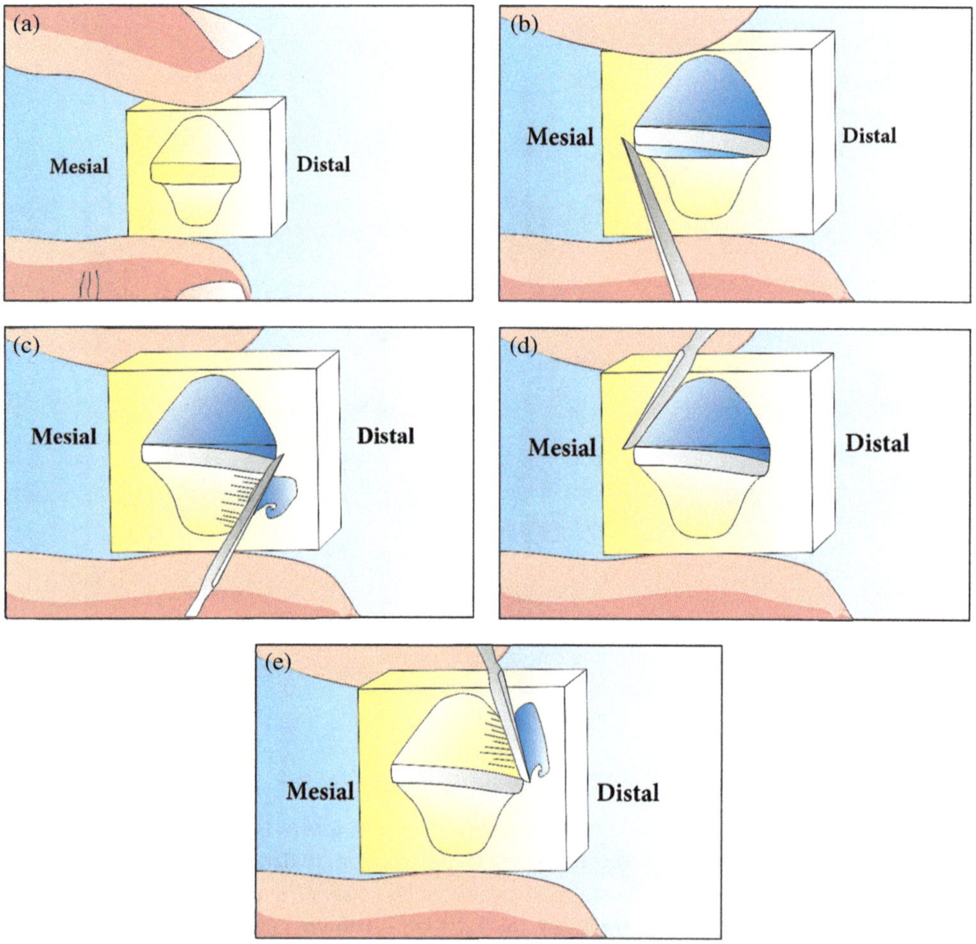

Figure 8.8 (a–e) Creating the distolingual twist of the crown.

References

1 Stanley, J.N. and Major, M.A.C. (2010). *Wheeler's Dental Anatomy and Occlusion*, 9e. Saunders Elsevier: St. Louis, MO.

2 Rickne, C.S. and Weiss, G. (2012). *Woelfel's Dental Anatomy*, 8e. Philadelphia: Lippincott Williams & Wilkins.

9

Permanent Maxillary Canine

LEARNING OBJECTIVE
At the end of the chapter, the student should have knowledge of the permanent maxillary canine and develop the psychomotor skills for carving and waxing the same.

Permanent Maxillary Right Canine

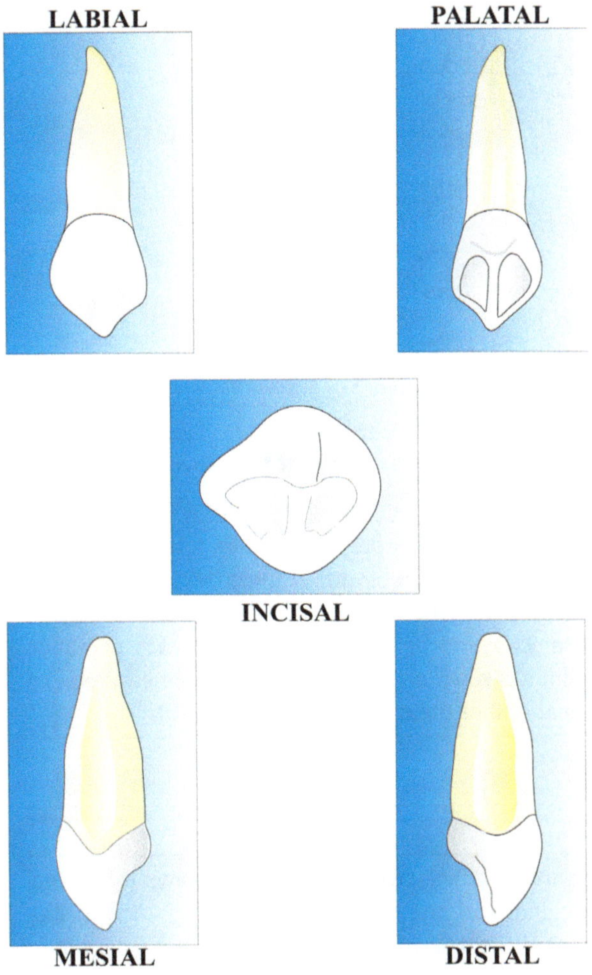

Labial Aspect

The maxillary canine is the third tooth from the midline (Figure 9.1). From this aspect, the crown appears pentagonal in shape [1]. The canine appears narrower mesiodistally than the central incisor [2]. Mesially, the crest of curvature is approximately at the junction of the middle and incisal third of the crown (Figure 9.2a). The crest of contour distally is in the middle of the middle third of the crown (Figure 9.2b) [1–3].

The mesial outline is convex from the cervical line to the crest of contour and concave from the crest of contour to the tip of the cusp. This concave part forms the mesial slope (Figure 9.2c). The distal outline of the crown is concave from the cervical line to the distal crest of contour. The outline from the distal crest of contour to the cusp tip is slightly concave (Figure 9.2d) [1, 2].

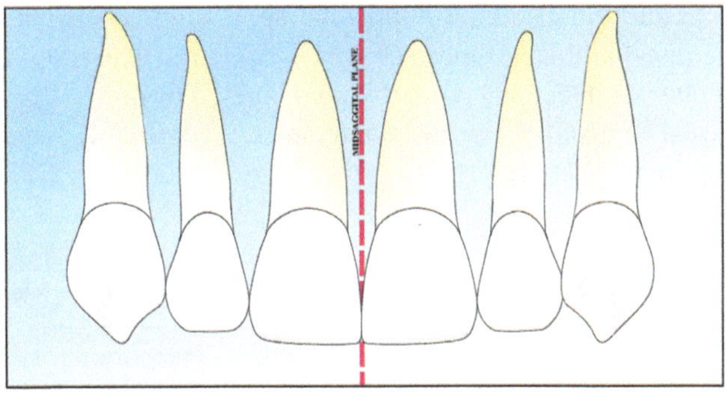

Figure 9.1 Position of the maxillary canine in relation to the midsagittal plane.

An Illustrated Atlas of Tooth Carving and Wax-Up Techniques, First Edition. Anil Bangalore Shivappa.

Companion website: www.wiley.com/go/bangalore/toothcarving

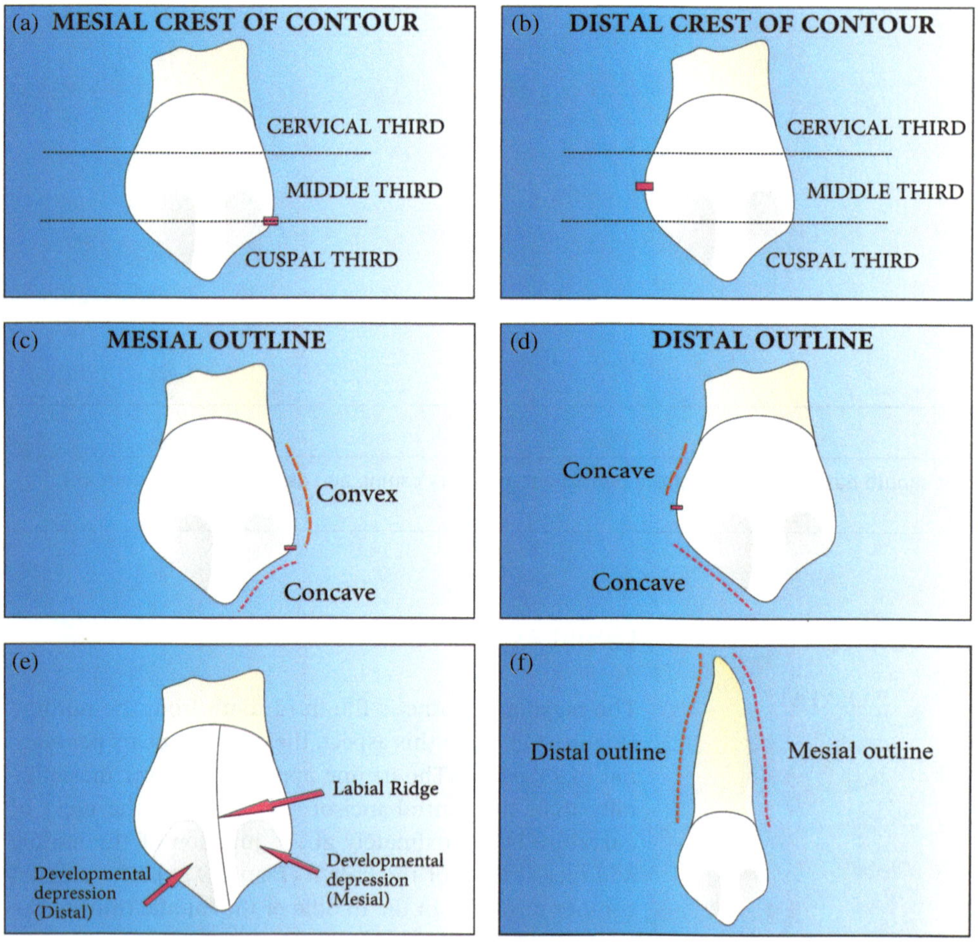

Figure 9.2 (a–f) Characteristic features of the crown and root of the maxillary canine from the labial aspect.

The labial surface shows three developmental lobes: mesial, distal, and labial [3]. The crest of the labial ridge that runs from the cervical line to the cusp tip is not straight; it is curved mesially [2]. Between these lobes there are developmental depressions; the mesial developmental depression is the one between the mesial and labial lobes and the distal developmental depression is between the distal and labial lobes (Figure 9.2e) [1, 2]. The root is slender and conical with blunted apex, curving either mesial or distally. The distal curvature is commonly seen (Figure 9.2f) [1–3].

Carving from the Labial Aspect

Exercise: Marking the Length of the Crown and Root on the Wax Block

After the pre-carve preparation of the wax block, measurement for the length of the crown about 10 mm is taken from the incisal edge of the wax block (Figure 9.3a and b) and length of the root of about 17.0 mm is taken from the end of the crown measurement (cervical end of the crown) (Figure 9.3c) [2].

Exercise: Marking the Mesiodistal Dimension of the crown

The mesiodistal diameter of the crown measurement is marked at the incisal edge, about 7.5 mm (3.75 mm on either side of the midline; Figure 9.3e), and the mesiodistal diameter of the crown at the cervix is marked at the cervix, about 5.5 mm (2.75 mm on either side of the midline; Figure 9.3f). The crown boundary is drawn by joining the markings on the mesial (Figure 9.3g) and distal (Figure 9.3h) sides of the midline of the wax block (Figure 9.3i). Excess, unwanted wax as indicated in blue colour as shown (Figure 9.3j–n) [2].

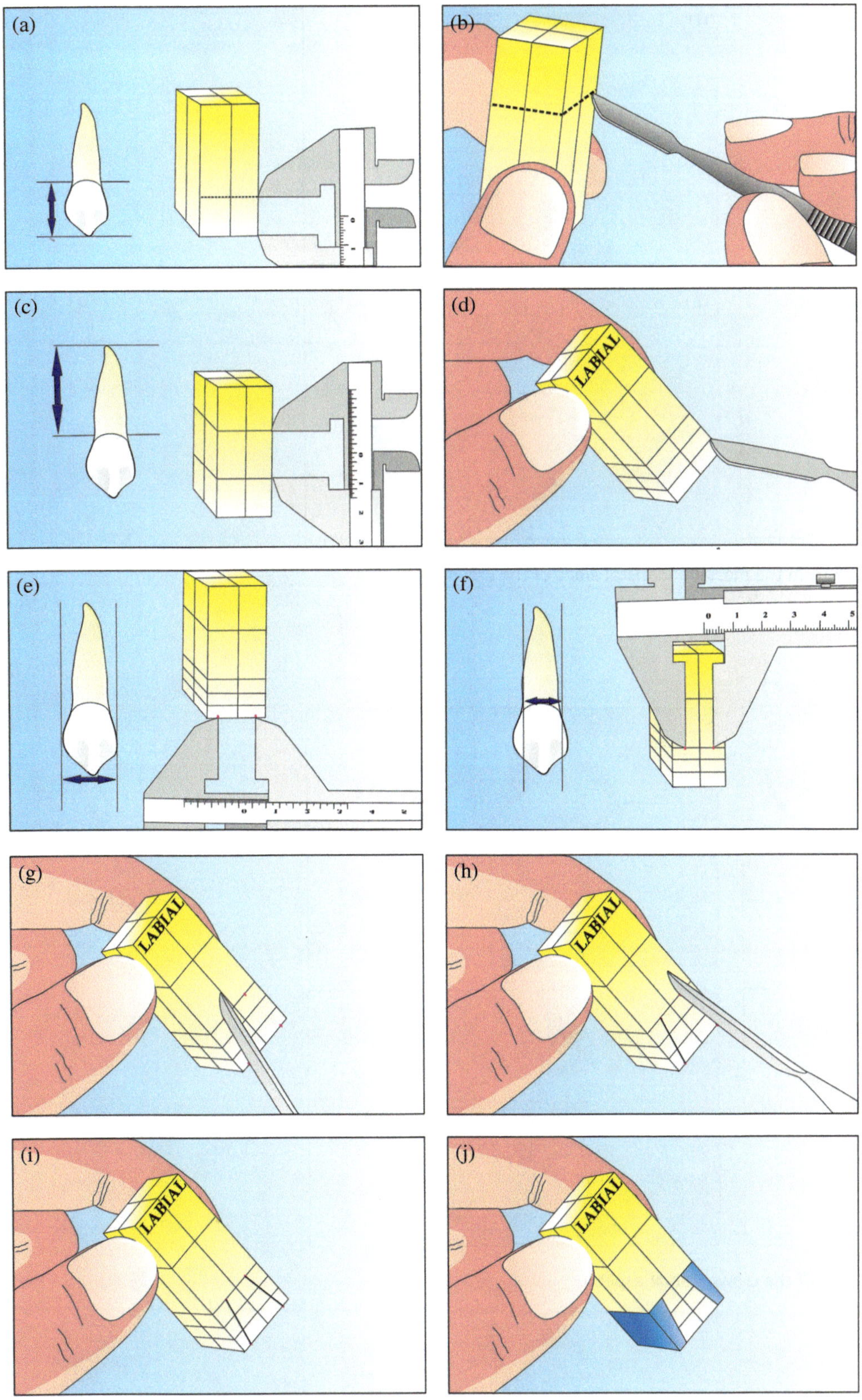

Figure 9.3 (a–j) Measuring and marking the crown dimension and root length on the labial aspect of the wax block.

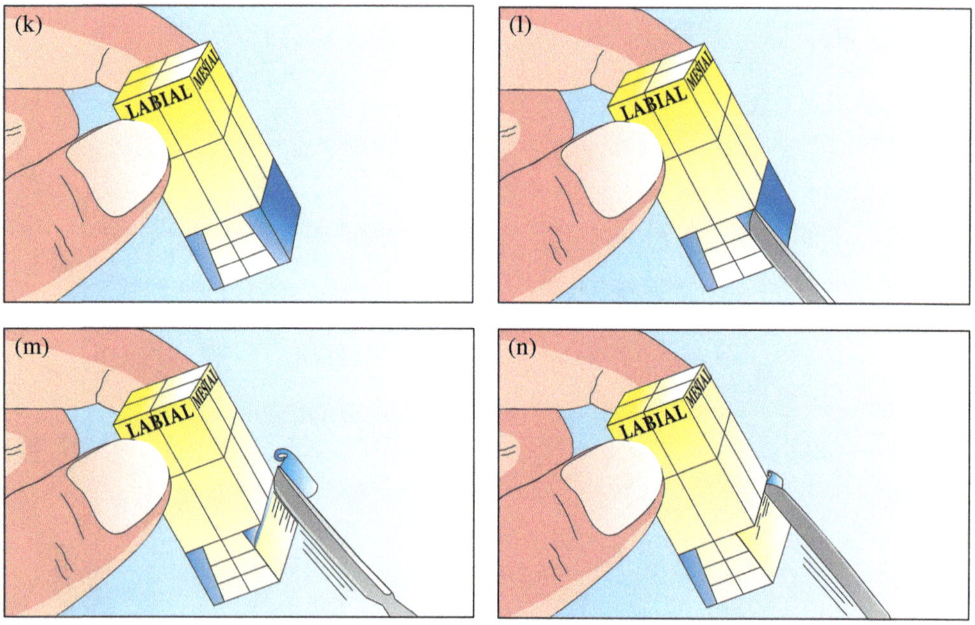

Figure 9.3 (k–n) Carving excess wax from the mesial and distal sides of the crown.

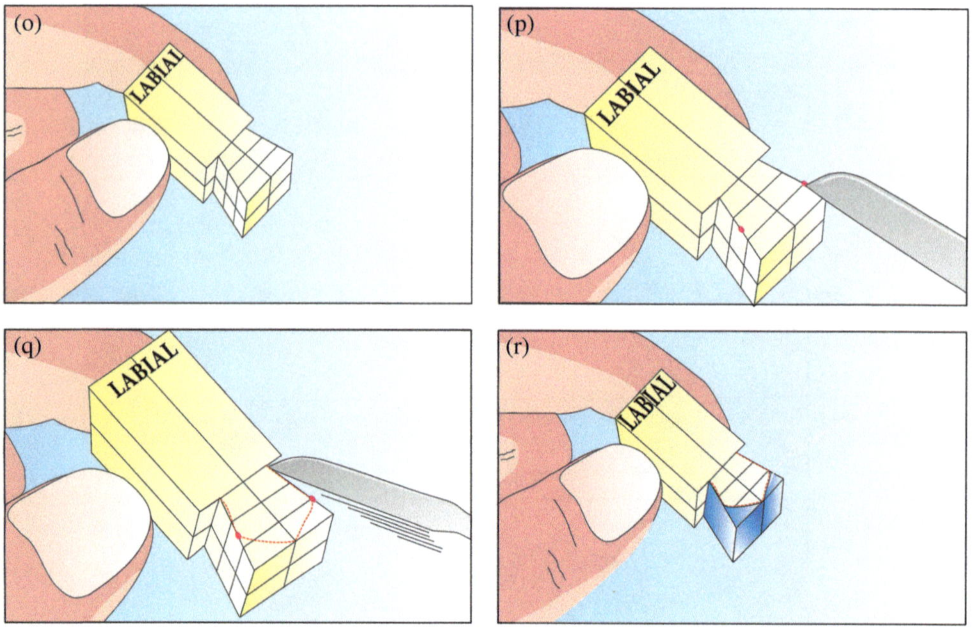

Figure 9.3 (o–r) Marking the outline of the crown (labial aspect).

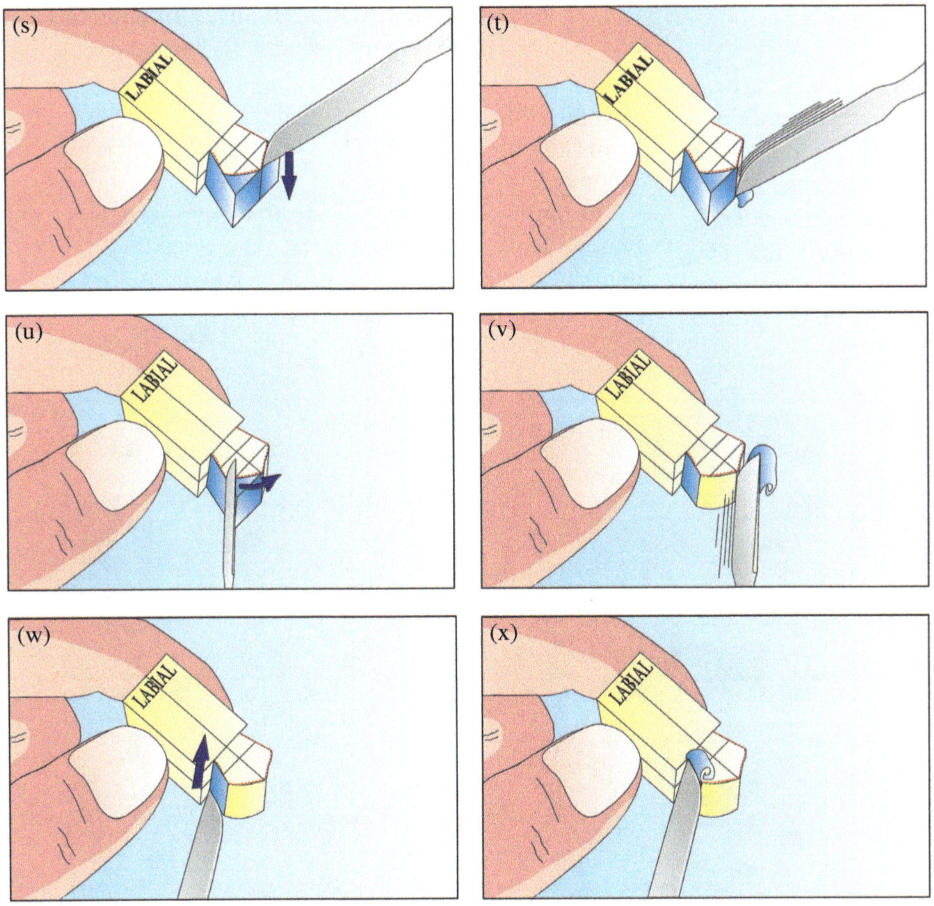

Figure 9.3 (s–x) Carving the outline of the crown (labial aspect).

Exercise: Steps to Carve Excess Wax from Mesial and Distal side

Excess wax on the middle and occlusal third of the mesial side is carved, by placing the anterior part of the cutting edge of the carver facing the wax (Figure 9.3l) and moving in a labiopalatal direction (Figure 9.3m). Then the wax near the cervical third is carved by placing the back of the carver facing the wax and the tip of the wax facing the cervix (Figure 9.3n). In a similar way, excess wax is also carved on the distal side.

Exercise: Marking the Outline of the Crown

After carving excess wax from both the mesial and distal sides (Figure 9.3o), the crest of contour of the mesial and distal outlines is marked, with the mesial crest of contour at the junction of the middle and incisal third and the distal crest of contour at the middle of the middle third (Figure 9.3p). The outline of the crown is drawn with features described (Figure 9.3q). The excess wax that needs to be carved is indicated in blue colour (Figure 9.3r).

Exercise: Carving Excess Wax to Create the Outline of the Crown

Excess wax at the mesial slope is carved by placing the convex part of the carver facing the wax (Figure 9.3s) and moving the carver labiopalatally, so that the concavity of the mesial slope is created (Figure 9.3t). To get the convex distal slope, the carver is placed in labiopalatal direction (Figure 9.3u) and moved from the distal contact to the cusp tip in a curvy manner (Figure 9.3v). To get the concave distal outline above the crest of curvature, the curved part of the cutting edge of the carver is placed in the cervico-occlusal direction (Figure 9.3w) and moved in the labiopalatal direction (Figure 9.3x).

Mesial Aspect

This tooth has greater bulk and labiopalatal measurement than any other anterior tooth [1–3]. The crown outline is wedge shaped or triangular shaped, with the tip of the wedge towards the cusp tip (Figure 9.4a). The crest of curvature labially is in the cervical third but placed more incisally because of well-developed lobes (Figure 9.4b). The crest of curvature palatally is also at the cervical third but placed more cervically than that of the labial outline (Figure 9.4b). The labial outline is convex from the cervical line to the cusp tip (Figure 9.4c and d). The palatal outline has convexity representing the cingulum (Figure 9.4e), the straight middle third (Figure 9.4f), and the convex incisal third (Figure 9.4g) [1–3]. The curvature of the cervical line is about 2 mm incisally [2, 3].

The outline of the root is conical with uniform taper and blunted root apex. The root surface shows shallow developmental depression. The cusp tip is labially placed to the long axis of the tooth (Figure 9.4h) [2, 3].

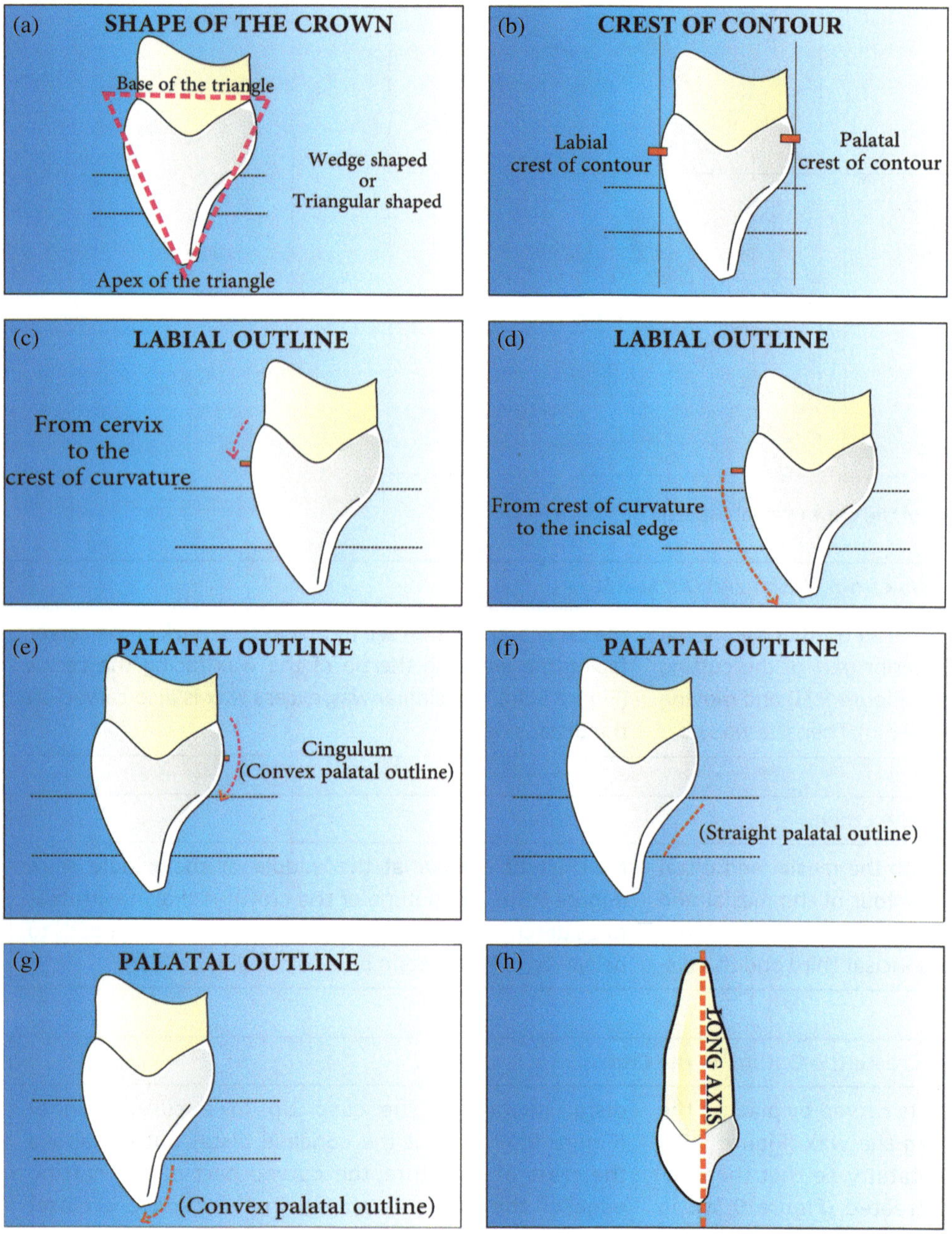

Figure 9.4 (a–h) Description of the right maxillary canine from the mesial aspect.

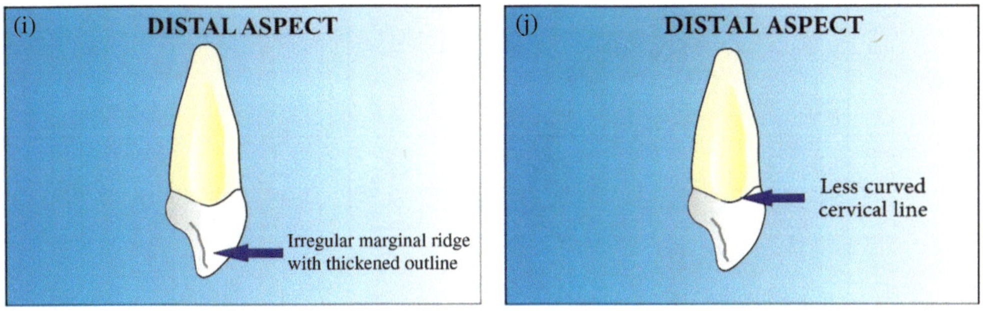

Figure 9.4 (i–j) Description of the right maxillary canine from the distal aspect.

Distal Aspect

The distal aspect appears similar to the mesial aspect, with the following variations: irregular outline with a thicker marginal ridge (Figure 9.4i) and the cervical line exhibiting less curvature. The root exhibits a more pronounced developmental depression (Figure 9.4j).

Carving from the Mesial/Distal Aspect

Exercise: Marking the Labiopalatal Dimension of Crown on the Distal Aspect
The labiopalatal dimension of the crown at the cervix of 7.0 mm (3.5 mm on either side of the midline) is marked at the cervix (Figure 9.5a and b). The labiopalatal dimension which is the bulkiest dimension of the crown measuring 8.0 mm (4.0 mm on either side of the midline) is marked at the occlusal edge of the crown (Figure 9.5c and d) [2].

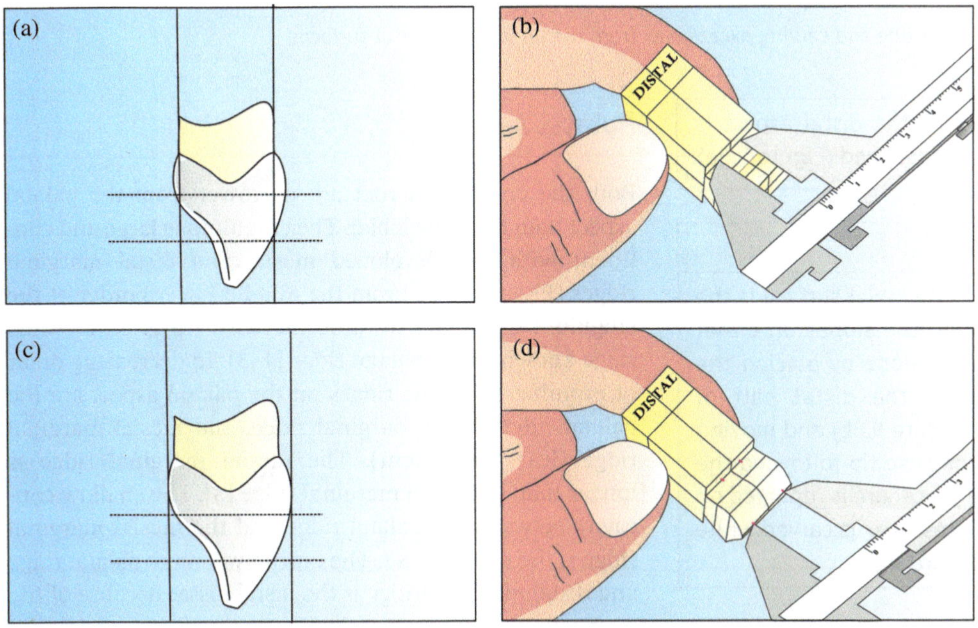

Figure 9.5 (a–d) Measuring and marking the crown dimension on the distal aspect of the wax block.

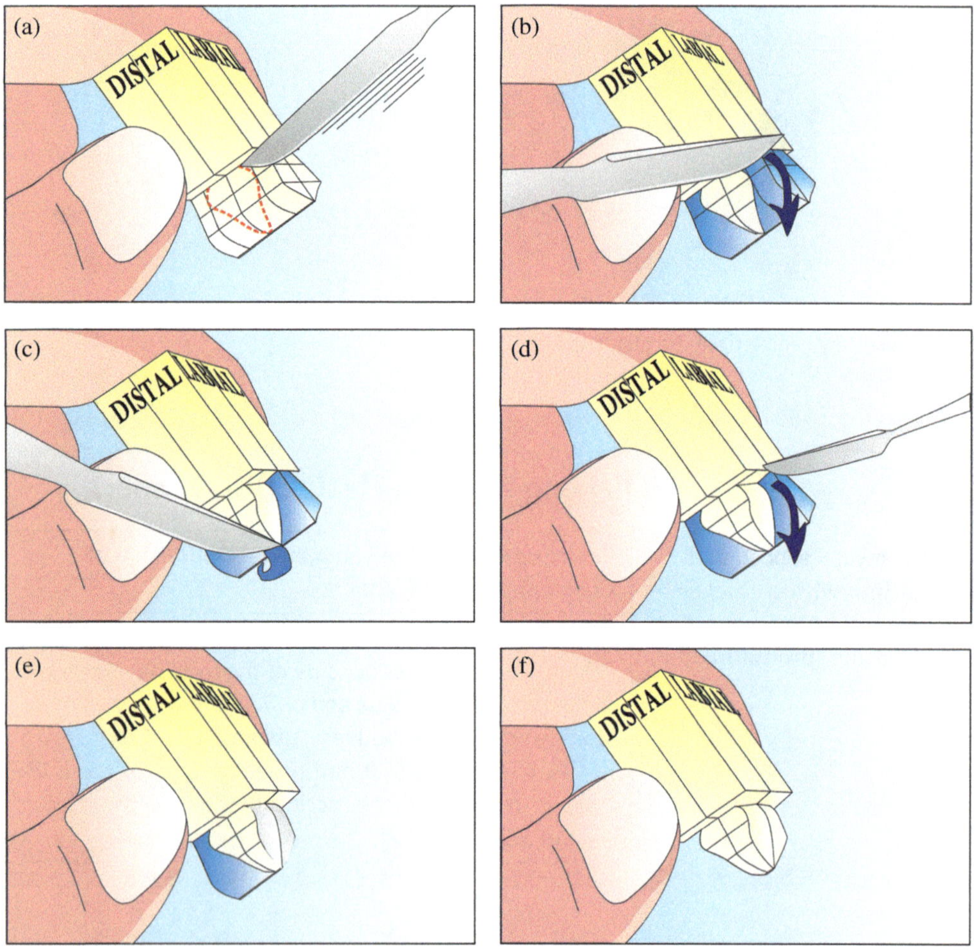

Figure 9.6 (a–f) Drawing the crown outline and carving excess wax from the labial and palatal surfaces.

The labial and palatal outline on the distal aspect is drawn with the features already described (Figure 9.6a).

Exercise: Carving the Labial Ridge

The most important feature on the labial surface is the labial ridge, obtained by creating the slopes on either side of the labial midline. This is done by placing the cutting edge of the carver on the distal half of the labial surface at an angle (Figure 9.6b) and moving the carver from the cervix to the cusp tip following the outline (Figure 9.6c). The same procedure is repeated on the mesial half (Figure 9.6d). Excess wax is carved while creating a slope as shown in Figure 9.6e.

Exercise: Carving Excess Wax from the Palatal Side

The palatal excess wax is carved by creating a flat and curved palatal surface following the outline (Figure 9.6f).

Palatal Aspect

Both the crown and root are narrower from the palatal aspect than from the labial. The cingulum is large and confluent with well-developed mesial and distal marginal ridges (Figure 9.7a). From the middle lower border of the cingulum extending towards the cusp tip is an elevated ridge known as the palatal ridge [1–3]. In decreasing order of prominence of the ridges on the palatal aspect are the palatal ridge, distal marginal ridge, and mesial marginal ridge (least prominent). The mesial marginal ridge is longer than the distal marginal ridge [3]. The shallow concavity between the palatal ridge and the mesial marginal ridge is the mesial fossa. The one between the palatal ridge and distal marginal ridge is the distal fossa. Because of the narrowness of the root palatally, most of the mesial and distal surfaces of the root are seen with respective developmental depressions (Figure 9.7b) [1–4].

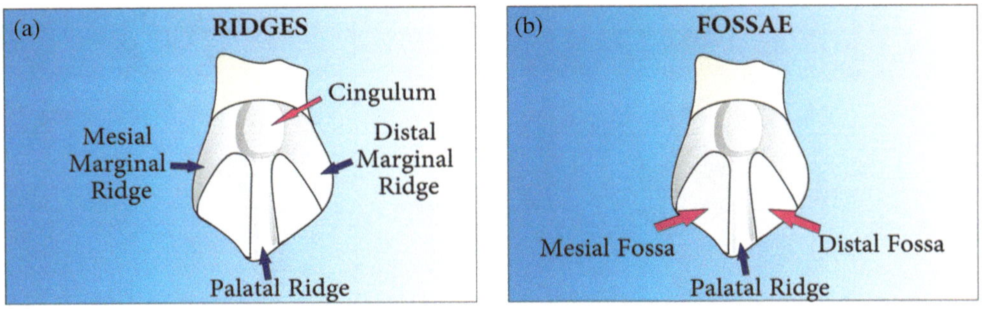

Figure 9.7 (a–b) Description of the maxillary right canine from the palatal aspect.

Carving from the Palatal Aspect

Features to be carved:

1) Palatal convergence of the mesial and distal surfaces
2) Carving the mesial and distal fossae
3) Creating the cingulum
4) Creating the marginal ridges – mesial and distal

Exercise: Creating the Palatal Convergence

The palatal convergence is created by drawing an outline on the palatal surface as shown in the Figure 9.8a. The outline should follow the mesial and distal outline labially, but narrower. The excess wax indicated by blue colour wax on the mesial side is carved by moving the carver in a palato-labial direction as shown without disturbing the outline labially (Figure 9.8b and c). The same procedure is repeated on the other side (Figure 9.8d).

Exercise: Carving the Mesial and Distal Fossae

The outline of the mesial and distal fossae is marked on the palatal surface such that the mesial fossa is greater than the distal fossa (Figure 9.8e). Using the excavating end of the Lecron carver, the wax is carved deeper near the cingulum and shallower as moved towards the cuspal ridge of the side respectively (Figure 9.8f and g). The same procedure is repeated for the distal fossa (Figure 9.8h).

Exercise: Creating the Cingulum and Marginal Ridges

While creating the palatal convergence and fossae, the cingulum is formed at the cervical portion and marginal ridges are formed near the middle and incisal portion. The cingulum and marginal ridges are then smoothed.

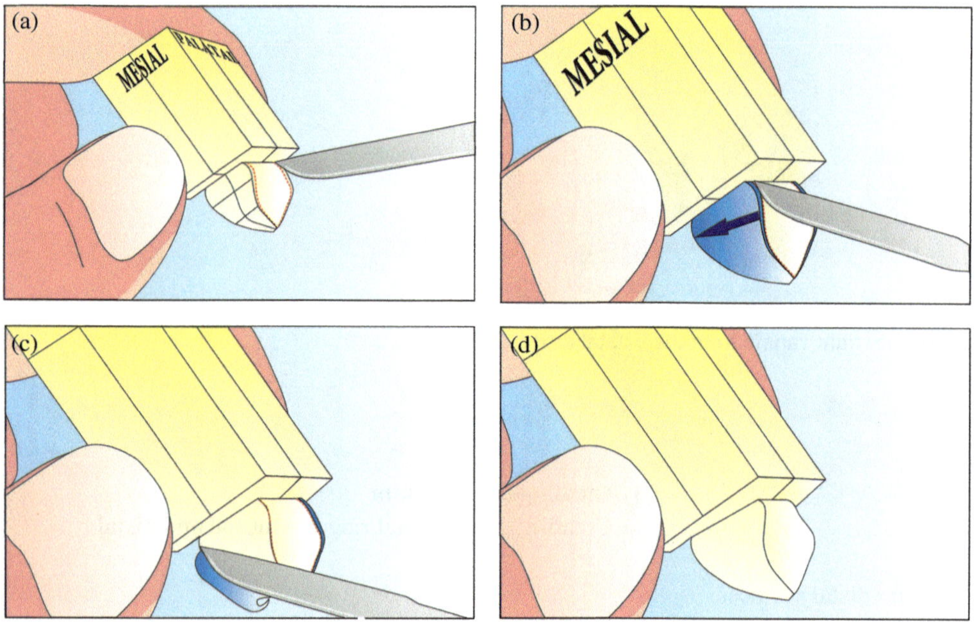

Figure 9.8 (a–d) Creating the palatal convergence.

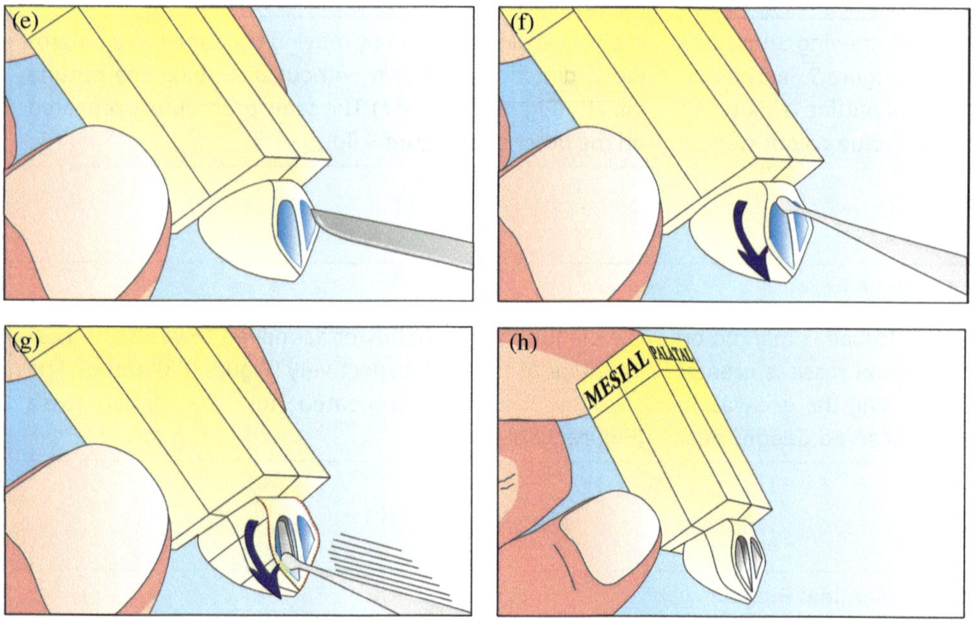

Figure 9.8 (e–h) Carving the mesial and distal fossae.

Incisal Aspect

The labiopalatal dimension of the crown is greater than the mesiodistal dimension (Figure 9.9a and b). The tip of the crown is placed more mesially and labially (Figure 9.9c). The cingulum occupies the palatal third of the crown (Figure 9.9d). The mesial half outline is semicircular (Figure 9.9e) and the distal half outline shows concavity both labially and palatally (Figure 9.9f). The line bisecting the cusp and cuspal ridges is always straight [1–3]

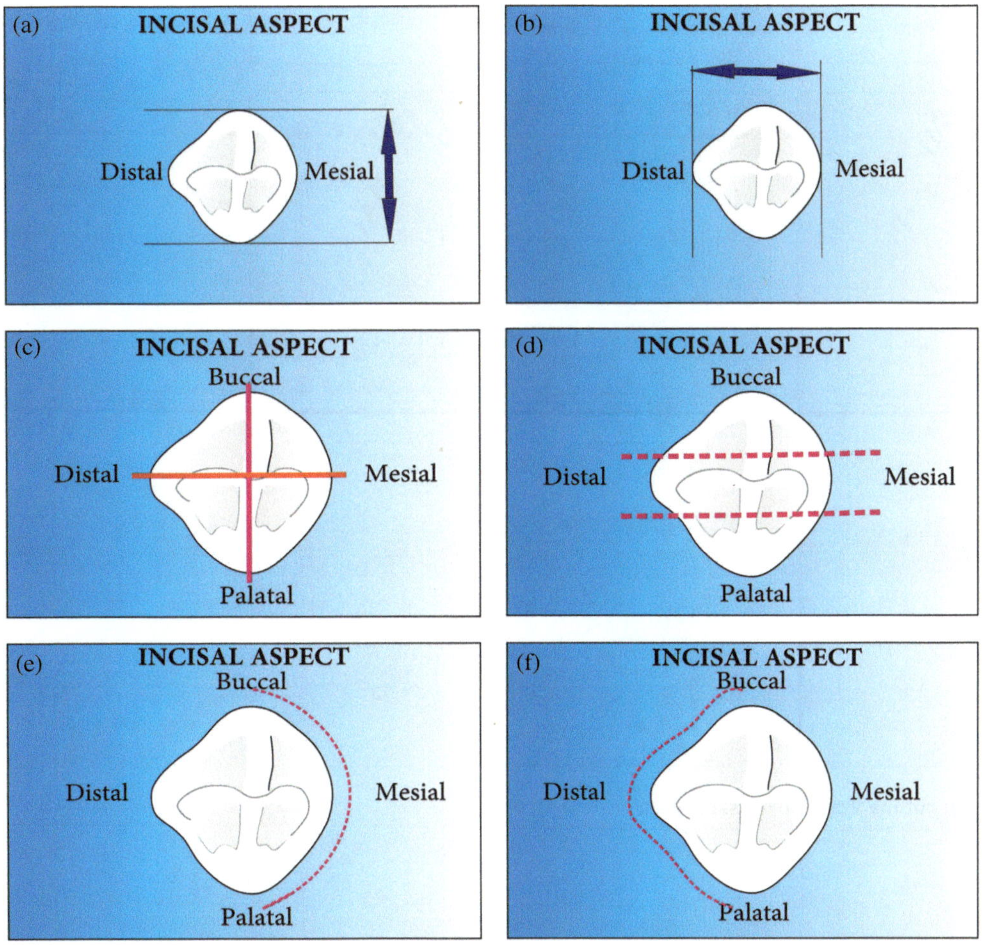

Figure 9.9 (a–f) Description of the permanent maxillary right canine from the incisal aspect.

Carving from the Incisal Aspect

Exercise: Creating the Mesial and Distal Outline from the Incisal Aspect
The mesial half of the crown is rounded to get a semicircular outline of the crown by moving the carver in the sequence of steps labially (Figure 9.10a and b) and palatally (Figure 9.10c and d). On the distal half of the crown, the concavities are created both labially and palatally, towards the cervical portion (Figure 9.10e and f).

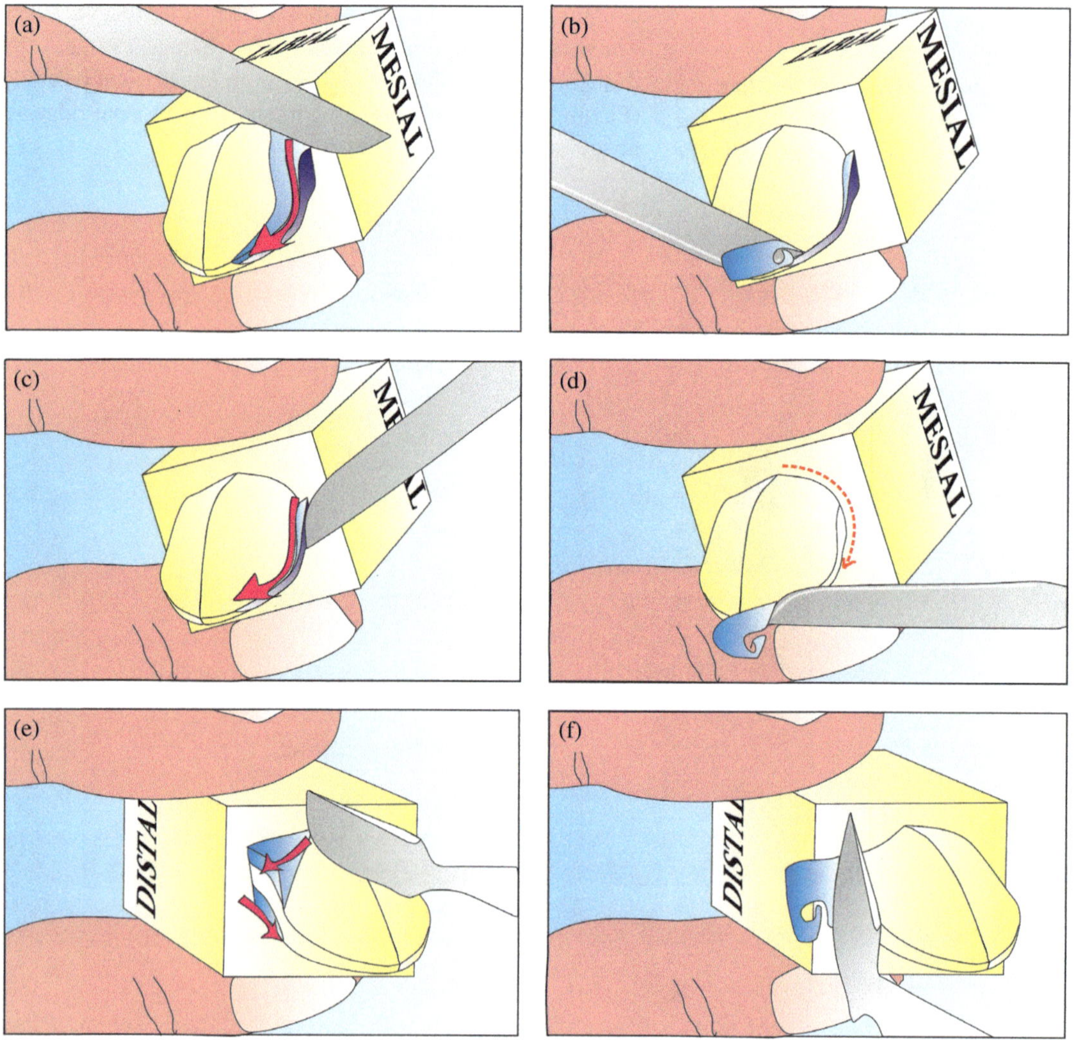

Figure 9.10 (a–f) Refining the crown outline from the incisal aspect.

Carving the Root

Exercise: Carving the Root from the Mesial Aspect

The labiopalatal outline of the root is drawn with its specific features on the mesial side, so that the excess wax outside the root outline indicated in blue needs to be carved out (Figure 9.11a). The carving on the palatal side is done in two steps. With the anterior half of the cutting edge of the carver facing the cervical half of the root portion of wax (Figure 9.11b), the carver is moved in a mesiodistal direction until the root outline is reached (Figure 9.11c). The carver is reverted so that the non-cutting side is facing wax at the apical half and follows the curved root outline. The carver is once again moved in a mesiodistal direction until the root outline is reached (Figure 9.11d). In a similar way, wax is carved on the labial side (Figure 9.11e).

Exercise: Carving the Root from the Labial Aspect

On the labial aspect, the mesiodistal outline of the root is drawn (Figure 9.11f) with its features. The excess wax on the distal side is carved in three steps as shown. At the apical end of the root near the distal curvature, the convex part of the carver is used to carve wax by moving it labiopalatally (Figure 9.11g–i). Wax near the cervical third is carved in a similar way (Figure 9.11j and k). Wax at the middle of the root is carved (Figure 9.11l). Wax on the mesial side is carved at the apical third with the anterior non-cutting part of the carver facing wax and the carver is moved in a labio-palatal direction. Remaining part of the wax is carved in a similar way as described for the distal side of the root (Figure 9.11l).

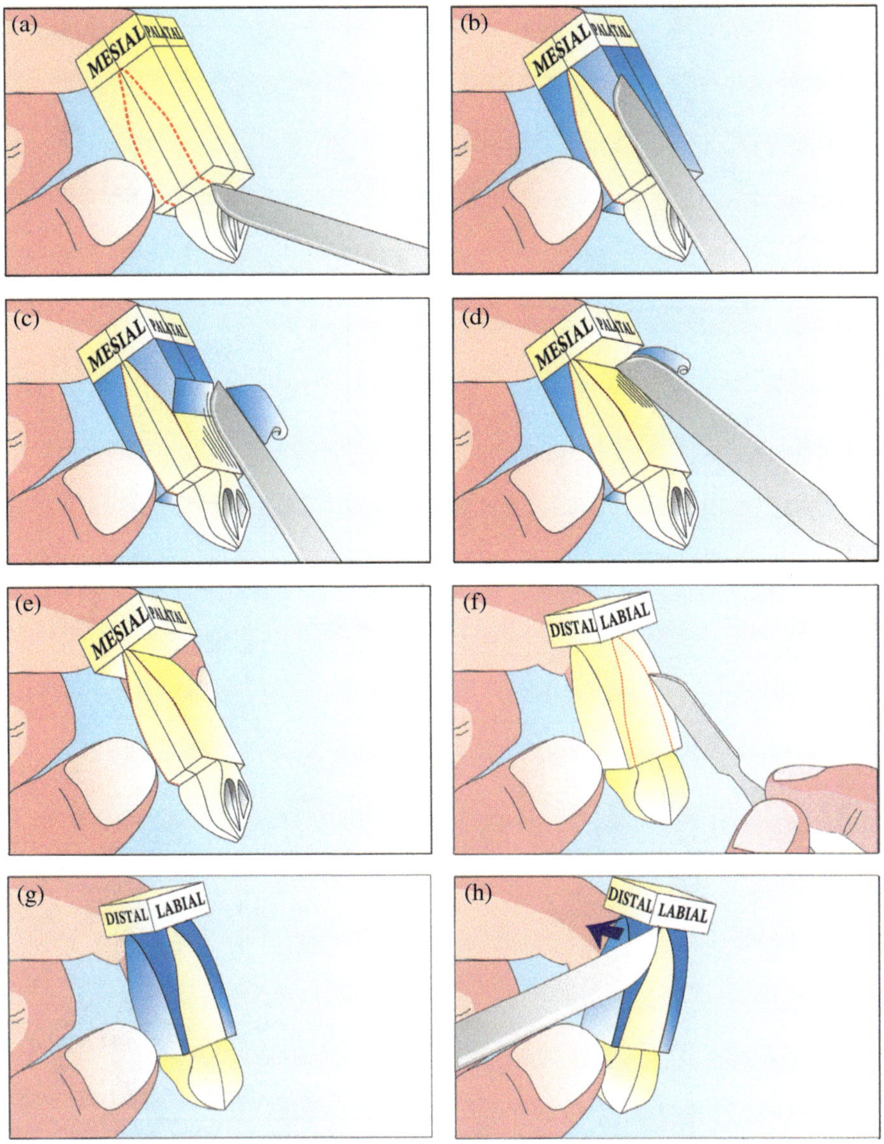

Figure 9.11 (a–o) Carving the root from the mesial and labial aspect.

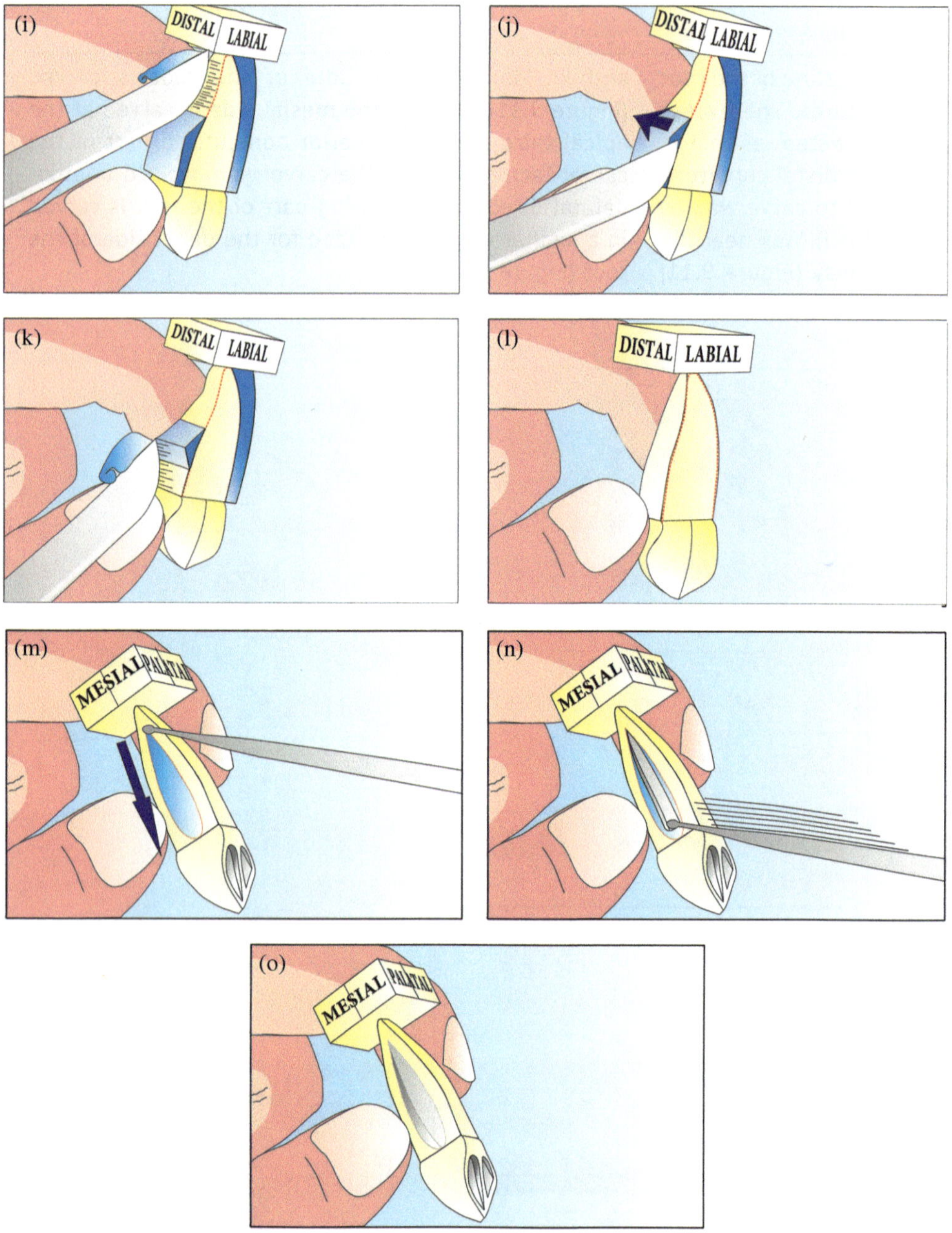

Figure 9.11 (Cont'd) (a-o)

Exercise: Creating the Developmental Depression on the Mesial and Distal Surface of the Root

The outline for the developmental depression is marked in the centre of the root. Using the excavating end of the carver, the wax is carved apicocervically (Figure 9.11m and n), shallow near the periphery and deep at the middle of the depression outline (Figure 9.11o)

Exercise: Marking the Cervical Line

After the completion of tooth carving, the cervical line is drawn at the junction between the crown and root. The curvature of the cervical line on the mesial side is 2.5 mm incisally, whereas on the distal side it is 1.5 mm [2].

References

1 James, L.F., Gerald, E.D., and Thomas, M. (2001). *Concise Dental Anatomy and Morphology*, 4e. Iowa City, IA: University of Iowa College of Dentistry.
2 Stanley, J.N. and Major, M.A.C. (2010). *Wheeler's Dental Anatomy and Occlusion*, 9e. Saunders Elsevier: St. Louis, MO.
3 Rickne, C.S. and Weiss, G. (2012). *Woelfel's Dental Anatomy*, 8e. Philadelphia: Lippincott Williams & Wilkins.
4 Geoffrey, C.B. (1983). *Dental Morphology. An Illustrated Guide*, 2e. Philadelphia: Wright Elsevier.

10

Permanent Mandibular Canine

LEARNING OBJECTIVE
At the end of the chapter, the student should have knowledge of the permanent mandibular canine and develop the psychomotor skills for carving and waxing the same.

Permanent Mandibular Right Canine

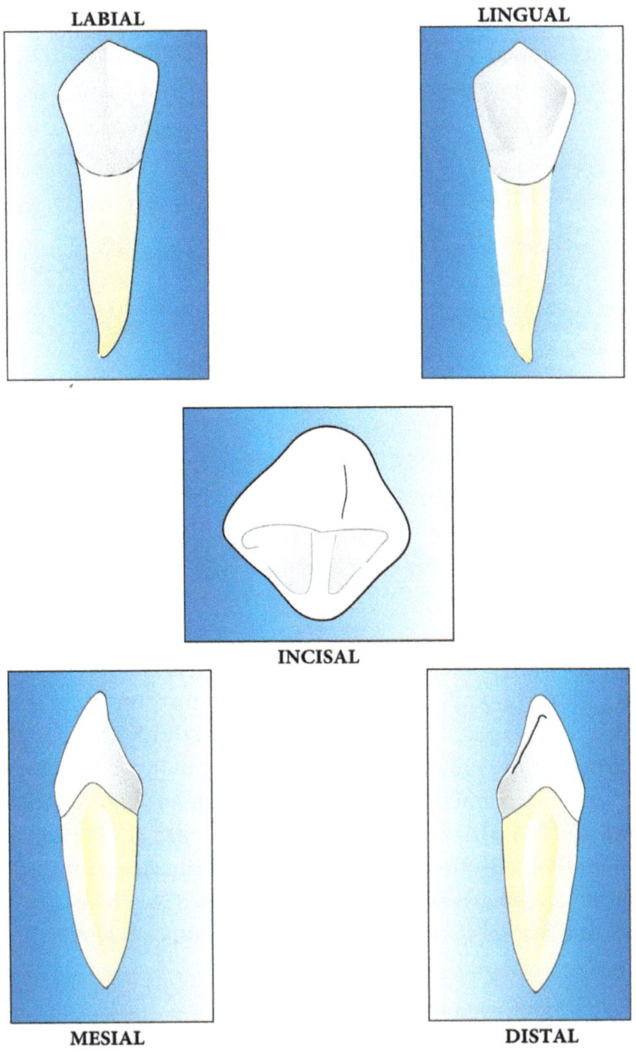

Labial Aspect

The permanent mandibular canine is the third tooth from the midline in the mandibular arch (Figure 10.1). The mesiodistal diameter of the crown of the mandibular canine is less than that of the maxillary canine. The crown is longer and narrower than that of the maxillary canine [1–3]. Contact areas on both the mesial and distal sides are placed more incisally, with the mesial contact placed more occlusally than the distal contact (Figure 10.2a) [1, 3, 4]. The mesial outline is straight with the mesial outline of root. The mesial cuspal ridge is shorter than the distal cuspal ridge (Figure 10.2b). The distal cuspal ridge is steeper than the mesial cuspal ridge [4]. The incisal half of the distal outline is convex whereas the cervical half is concave. Bulk is added on the distal half of the crown rather than the mesial, so the crown appears tilted distally on the root. The cervical line is semicircular with curvature apically.

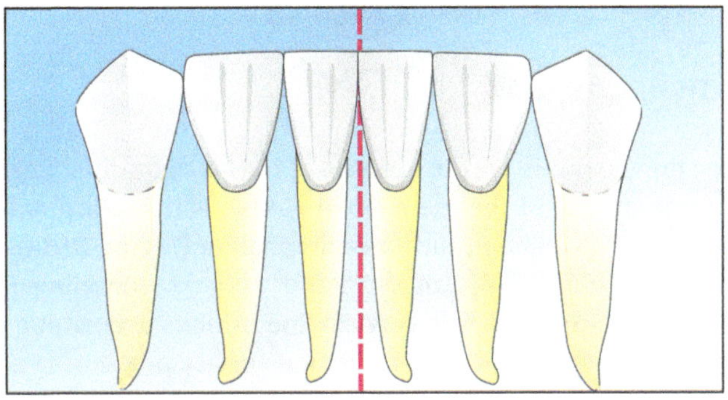

Figure 10.1 Position of the mandibular canine in relation to the midsagittal plane.

An Illustrated Atlas of Tooth Carving and Wax-Up Techniques, First Edition. Anil Bangalore Shivappa.

Companion website: www.wiley.com/go/bangalore/toothcarving

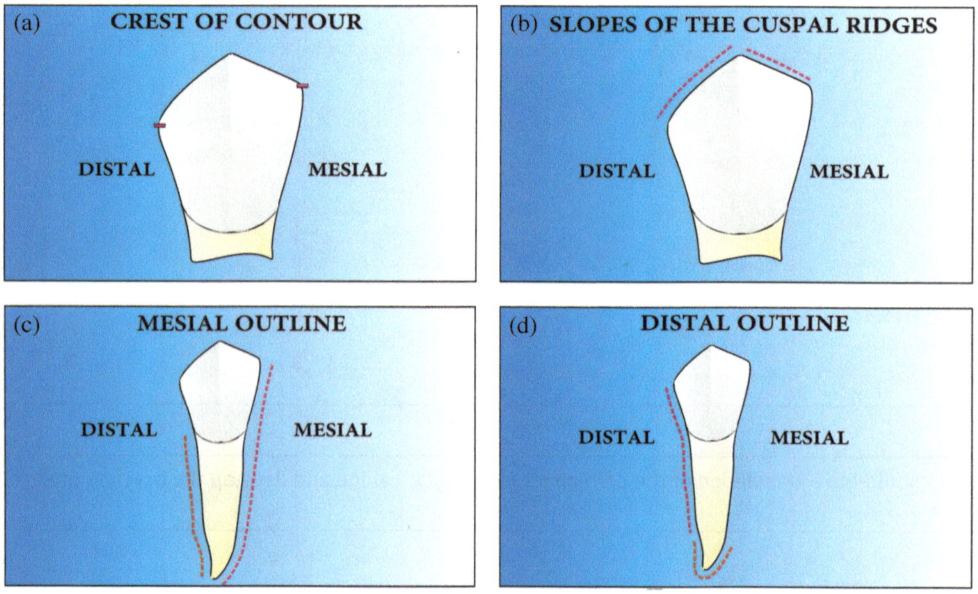

Figure 10.2 (a–d) Characteristic features of the permanent mandibular right canine from the labial aspect.

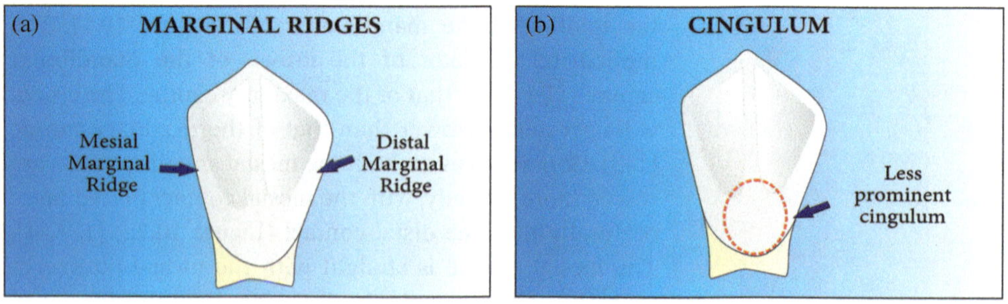

Figure 10.3 (a–b) Description of the permanent mandibular right canine from the lingual aspect.

The labial surface is smooth and the labial ridge is not as prominent as that of the maxillary canine. The root appears to bend distally and is shorter than that of the maxillary canine [1–4]. The apical end of the root is sharply pointed (Figure 10.2c and d) [2].

Lingual Aspect

The lingual outline is the opposite of the labial outline. The lingual surface of the mandibular canine is flat. Marginal ridges are less distinct, and fossae are shallow (Figure 10.3a). The cingulum is smooth and poorly developed (Figure 10.3b) [1–4]. The cervical line exhibits deeper curvature offset to distal [4]. The lingual surface of the crown and root are slightly narrower than the labial portion (Figure 10.3a and b) [2–4].

Mesial Aspect

The crown has less curvature labially with a less prominent cingulum lingually. The crest of curvature on both the labial and lingual outline is at the cervical third. The incisal portion of the crown is reduced labiolingually, so the cusp tip appears pointed and the ridges are slender (Figure 10.4a and b) [2–4]. In most of the cases, the cusp tip is placed lingually [2, 3]. In a few cases the tip of the cusp is in line with the long axis of the tooth [3] (Figure 10.4c). The cervical line curves more incisally. The root appears similar to

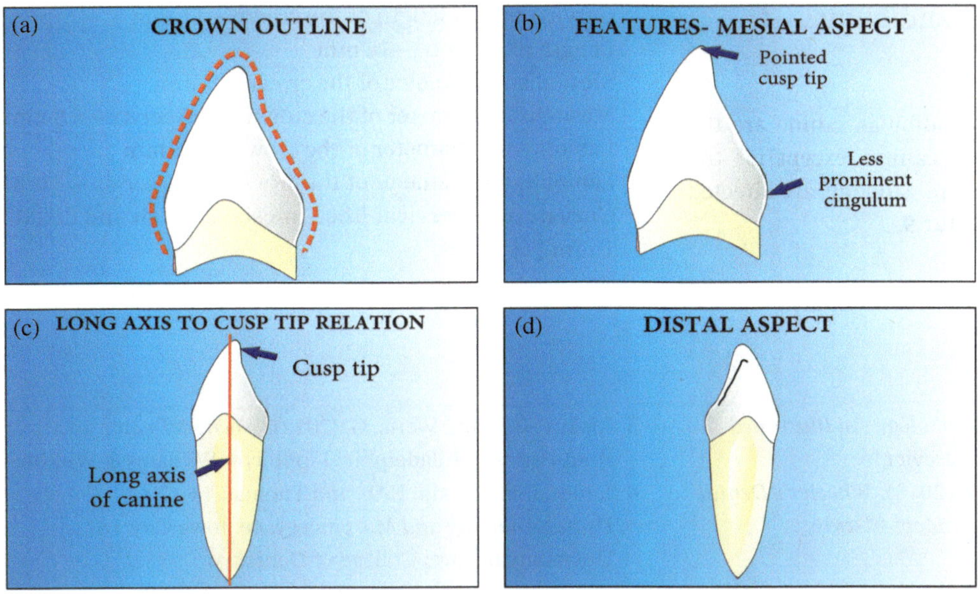

Figure 10.4 (a–d) Description of the permanent mandibular right canine from the mesial and distal aspects.

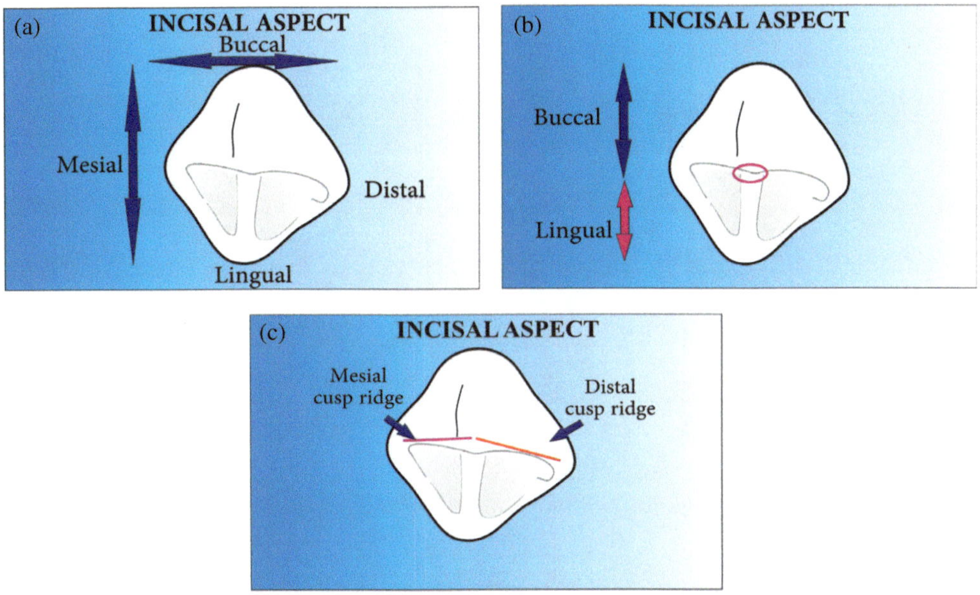

Figure 10.5 (a–c) Description of the mandibular right canine from the incisal aspect.

that of the maxillary canine with a more pointed root tip. The developmental depression is more pronounced [1–3].

Distal Aspect

The distal aspect of the tooth has similar features to the mesial aspect with the crest of contour placed more cervically (Figure 10.4d). The cervical line has less curvature towards the incisal edge compared to the mesial side. The developmental depression on the distal root surface is more distinct than on the mesial [2, 3].

Incisal Aspect

The tooth is similar to the maxillary canine in this aspect. The crown is wider labiolingually than mesiodistally (Figure 10.5a) [3, 4]. The cusp tip is placed either at the centre labiolingually or lingual to the centre (Figure 10.5b). The distolingual tilt of the crown can be seen from this aspect (Figure 10.5c). The mesial half of the labial outline is convex, and the distal half of the crown is flat. The cingulum is convex, either placed at centre or slightly distally[3].

Carving the Permanent Mandibular Right Canine

NOTE: Steps for carving the mandibular canine are the same as those for the maxillary canine, except for the difference in features described here. Students are directed to refer the carving steps of **Chapter 9**.

Measurements:

Cervico-incisal length of the crown – 11 mm
Length of the root – 16 mm
Mesiodistal diameter of the crown – 7 mm
Mesiodistal diameter of the crown at the cervix – 5.5 mm
Labiolingual diameter of the crown – 7.5 mm
Labiolingual diameter of the crown at the cervix – 7 mm
Curvature of cervical line – mesial 2.5 mm and distal 1 mm [2]

References

1 Geoffrey, C.B. (1983). *Dental Morphology. An Illustrated Guide*, 2e. Philadelphia: Wright Elsevier.
2 Stanley, J.N. and Major, M.A.C. (2010). *Wheeler's Dental Anatomy and Occlusion*, 9e. Saunders Elsevier: St. Louis, MO.
3 Rickne, C.S. and Weiss, G. (2012). *Woelfel's Dental Anatomy*, 8e. Philadelphia: Lippincott Williams & Wilkins.
4 James, L.F., Gerald, E.D., and Thomas, M. (2001). *Concise Dental Anatomy and Morphology*, 4e. Iowa City, IA: University of Iowa College of Dentistry.

11

Permanent Maxillary First Premolar

LEARNING OBJECTIVE
At the end of the chapter, the student should have knowledge of the permanent maxillary first premolar and develop the psychomotor skills for carving and waxing the same.

Permanent Maxillary Right First Premolar

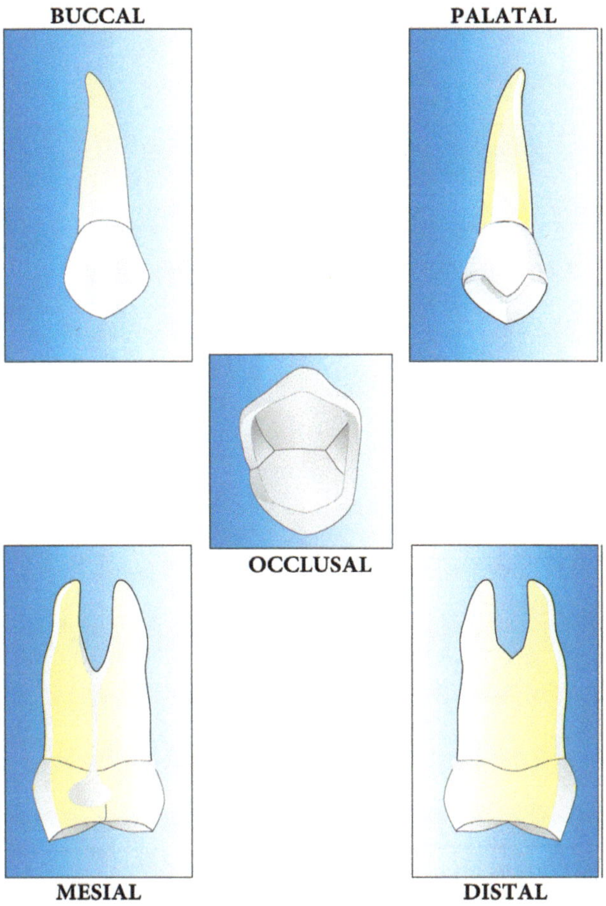

Buccal Aspect

The maxillary first premolar is the fourth tooth from the midline (Figure 11.1). The shape of the crown from this aspect is trapezoidal (with four unequal sides) (Figure 11.2a) [1]. The mesial crest of contour is broader, in the middle third near the junction of the middle and occlusal third. The distal crest of contour is also broader and is placed in the middle third, more cervically than the mesial crest of contour (Figure 11.2b). The outline of the crown cervical to both the mesial and distal crest of contour is concave, the distal being more concave than the mesial [2, 3]. From the contact the outline slopes on both the mesial and distal sides to unite at the cusp tip. The mesial slope (mesial cuspal ridge) is wider than the distal slope or distal cuspal ridge (Figure 11.2c). Because of this the cusp tip is placed slightly distally (Figure 11.2d) [3, 4]. The cervical line is less convex with convexity facing the root [1]. The buccal surface of the crown is convex with a well-developed midbuccal lobe represented by the buccal ridge running from the cervical line to the cusp tip. Developmental depressions can be seen on either side of the buccal ridge occlusal to the middle third (Figure 11.2e) [3, 4]. The buccal root bears close resemblance to that of the maxillary canine with the distal tilt of apex (Figure 11.2f).

An Illustrated Atlas of Tooth Carving and Wax-Up Techniques, First Edition. Anil Bangalore Shivappa.

Companion website: www.wiley.com/go/bangalore/toothcarving

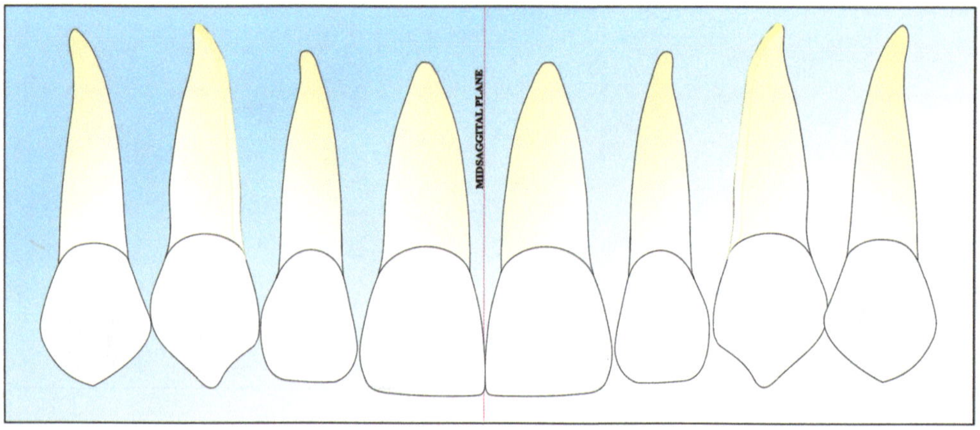

Figure 11.1 Position of the permanent maxillary first premolar in relation to the midsagittal plane.

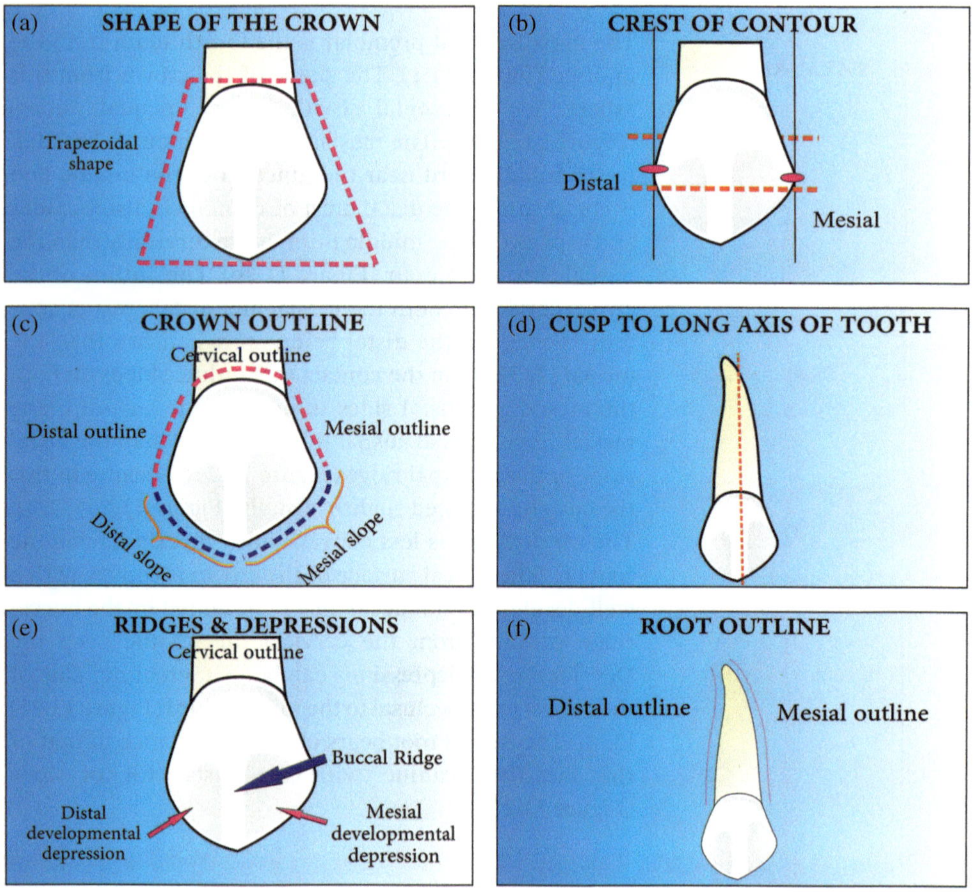

Figure 11.2 (a–f) Descriptive features of the permanent maxillary right first premolar from the buccal aspect.

Carving from the Buccal Aspect

Exercise: Marking the Length of the Crown and the Root

After the preparation of the wax block, each side of the wax block is divided into two equal parts. Then the length of the crown about 8.5 mm is taken from the occlusal edge of the crown (Figure 11.3a). The same measurement is marked on all other sides (Figure 11.3b). From the cervical end of the crown, the length of the root about 14.0 mm is marked on all four sides of the wax block (Figure 11.3c) [1].

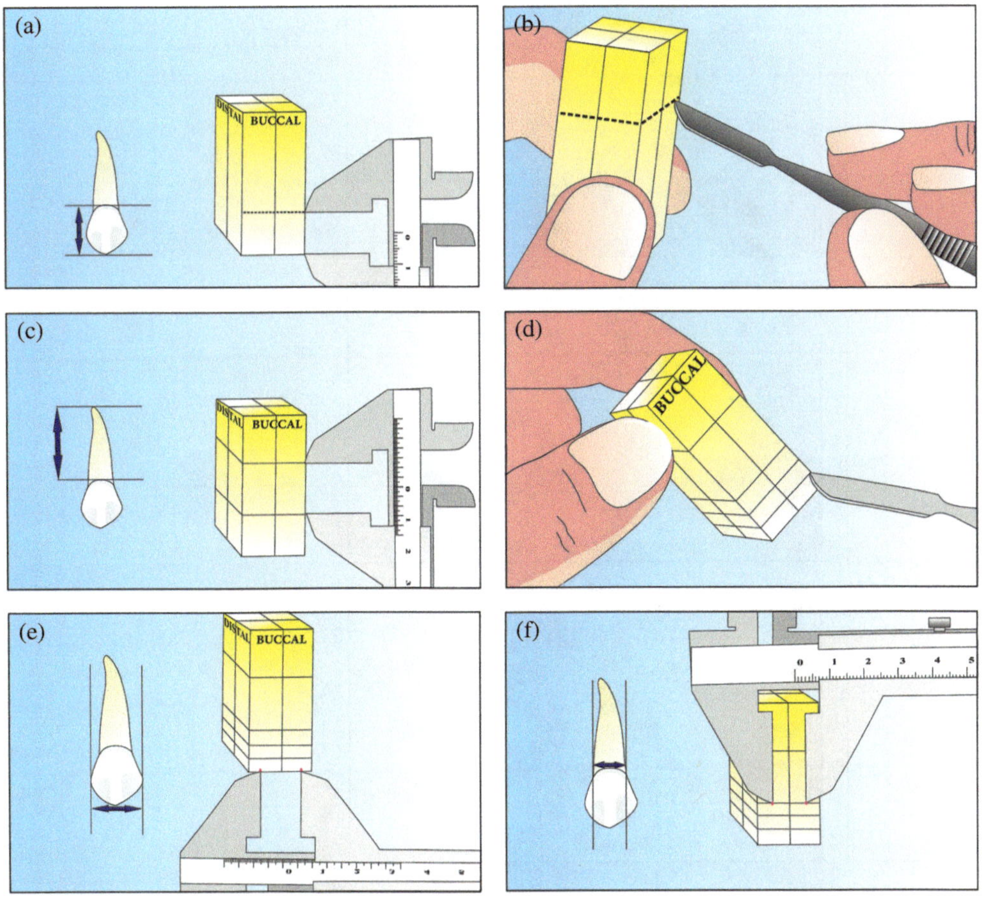

Figure 11.3 (a–f) Measuring and marking the crown dimension and root length on the buccal aspect.

Exercise: Marking the Mesiodistal Dimensions

After marking the length of the root and crown, the crown part is divided into three equal parts: occlusal third, middle third, and cervical third starting from the occlusal towards the cervical line (Figure 11.3d). The mesiodistal diameter of the crown about 7.0 mm (3.5 mm on either side of the midline) is marked on the buccal surface (Figure 11.3e). The mesiodistal diameter of the crown at the cervix about 5 mm (2.5 mm on either side of the midline) is marked at the cervical line on the buccal surface (Figure 11.3f) [1].

Exercise: Marking the border of the Crown and Carving Excess Wax

The mesial and distal border of the crown, within which the crown outline to be drawn, is marked on either side of the midline (Figure 11.3g–i). Excess wax indicated in blue colour is carved (Figure 11.3j and k). The bulk of the wax in the occlusal and middle third on the mesial and distal side is carved using the anterior part of the cutting edge of the carver, moving it buccopalatally (Figure 11.3l and m). Remaining wax near the cervical third is carved with the tip of the carver facing the cervix and the anterior part of the non-cutting edge of the carver facing excess wax (Figure 11.3n).

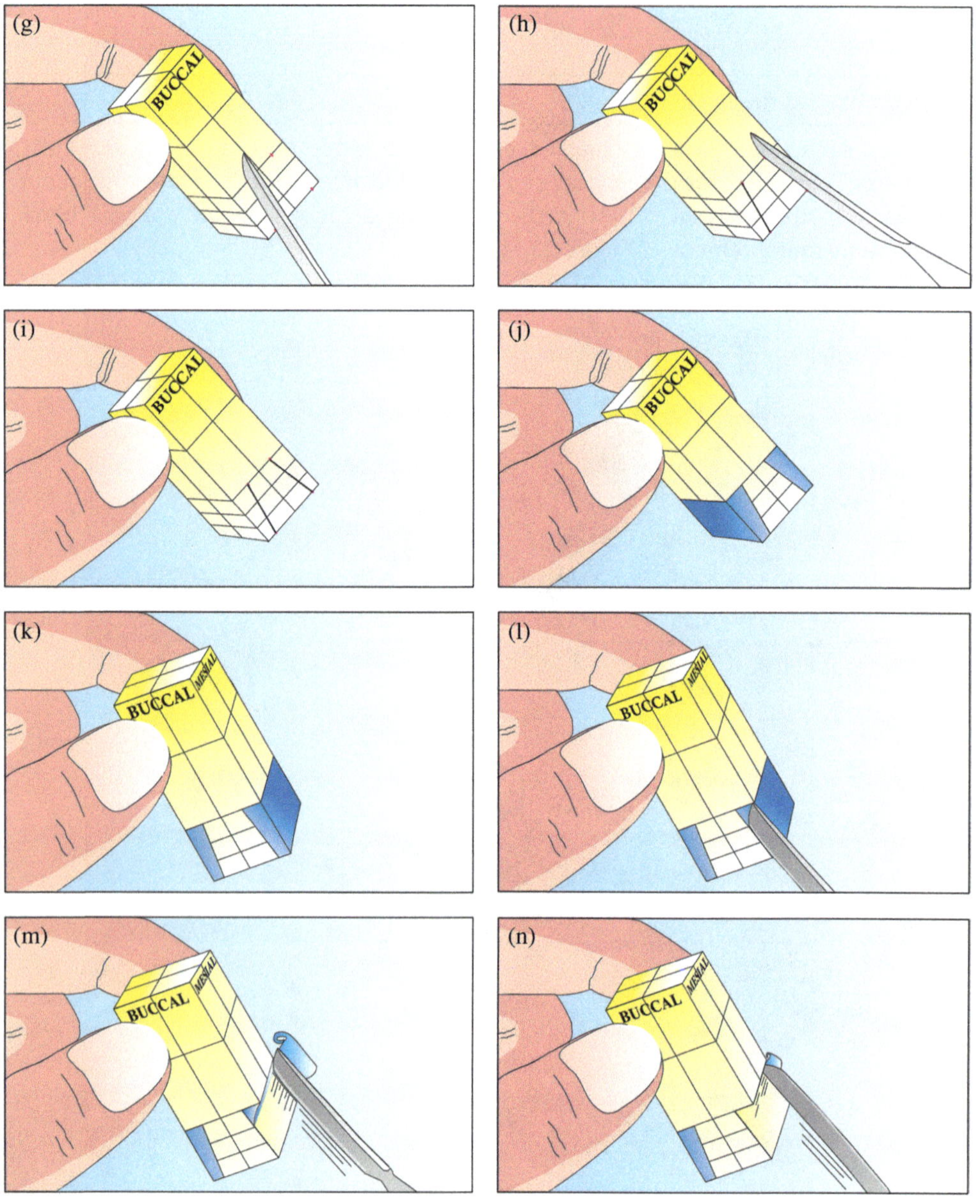

Figure 11.3 (g–n) Marking the crown dimension and carving excess wax from the mesial and distal side of the crown.

Palatal Aspect

The palatal cusp is narrower mesiodistally than the buccal cusp. Because of this narrowness palatally, most of the mesial and distal surfaces are seen from this side (Figure 11.4a) [1–3]. The palatal cusp is smooth and spheroidal from the cervical portion to the area near the cusp tip (Figure 11.4b) [1]. The cusp tip is pointed and is placed mesial to the long axis of the tooth (Figure 11.4c) [2, 3]. The mesial and distal outlines from this aspect are smooth and convex from the cervical lines that are continuous with their slopes respectively [3]. The cervical line appears regular and curved towards the root slightly. Because the root along with the crown tapers palatally, the mesial and distal sides of the roots can be seen. The palatal root is smooth and convex with the blunt root apex [2, 3].

Mesial Aspect

The crown from this aspect is trapezoidal in shape, with the longest side towards the cervical and the shortest towards the occlusal (Figure 11.5a) [1, 3]. The crest of curvature on the buccal outline is located at the cervical

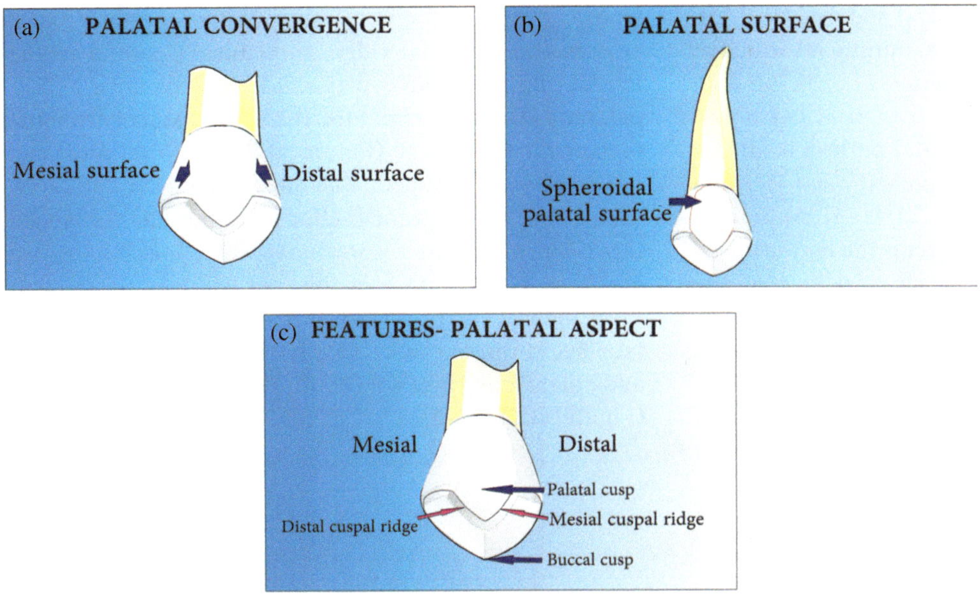

Figure 11.4 (a–c) Description of the maxillary right first premolar from the palatal aspect.

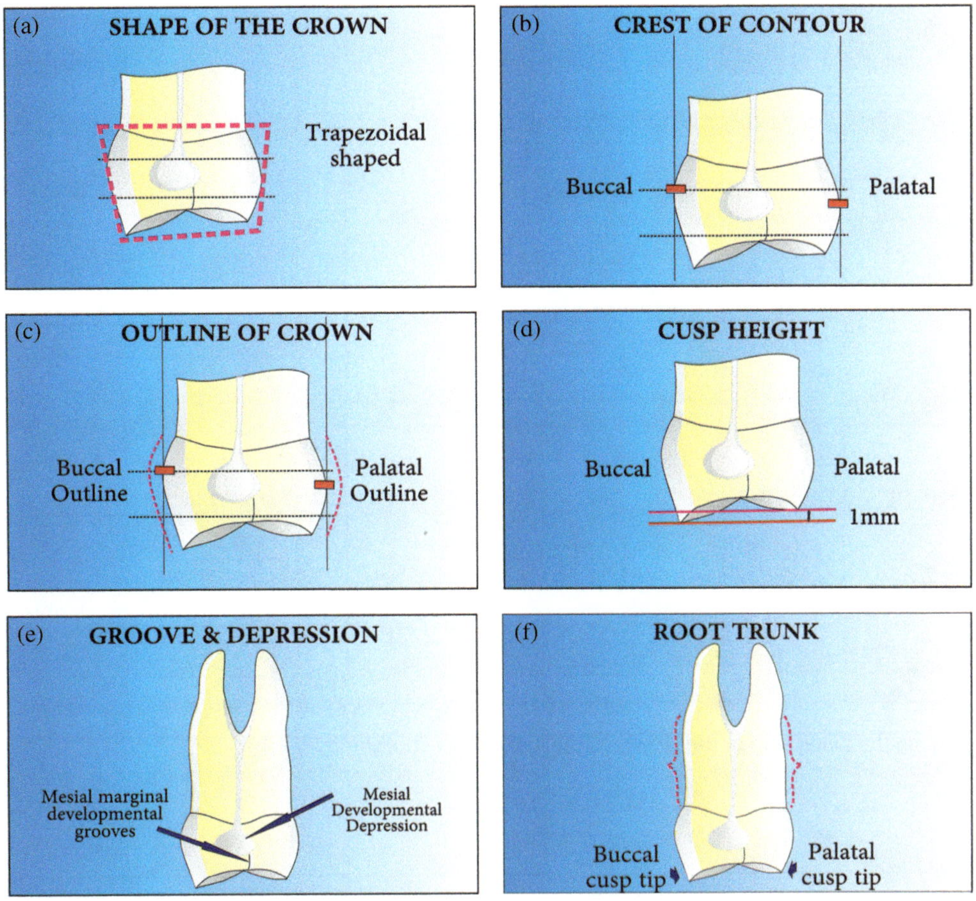

Figure 11.5 (a–f) Description of the permanent maxillary right first premolar from the mesial aspect.

third near the junction of the cervical and middle third. The crest of curvature on the palatal outline is located at the middle of the middle third (Figure 11.5b). The buccal outline from the crest of curvature runs as smooth convex until the cusp tip. The palatal outline is almost semicircular (Figure 11.5c). The palatal cusp is 1 mm short of the buccal cusp (Figure 11.5d) [1–3]. An important feature seen on the mesial aspect is the *mesial developmental depression*, seen in the cervical half of the crown. It is also known as fossa canina or canine fossa. The depression extends into the mesial furcation of the root [1, 4]. Another important feature of the maxillary first premolar is the *mesial marginal developmental groove*, which is the continuity of the central groove, crosses the marginal ridge immediately palatal to the mesial contact or at two thirds of the distance buccopalatally [1–4]. It terminates at a short distance from the mesial marginal ridge (Figure 11.5e) [1]. Two roots can be seen from this aspect. The buccal root from the cervical line is straight and inclines palatally at the apical third. The palatal root is straight and inclines buccally in most cases. The length of the root trunk is almost half the length of the root, with furcation on the mesial surface beginning more cervically than distal. The buccal and palatal cusps are well confined within the root trunk (Figure 11.5f) [1, 3].

Carving from the Mesial Aspect

Exercise: Marking the Buccopalatal Dimension of the Crown

The buccopalatal diameter of the crown at the cervix, measuring 8.0 mm (4.0 mm on either side of the midline) is marked near the cervix of the crown (Figure 11.6a and b). In a similar way, the buccopalatal diameter of the crown, measuring 9.0 mm (4.5 mm on either side of the midline) is marked at the occlusal edge (Figure 11.6c and d) [1]. Now, a vertical reference line is drawn at the outer diameter dimension (Figure 11.6e).

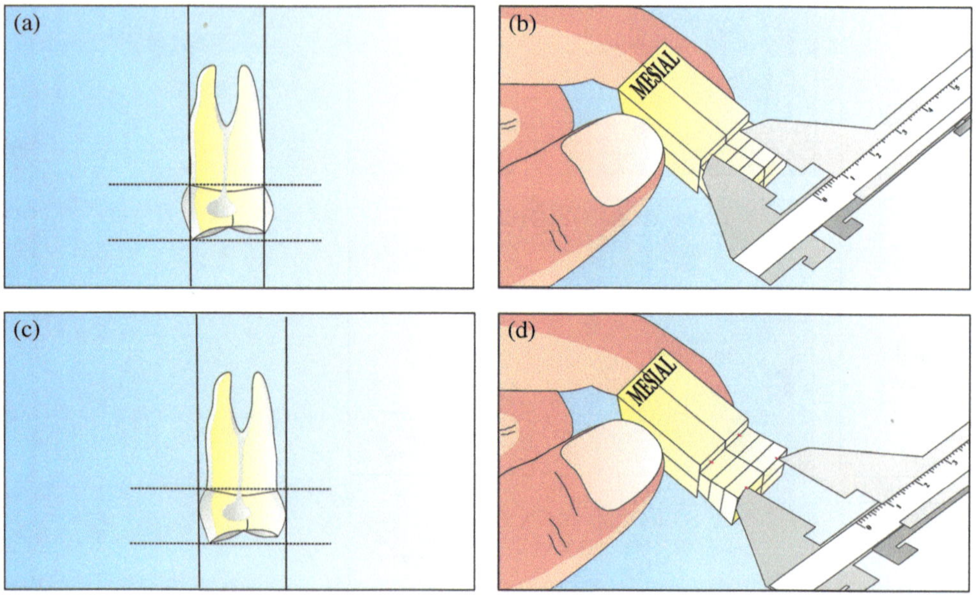

Figure 11.6 (a–d) Measuring and marking the dimension of the crown on the mesial aspect of the wax.

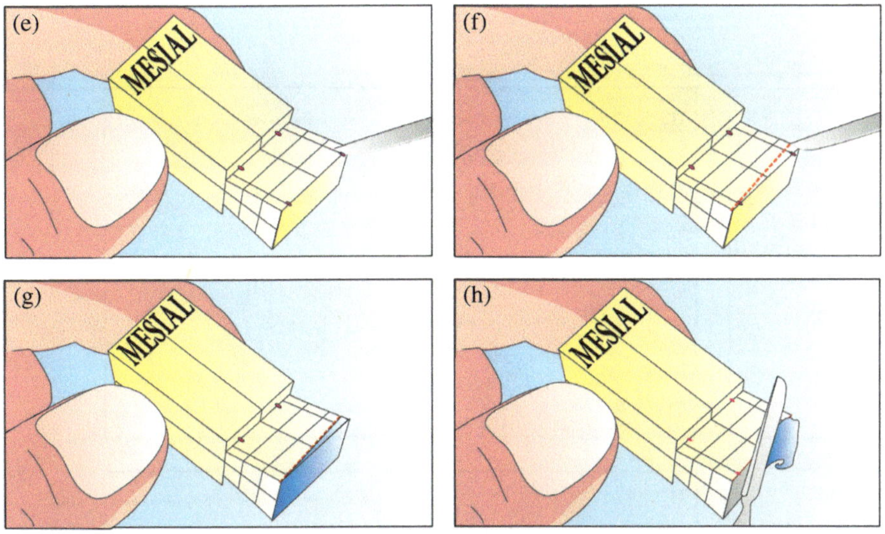

Figure 11.6 (e–h) Steps to show reduction of the height of the crown palatally.

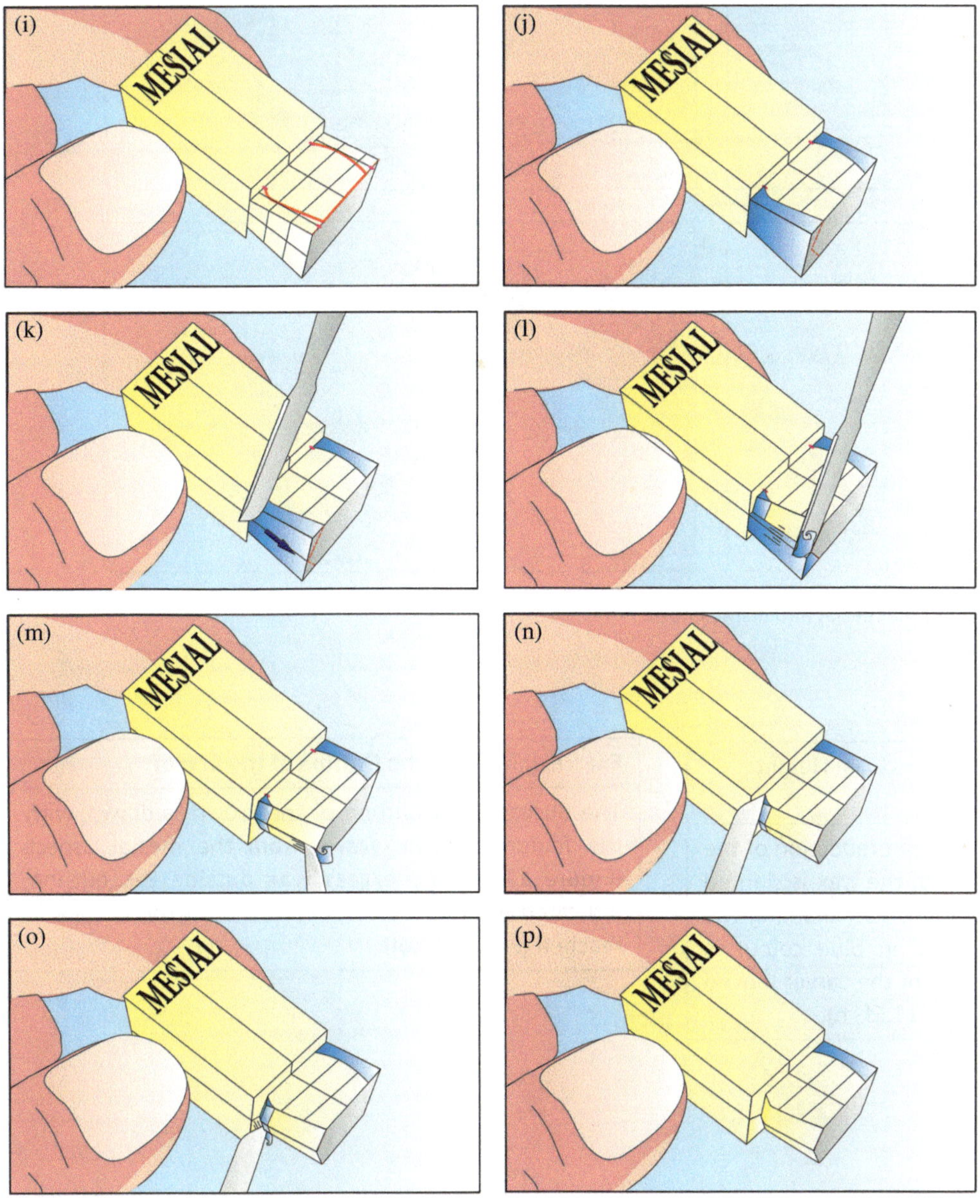

Figure 11.6 (i–p) Drawing the crown outline and carving excess wax from the buccal and palatal surfaces.

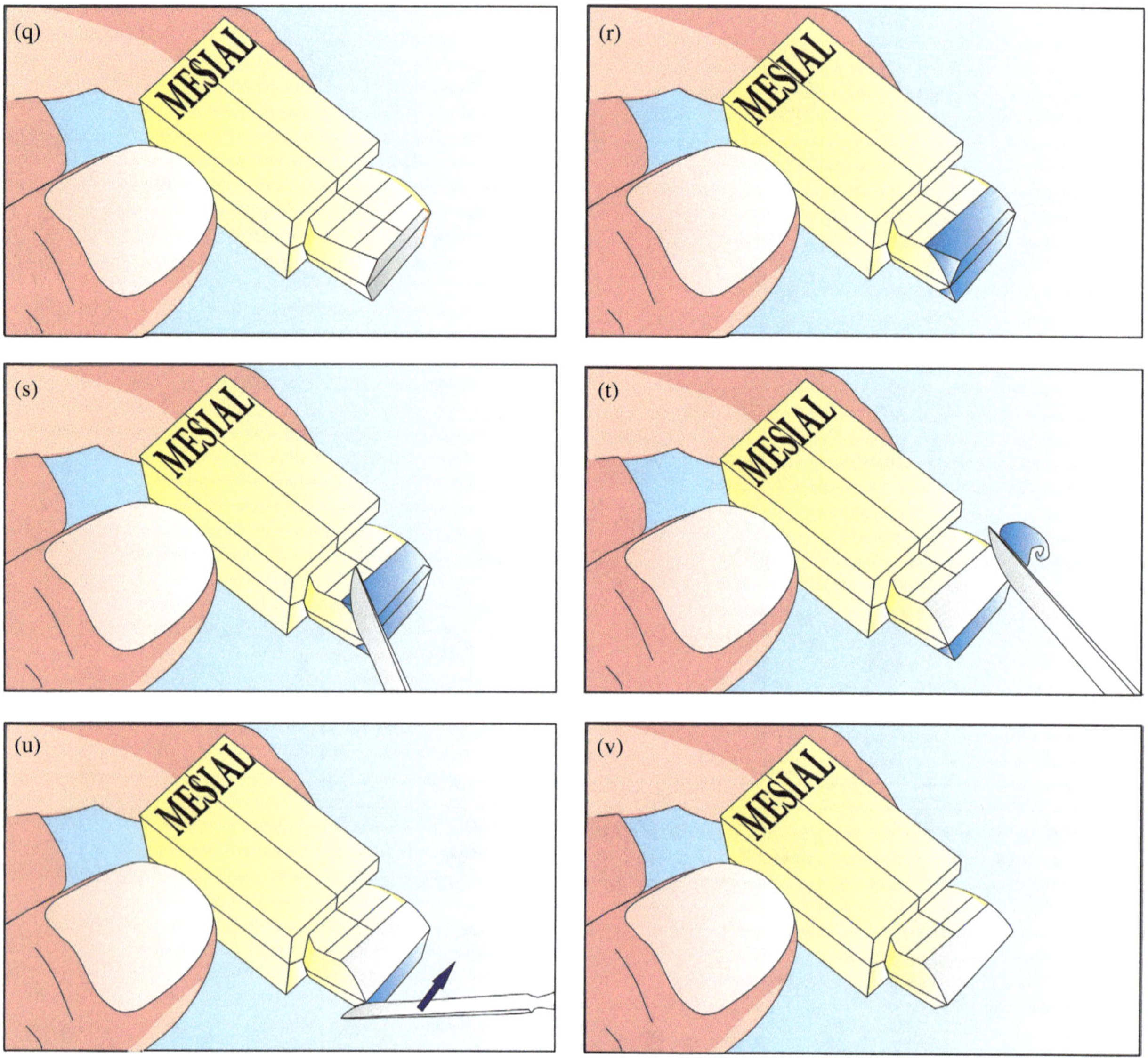

Figure 11.6 (q–v) Marking and carving the mesial and distal slopes.

Exercise: Reduction of the Cervico-occlusal Height Palatally

As a part of preparation for the height reduction of the palatal cusp, the occlusal surface of the wax is slanted towards palatal side of about 1 mm. After marking the outline, the excess wax indicated in blue colour is carved out using the cutting edge of the carver moved in a buccopalatal direction (Figure 11.6f–h).

Exercise: Marking the Outline of the Crown

The buccopalatal outline of the crown is drawn, with the features of the crown from the mesial aspect (Figure 11.6i). The excess wax outside the outline, indicated in blue colour, is carved until the outline is reached (Figure 11.6j).

Exercise: Carving Excess Wax from the Buccal Surface

The buccal wax reduction is done in two planes to create the buccal ridge. The mesial half of the buccal surface is carved with the cutting edge of the carver facing the wax at an angle and the carver is moved in a cervico-occlusal direction, following the buccal outline (Figure 11.6k and l). The same steps are followed on the distal half of buccal surface of the wax (Figure 11.6m). The wedge of wax at the cervical third is carved with the non-cutting side of the carver facing wax and the tip pointing at cervix. The carver is then moved in a mesiodistal direction. With this the crest of contour on the buccal surface of the wax is created (Figure 11.6n–p).

Exercise: Carving Excess Wax from the Palatal Surface

The excess wax is also carved from the palatal side following the aforementioned steps, except the crest of contour should be at the centre of the outline and the palatal ridge is smoothed (Figure 11.6q).

Exercise: Marking and Carving the Mesial and Distal Slopes of the Occlusal Surface

Now the mesial and distal slopes are created on the occlusal surface. The slopes are drawn on the buccal surface from the mesial and distal crest of contour (Figure 11.6r). The excess wax in blue is carved by placing the curved part of the carver facing the mesio-incisal edge of the wax at an angle and moving in a buccopalatal direction until the outline is reached (Figure 11.6s and t). The same steps are repeated to create the distal slope (Figure 11.6u and v).

Distal Aspect

The crown from this aspect has an outline similar to that of the mesial. The distal marginal ridge is placed more cervically than the mesial. The curvature of the cervical line is less and almost a straight line running buccopalatally. Developmental grooves are not evident from this aspect [2, 3]. Distal surface shows the flattened root trunk. Bifurcation of the root takes place near the apical third without the presence of any developmental grooves [1].

Occlusal Aspect

From this aspect, the crown is wider buccopalatally than mesiodistally. The occlusal outline of the tooth is roughly hexagonal with six sides, varying in length (Figure 11.7a) [1–3]. For the sake of convenience, from this aspect, six reference points are taken: buccal ridge, mesiobuccal line angle, mesiopalatal line angle, palatal ridge, distopalatal line angle, and distobuccal line angle [1]. The cuspal ridge between the buccal ridge and the mesiobuccal line angle is the *mesiobuccal cuspal ridge*. One between the mesiobuccal line angle and the mesiopalatal line angle is the *mesial marginal ridge*. The cuspal ridge between the mesiopalatal line angle and the palatal ridge is the *mesiopalatal cuspal ridge*. The ridge between the palatal ridge and the distopalatal line angle is the *distopalatal cuspal ridge*. The one between the distopalatal line angle and the distobuccal line angle is the *distal marginal ridge. The ridge between* the distobuccal line angle and buccal ridge is the distobuccal cuspal ridge (Figure 11.7b) [2, 3].

The mesiobuccal ridge is wider than the distobuccal ridge; because of this the mesial marginal ridge appears smaller than the distal marginal ridge. The mesiopalatal ridge is shorter than the distopalatal ridge. The mesiobuccal line angle is nearly a right angle, whereas the distobuccal line angle is acute (Figure 11.7b) [1–3].

The occlusal surface has two cusps with respective triangular ridges, the buccal triangular ridge and the palatal triangular ridge (Figure 11.7c). The two ridges are separated equally by the central developmental groove that runs mesiodistally. Mesially, the groove ends in a pit called the mesial pit and distally ends in the distal pit (Figure 11.7d). The triangular fossa that harbours the mesial pit is the mesial triangular fossa and the one that harbours the distal pit is the distal triangular fossa. In the mesial triangular fossa, the central developmental groove joins the mesial marginal developmental groove, which crosses the mesial marginal ridge and ends on the mesial surface. The mesial marginal ridge appears concave because of the depression created by the mesial developmental groove. The palatal cusp is sharper than the buccal cusp, even though the palatal triangular ridge is less prominent (Figure 11.7e). The palatal cusp is placed mesial to the long axis of the tooth [1–4].

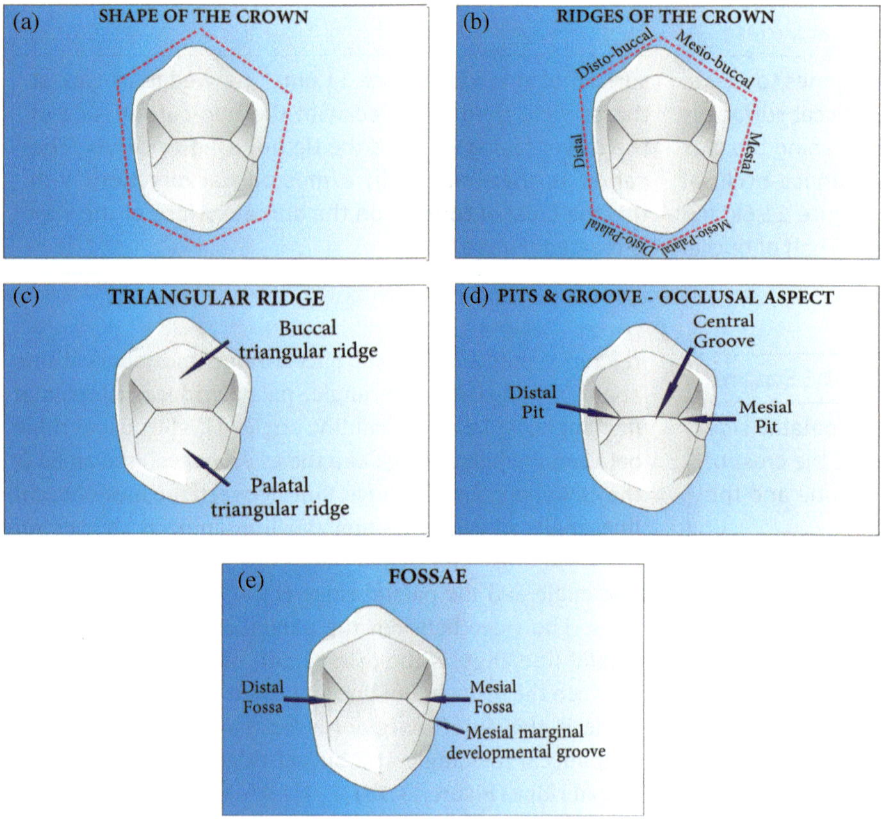

Figure 11.7 (a–e) Description of the maxillary right first premolar from the occlusal aspect.

Carving from the Occlusal Aspect

Exercise: Creating the Palatal Convergence
The initial step in carving the occlusal aspect is creating the palatal convergence,This is done by marking lines on both mesial and distal sides on the occlusal surface, with their palatal convergence (Figure 11.8a). Excess wax is carved by placing the cutting edge of the carver facing the occlusal surface of wax and moved it in an occluso-cervical direction, until the outline is reached (Figure 11.8b–d).

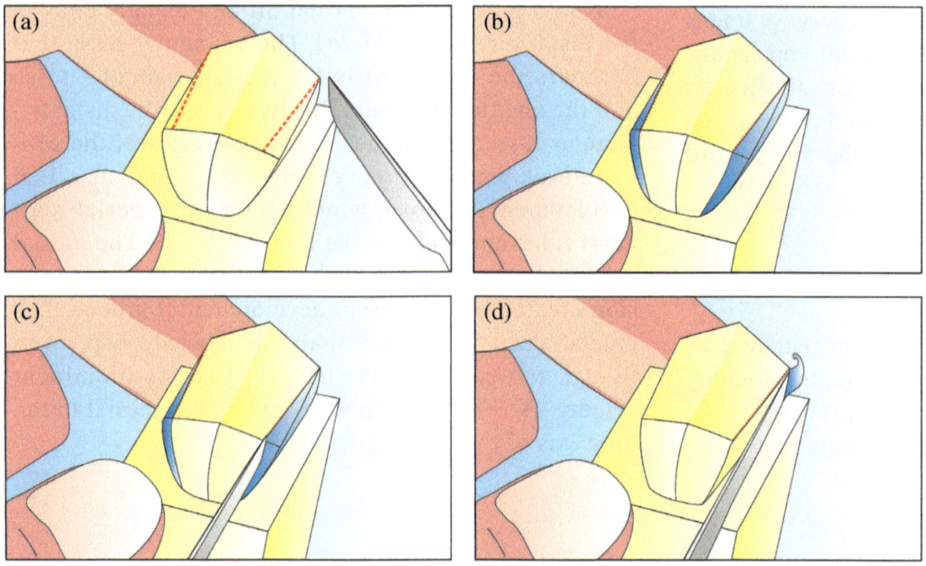

Figure 11.8 (a–d) Creating the palatal convergence of the mesial and distal surfaces.

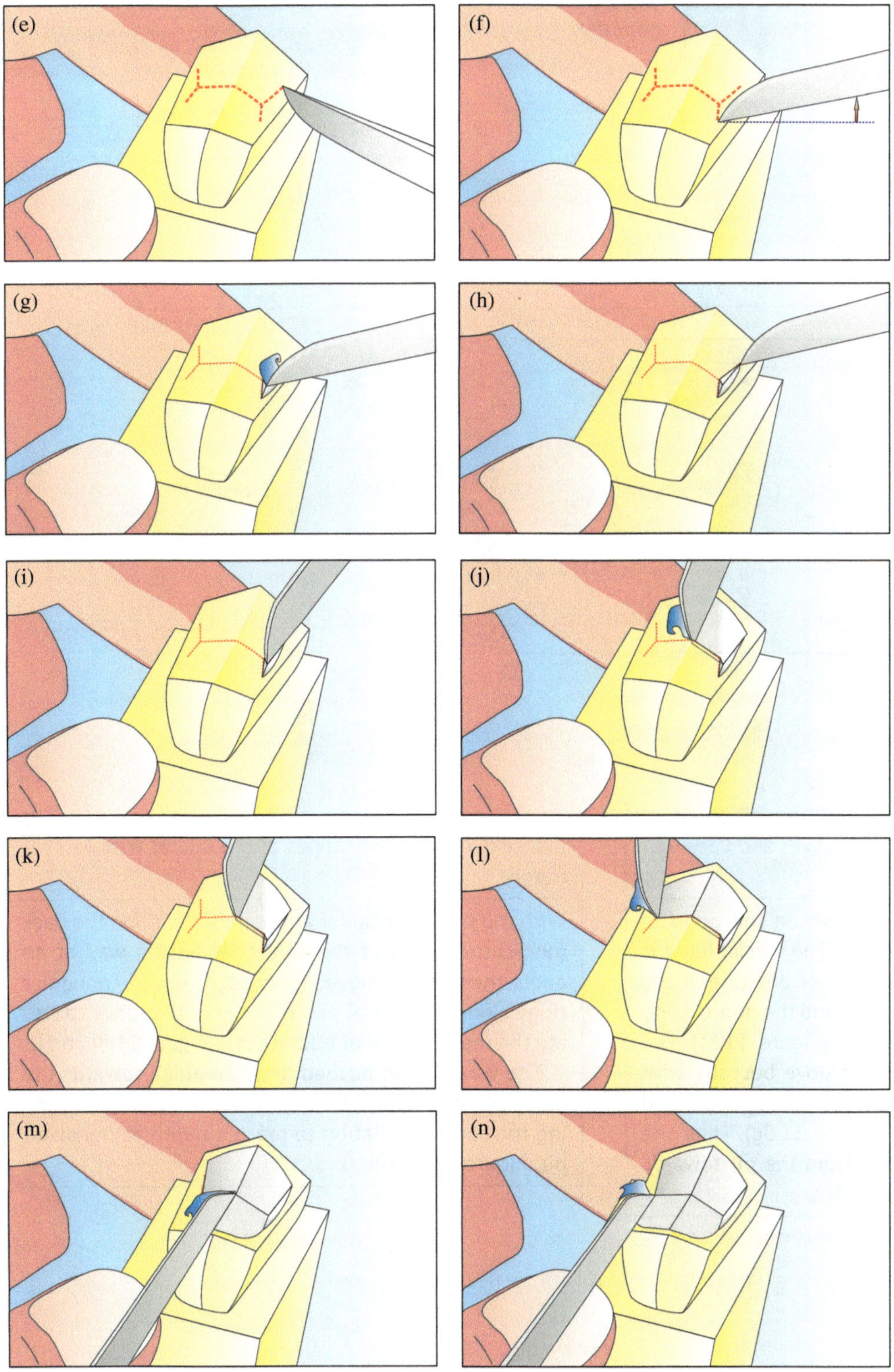

Figure 11.8 (e–q) Step sequence to carve occlusal features of the maxillary right first premolar.

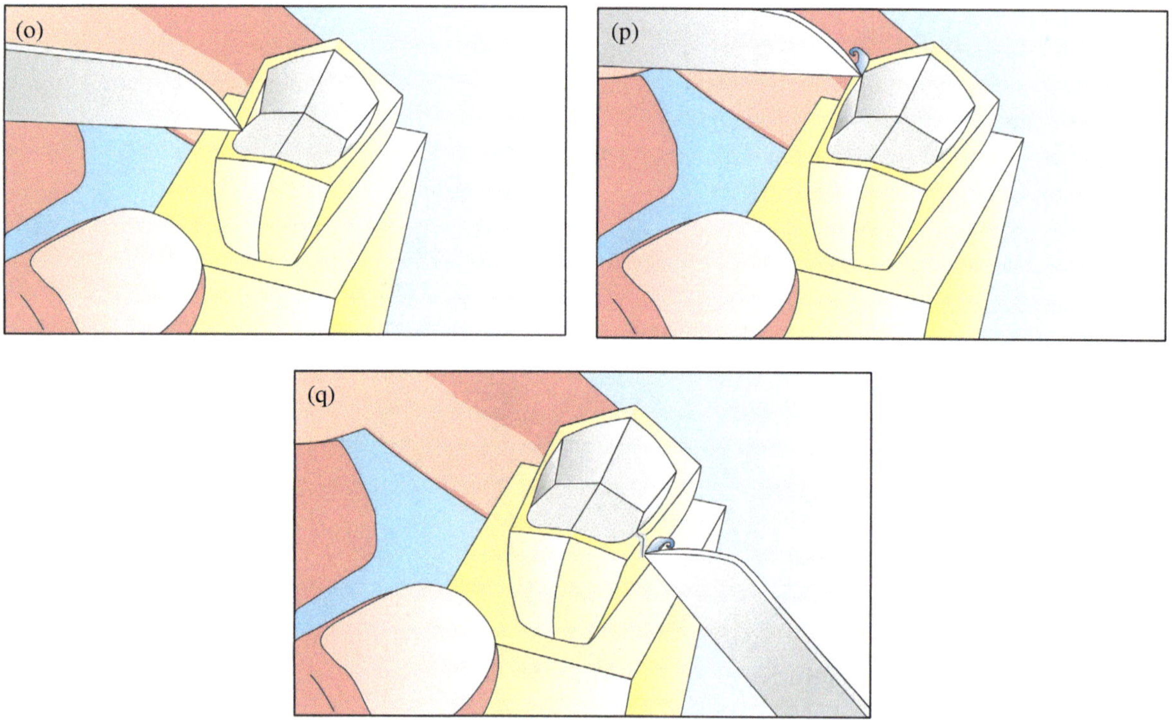

Figure 11.8 (Cont'd) (e–q)

Exercise: Marking the Outline of Grooves and Carving the Mesial Triangular Fossa

The outline of the grooves is drawn on the occlusal surface of the crown (Figure 11.8e). The mesial fossa is carved by placing the tip of the carver pointing at the palatal end of 'V' part of the groove and the non-cutting side of the carver facing the wax (Figure 11.8f). The carver is then moved along the groove buccally with application of pressure so that the carver is pushed deep into the wax at the pit (Figure 11.8g). Then the carver is pulled out as it moves from the pit towards the other end of the 'V' (Figure 11.8h).

Exercise: Carving the Slopes of the Buccal Triangular Ridge

With the tip of the carver at the mesial pit and the back (non-cutting end) of the carver facing the wax at an angle, the carver is moved towards the buccal triangular ridge along the mesial part of the central groove to create the mesial slope of buccal cusp (Figure 11.8i and j).

The wax is then pushed from the ridge towards the distal pit with application of pressure, while maintaining the same angulation to reach a depth at the distal pit (Figure 11.8k and l).

Exercise: Carving the Slopes of the Palatal Triangular Ridge

The same steps are repeated on the palatal part of the wax block to create the mesial and distal slopes of the palatal ridge (Figure 11.8m and n).

Exercise: Carving the Distal Triangular Fossa

The distal fossa is then refined by moving the carver buccopalatally along the groove (Figure 11.8o and p).

Exercise: Carving the Mesial Developmental Groove

Mesial marginal developmental groove is carved by extending the central groove on the mesial side to cross the mesial marginal ridge and extend to the mesial surface (Figure 11.8q).

Carving the Root

Exercise: Carving the Root from the Buccal & Palatal Aspect

The root outline is drawn with its features described previously (Figure 11.9a). The cervical and middle third of the mesial side of the root is carved with the anterior part of the cutting edge of the carver facing the wax surface, moving it buccopalatally until the outline is reached (Figure 11.9b and c). The apical part of the wax is carved with the back of the carver facing the wax and the tip of the carver facing the apex. The carver is moved buccopalatally (Figure 11.9d and e). The excess wax on the distal side of the root is carved up to the root outline (Figure 11.9f–h).

Exercise: Carving the Root from the Proximal (Mesial) Aspect

Now the buccopalatal root outline is drawn on the mesial side (Figure 11.9i) and excess wax is carved from the buccal and palatal surfaces, until the outline is reached (Figure 11.9j and k).

Exercise: Carving the Furcal Part of the Root from the Proximal Aspect

The wax in the furcal part of the root is removed by carving along the outline of furcation using the anterior curved part of the carver and removing a wedge of wax (Figure 11.9l–p). The same steps are repeated on the distal furcal outline to carve the wax completely (Figure 11.9q).

Exercise: Marking and Creating the Mesial Developmental Depression

The mesial developmental depression outline is drawn cervical to the mesial contact that ends at the furcation. The depression is created using the excavating end of the carver moved in a cervico-apical direction. The depression is made deep at the centre of the root (Figure 11.9r–u).

Exercise: Drawing the Cervical Line on the Mesial and Distal Aspects

The cervical line is marked with its curvature of 1 mm, facing occlusally on the mesial aspect. On the distal surface, the cervical line is drawn straight without any curvature [1].

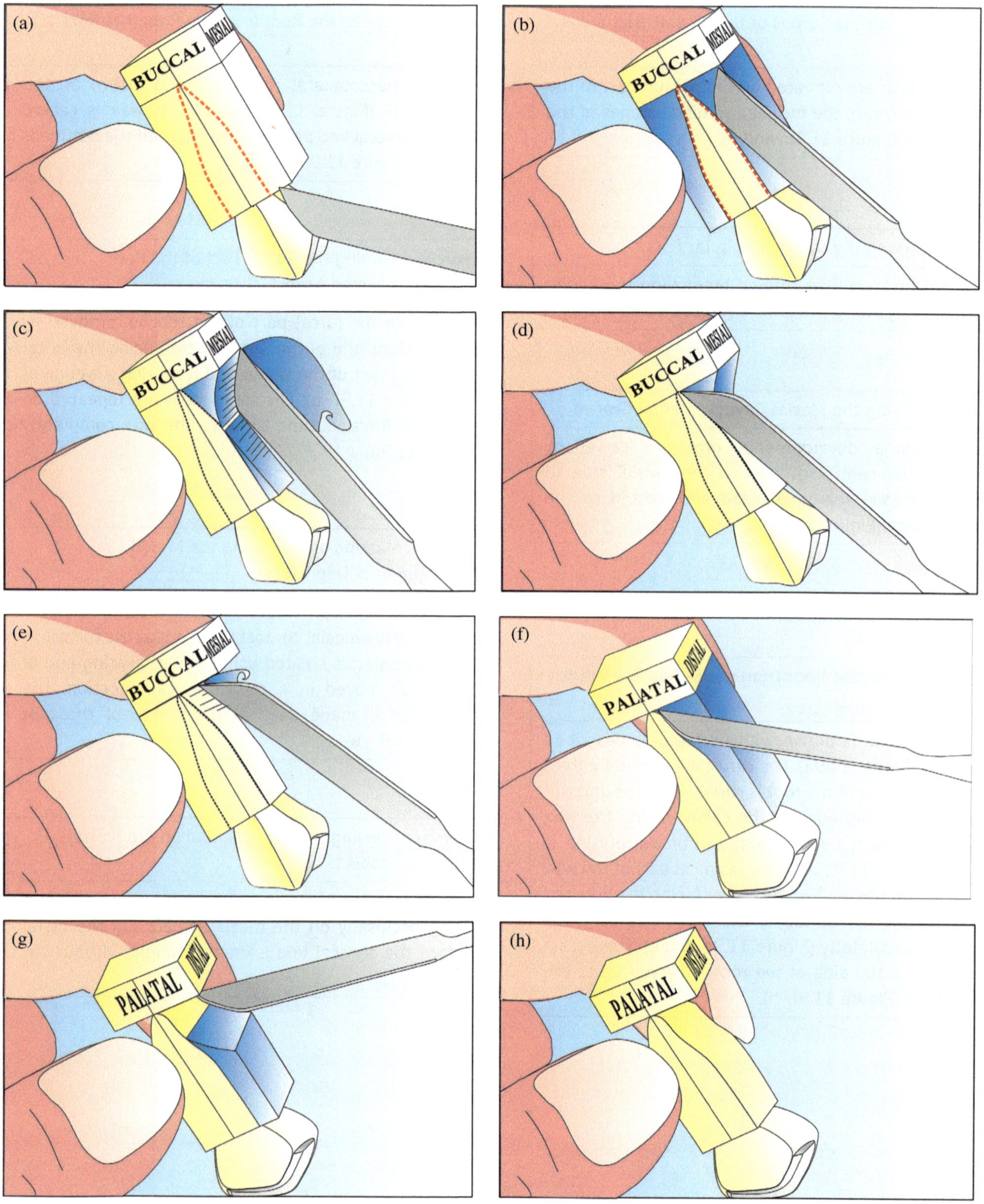

Figure 11.9 (a–u) Step sequence to carve the root from the buccal, palatal and mesial aspects.

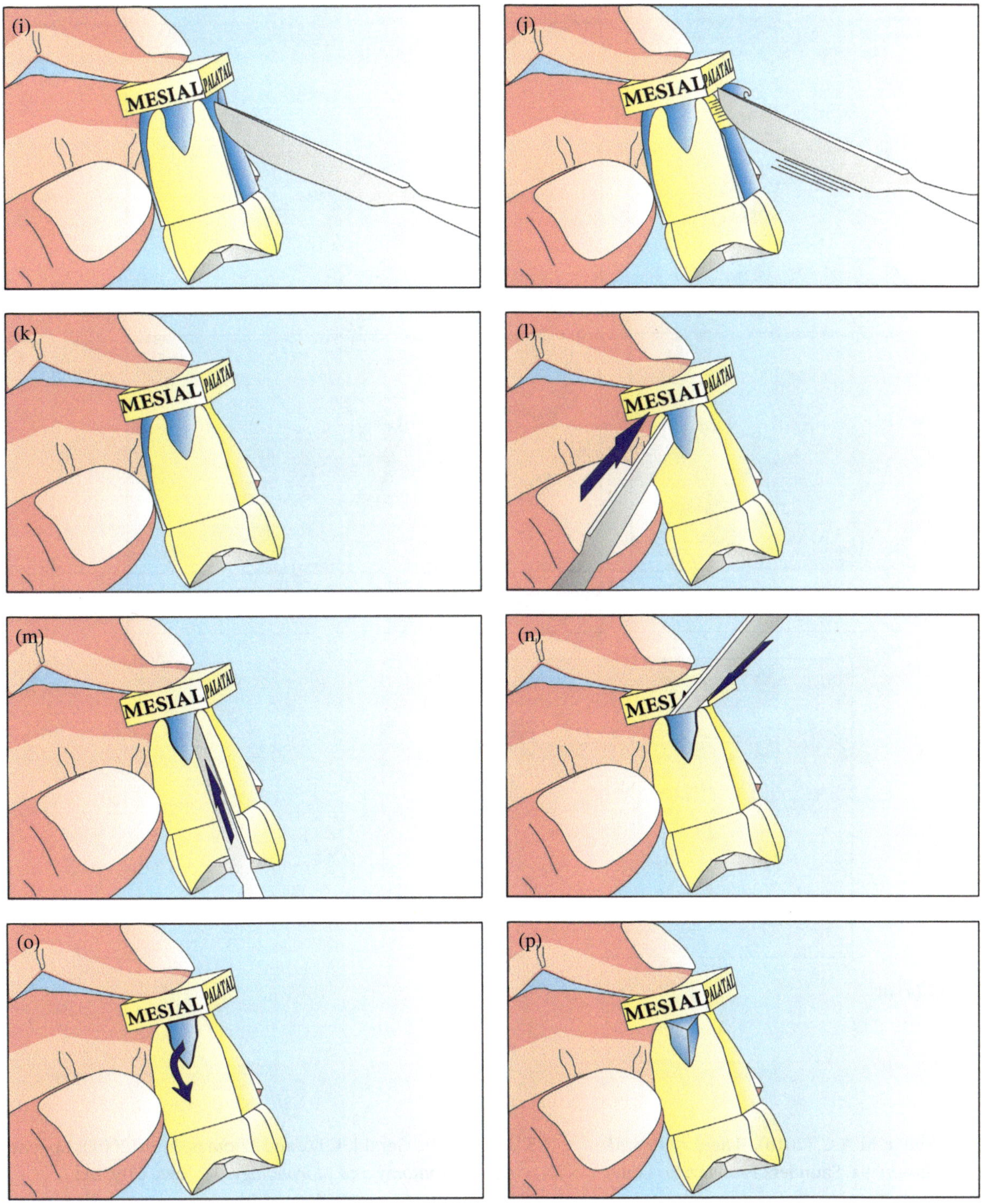

Figure 11.9 (Cont'd) (a–u)

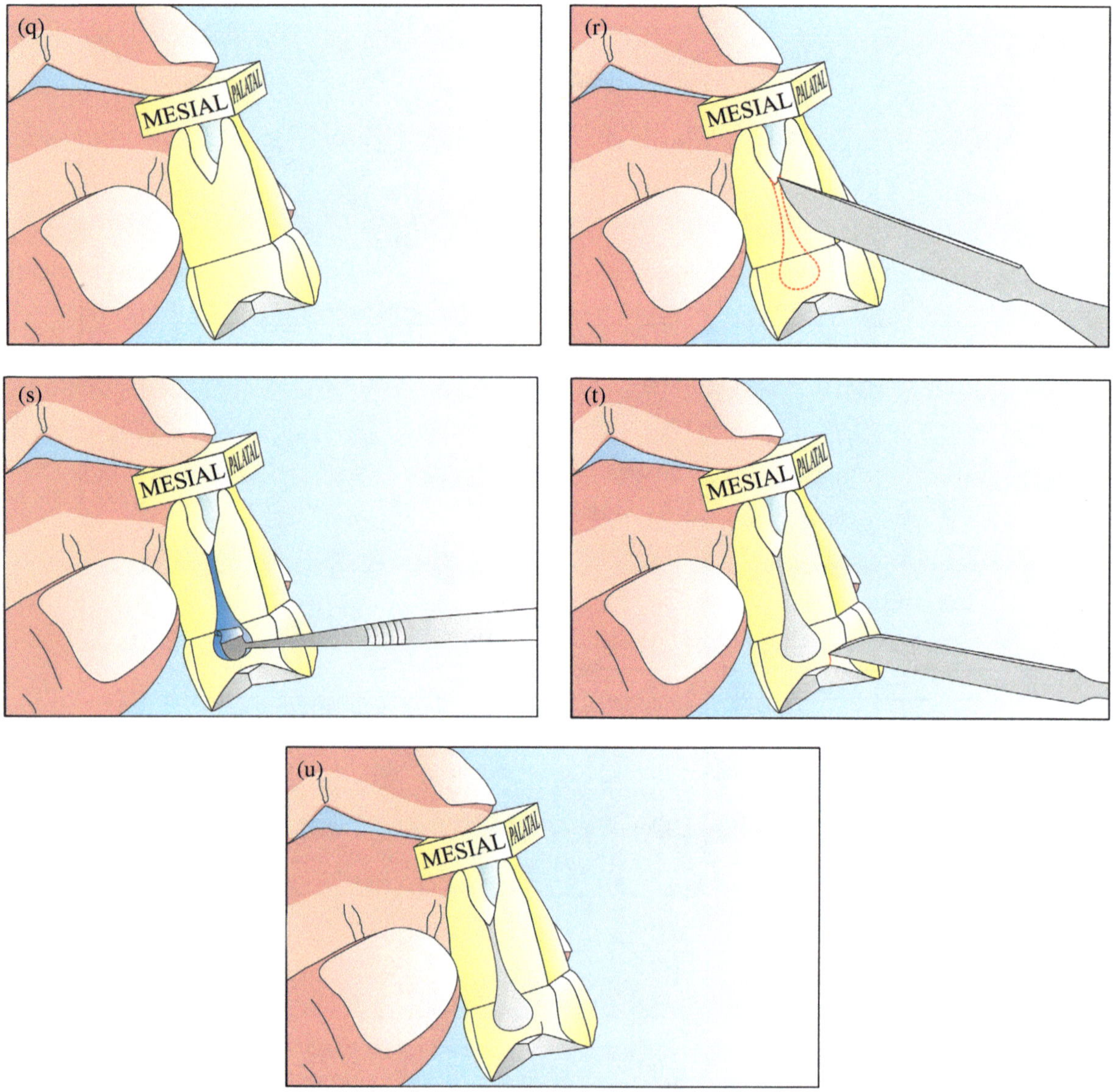

Figure 11.9 (Cont'd) (a–u)

References

1 Stanley, J.N. and Major, M.A.C. (2010). *Wheeler's Dental Anatomy and Occlusion*, 9e. Saunders Elsevier: St. Louis, MO.

2 Rickne, C.S. and Weiss, G. (2012). *Woelfel's Dental Anatomy*, 8e. Philadelphia: Lippincott Williams & Wilkins.

3 James, L.F., Gerald, E.D., and Thomas, M.S. (2001). *Concise Dental Anatomy and Morphology*, 4e. Iowa City, IA: University of Iowa College of Dentistry.

4 Geoffrey, C.V.B. (1983). *Dental Morphology. An Illustrated Guide*, 2e. Philadelphia: Wright Elsevier.

12

Permanent Maxillary Second Premolar

LEARNING OBJECTIVE
At the end of the chapter, the student should have knowledge of the permanent maxillary second premolar and develop the psychomotor skills for carving and waxing the same.

Permanent Maxillary Right Second Premolar

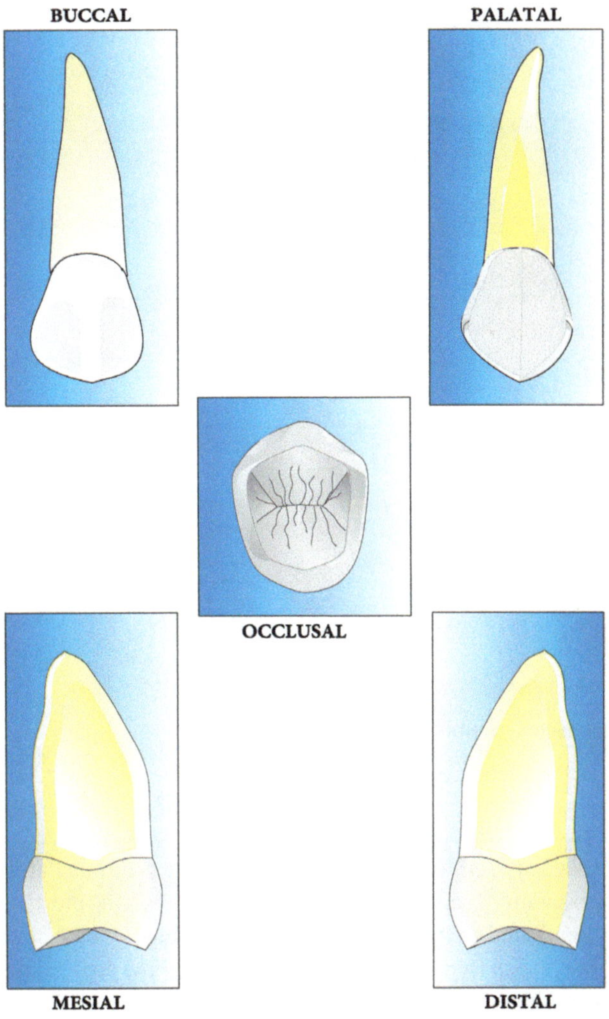

Buccal Aspect

The permanent maxillary second premolar is the fifth tooth from the midsagittal plane (Figure 12.1). The cervico-occlusal length of the crown is less compared to that of the first premolar. The mesial crest of contour is in the occlusal third, and the distal crest of contour is in the middle third but more occlusally placed (Figure 12.2a). The buccal cusp is less pointed with the mesial cuspal ridge smaller than the distal cuspal ridge (Figure 12.2b) [1–3]. The tip of the buccal cusp is placed mesial to the long axis of the tooth (Figure 12.2d) [4]. The buccal ridge is not as prominent as that seen in the first premolar (Figure 12.2c). The root tapers uniformly from the cervix to the apex. The root appears thicker at the cervical portion (Figure 12.2e) [1, 2].

Carving from the Buccal Aspect

Steps to carve from this aspect are the same as those for the maxillary first premolar. Students are requested to refer to Chapter 11 for the step sequences.

Measurements:
Length of the crown – 8.5 mm
Length of the root – 14.0 mm
Mesiodistal diameter of the crown – 7.0 mm
Mesiodistal diameter of the crown at the cervix – 5.0 mm [1]

Palatal Aspect

From this aspect, the palatal cusp is longer compared to that of the first premolar, equal in height to that of the buccal cusp. Other features are similar to those of the palatal aspect of the first premolar (Figure 12.3a and b) [1, 2].

An Illustrated Atlas of Tooth Carving and Wax-Up Techniques, First Edition. Anil Bangalore Shivappa.

Companion website: www.wiley.com/go/bangalore/toothcarving

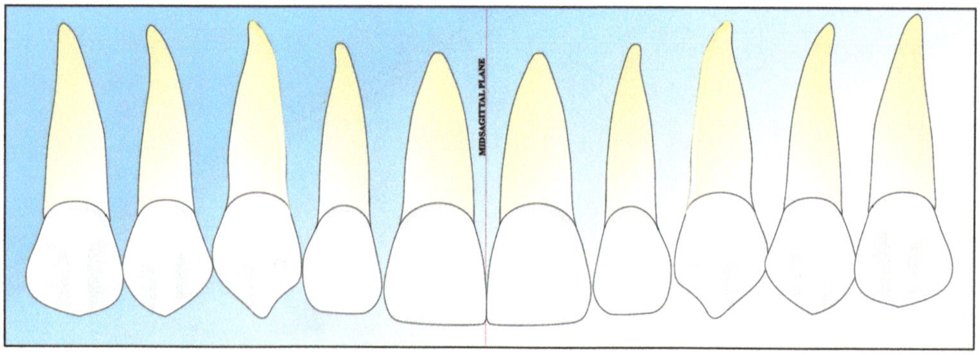

Figure 12.1 Position of the maxillary second premolar in relation to the midsagittal plane.

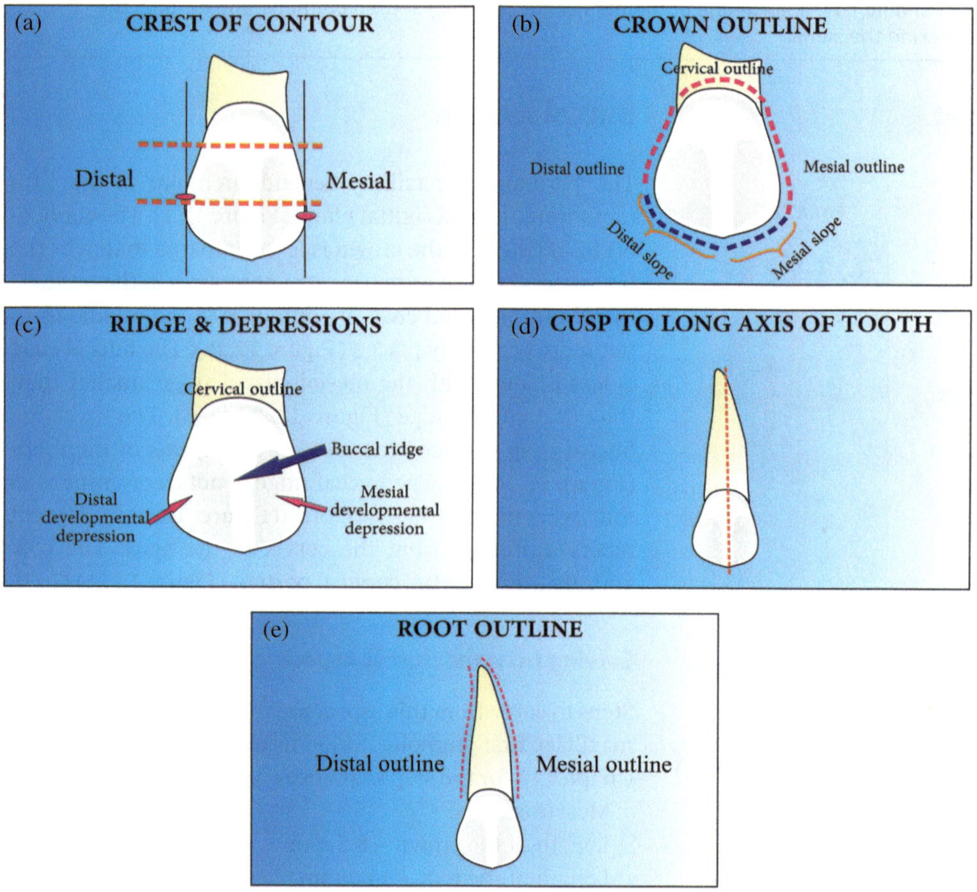

Figure 12.2 (a–e) Characteristic features of the permanent maxillary right second premolar from the buccal aspect.

Mesial Aspect

From the mesial aspect, the crown of the permanent maxillary right second premolar appears shorter. The buccal and palatal cusp heights are nearly equal [1–4]. The cusps exhibit greater distance between them [1]. The crown appears rounded and convex, with absence of developmental depression and the developmental groove crossing the marginal ridge [1, 2]. A single root is seen from this aspect that shows shallow depression at the middle of the root (Figure 12.4a–e)[2].

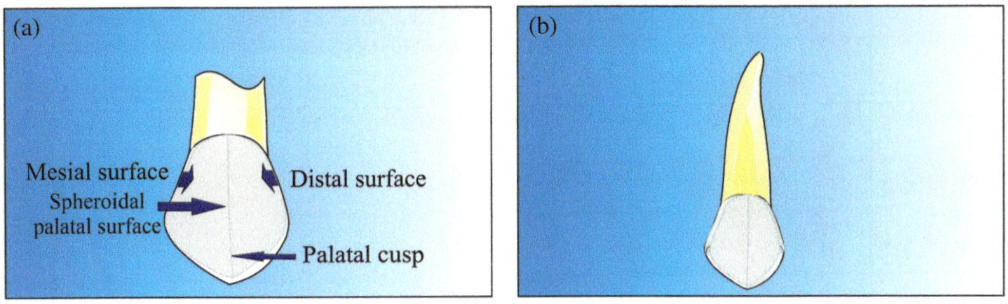

Figure 12.3 (a–b) Description of the permanent maxillary right second premolar from the palatal aspect.

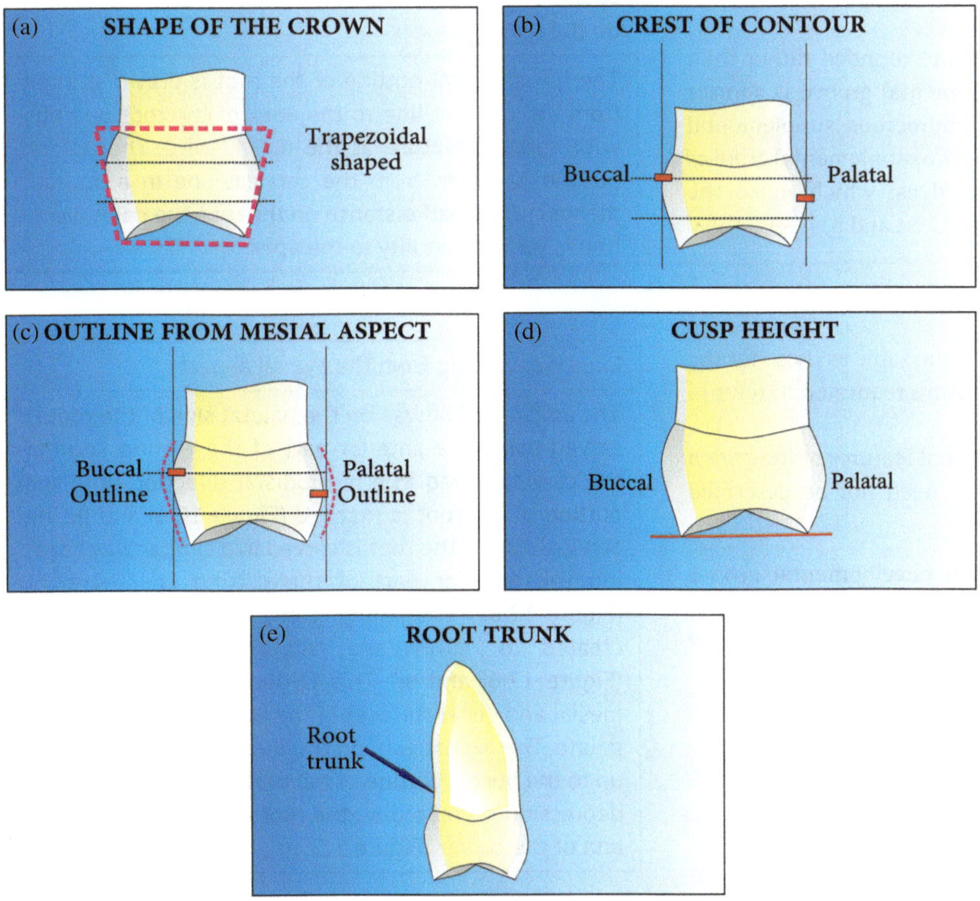

Figure 12.4 (a–e) Description of the permanent maxillary right second premolar from the mesial aspect.

Carving from the Mesial Aspect

Steps to carve from this aspect are same as those for the maxillary first premolar. Students are requested to refer to Chapter 11 for the step sequence.

NOTE: The step to create occlusal sloping (Figure 11.6f–h) is eliminated for this tooth (maxillary second premolar).

Measurements:

Buccopalatal diameter of the crown – 9.0 mm

Buccopalatal diameter of the crown at the cervix – 8.0 mm [1].

Distal Aspect

The crown from this aspect is similar to that of the mesial aspect, and the developmental depression on the root is more pronounced than that of the mesial [1, 2].

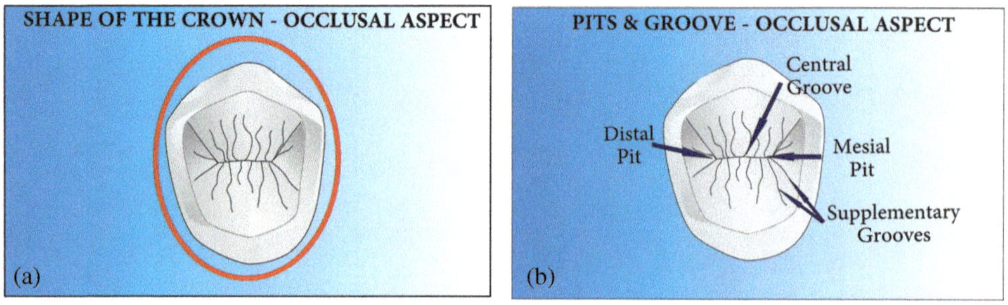

Figure 12.5 (a–b) Description of the permanent maxillary right second premolar from the occlusal aspect.

Occlusal Aspect

The crown from this aspect is more rounded rather than angular, and the central developmental groove is shorter and more irregular. There are numerous supplemental grooves along the central groove. The supplemental grooves may extend up to the cuspal ridges, which make the occlusal surface irregular (Figure 12.5a and b) [1–3, 5].

Carving from the Occlusal Aspect

Steps to carve from this aspect are the same as those for the maxillary first premolar. Students are requested to refer to Chapter 11 for the step sequence.

NOTE 1: A few steps for additional features of the crown (of the maxillary first premolar) need not be described here. They are

i) Carving the mesial marginal developmental groove (Figure 11.8q)
ii) Mesial developmental depression of the crown part (Figure 11.9r and s)

NOTE 2: Features of second premolar included are

i) All the line angles of the crown from this aspect are kept rounded.
ii) The central groove should be kept short.
iii) Supplemental grooves are drawn on the occlusal surface from the central groove radiating on the slopes of the triangular ridges towards the cuspal ridges.

Carving the Root

Exercise: Carving from the Buccal Aspect

The outline of the root is drawn on the buccal surface of the wax (Figure 12.6a). Excess wax (in blue colour) is carved on the mesial (Figure 12.6b–e) and distal sides throughout the buccopalatal length (Figure 12.6f–h).

Exercise: Marking the Buccopalatal Outline of the Root on the Mesial Aspect

The buccopalatal outline of the root is drawn straight from the cervical line to the apex of the root buccally, with some curvature at the apical third. The palatal outline is drawn from the cervical line in a straight manner; at its half distance on the root, the palatal outline is turned buccally to the apex.

Exercise: Carving from the Mesial Aspect

The apical half of wax on the palatal side of the root is carved using the anterior part of the cutting edge of the carver, moved in a mesiodistal direction until the outline of the root is reached (Figure 12.6i and j). The cervical half of the root is carved in a similar way keeping the anterior part of the cutting edge straight (Figure 12.6k). The palatal convergence of the root is created to narrow the palatal side of the root (Figure 12.6l and m). This is done by carving on the mesial and distal surfaces of the root, more towards the palate. The excess wax on the buccal surface is carved up to the buccal outline of the root. The developmental depression is created on the root using the excavating end of the carver (Figure 12.6n).

Exercise: Drawing the Cervical Line on the Mesial and Distal Aspect

The cervical line is marked with its curvature of 1 mm, facing occlusally on the mesial aspect. On the distal surface, the cervical line is drawn straight without any curvature.

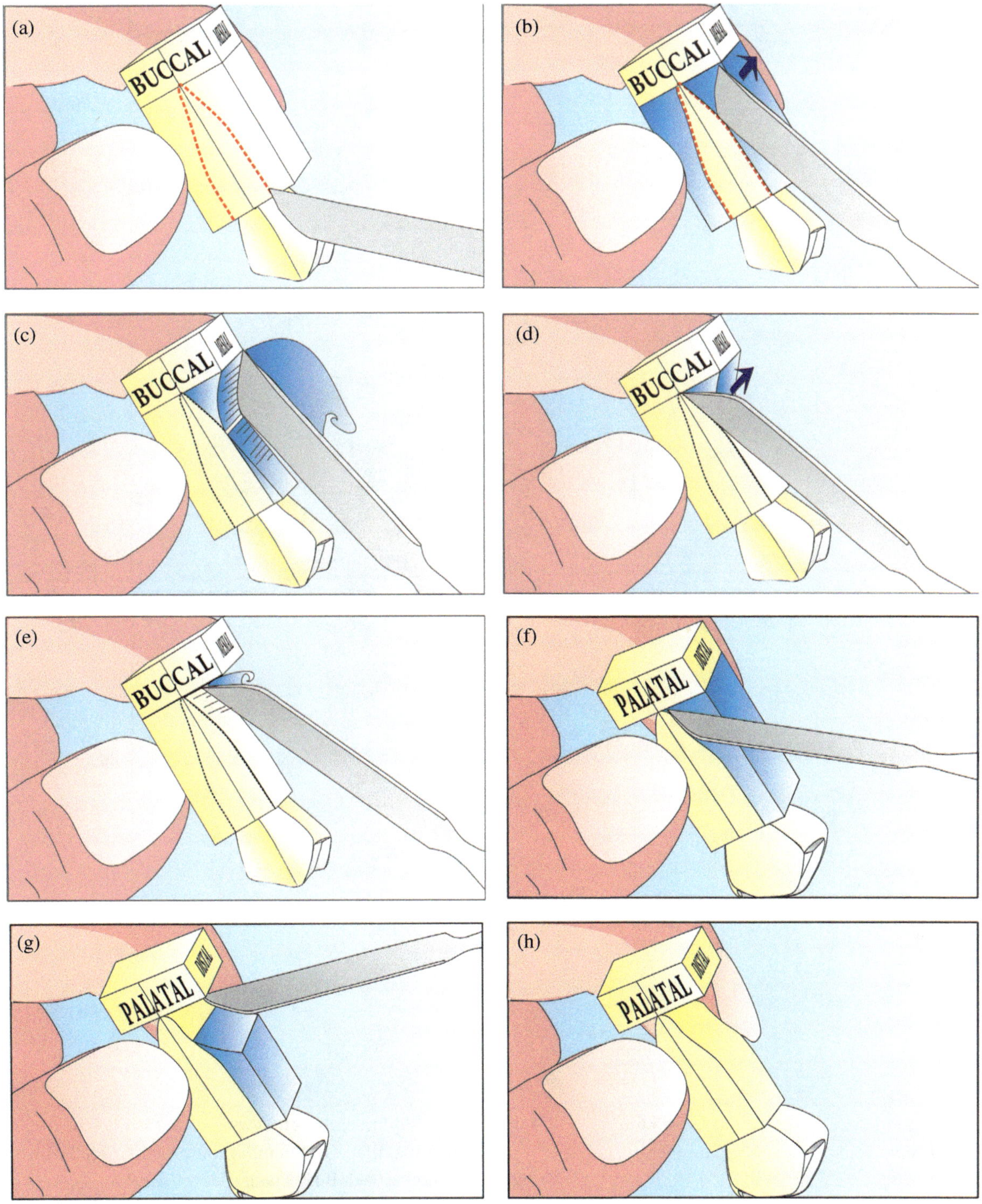

Figure 12.6 (a–n) Step sequence in carving the root of the permanent maxillary right second premolar.

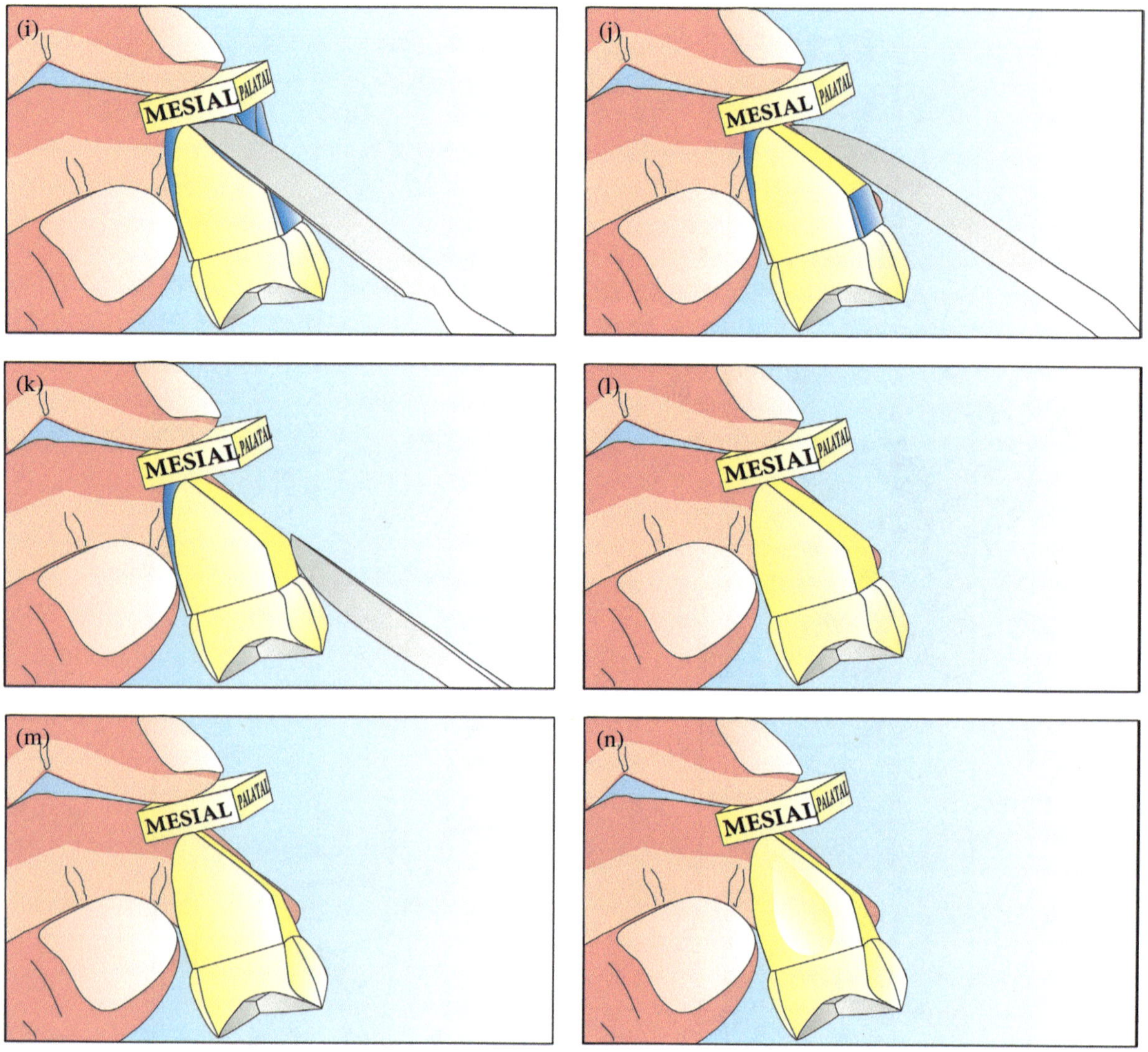

Figure 12.6 (Cont'd) (a–n)

References

1 Stanley, J.N. and Major, M.A.C. (2010). *Wheeler's Dental Anatomy and Occlusion*, 9e. St. Louis, MO: Saunders Elsevier.

2 Rickne, C.S. and Weiss, G. (2012). *Woelfel's Dental Anatomy*, 8e. Philadelphia: Lippincott Williams & Wilkins.

3 James, L.F., Gerald, E.D., and Thomas, M. (2001). *Concise Dental Anatomy and Morphology*, 4e. Iowa City: IA: University of Iowa College of Dentistry.

4 Nagaş, I.C., Eğilmez, F., and Kivanç, B.H. (2018). The permanent maxillary and mandibular premolar teeth. In: *Dental Anatomy* (ed. B.H. Kivanç). http://dx.doi.org/10.5772/intechopen.79464 (accessed 23 March 2020).

5 Geoffrey, C.B. (1983). *Dental Morphology. An Illustrated Guide*, 2e. Philadelphia: Wright Elsevier.

13

Permanent Mandibular First Premolar

LEARNING OBJECTIVE
At the end of the chapter, the student should have knowledge of the permanent mandibular first premolar and develop the psychomotor skills for waxing and carving the same.

Permanent Mandibular Right First Premolar

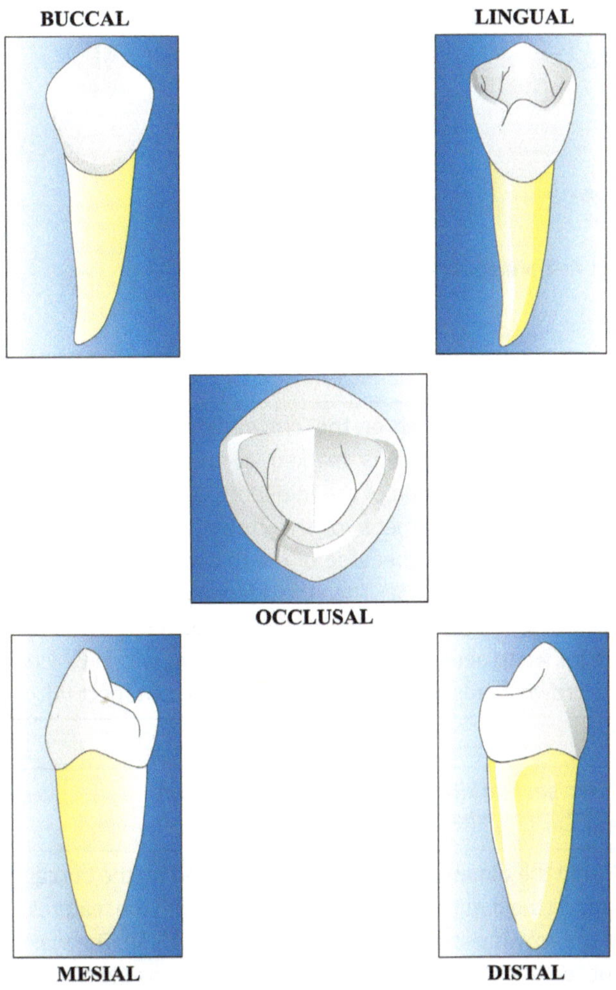

Buccal Aspect

The permanent mandibular first premolar is the fourth tooth from the midline (Figure 13.1). The crown appears roughly pentagonal in shape (Figure 13.2a) [1]. The crown is nearly symmetrical bilaterally. The crest of contour on the mesial side is near the junction of the middle and occlusal third [2]. The distal crest of contour is placed slightly occlusal compared to the mesial crest of contour (Figure 13.2b). Both the mesial and distal outlines of the crown are concave above and below the crest of contour (Figure 13.2c). The mesial cuspal ridge is shorter than the distal one (Figure 13.2d). The cusp tip is placed slightly mesial to the long axis of tooth. The cervical line shows little curvature with the crest at the centre of the root. The cervical part of the crown is much narrower. The buccal surface appears more convex. It shows development of three lobes:

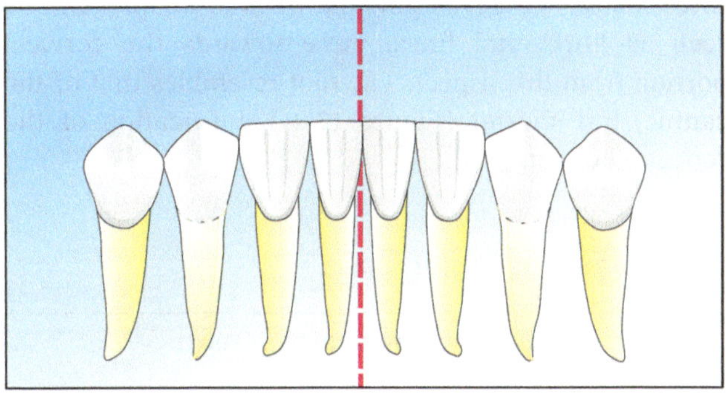

Figure 13.1 Position of the mandibular first premolar in relation to the midsagittal plane.

An Illustrated Atlas of Tooth Carving and Wax-Up Techniques, First Edition. Anil Bangalore Shivappa.

Companion website: www.wiley.com/go/bangalore/toothcarving

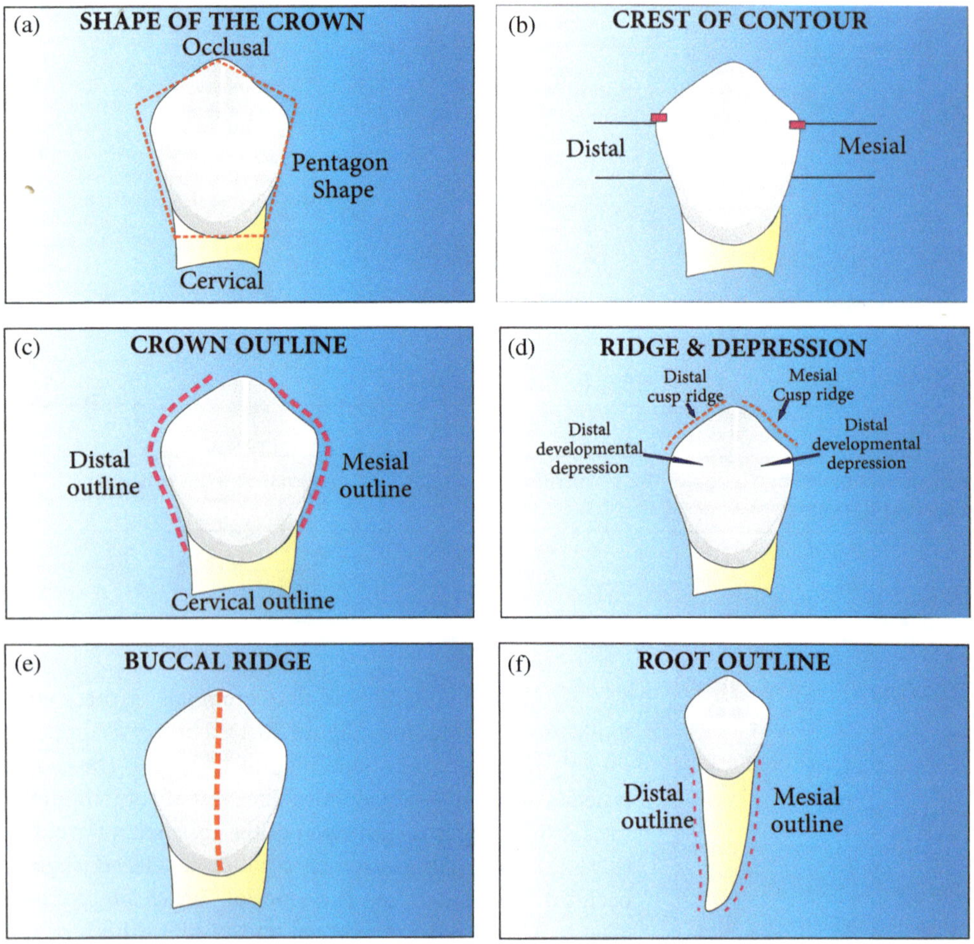

Figure 13.2 (a–f) Descriptive features of the permanent mandibular right first premolar from the buccal aspect.

the buccal lobe, the mesial lobe, and the distal lobe. Of the three, the buccal lobe is well developed, ending as a pointed cusp tip. The buccal ridge runs from the cervical line to the cusp tip (Figure 13.2e). Developmental depressions can be seen from this aspect between the three lobes. The developmental lines of enamel can be seen as horizontal lines, more towards the cervical portion from this aspect. The root resembles that of the canine, but shorter (Figure 13.2f). Bifurcation of the root can be seen [2,3].

Carving from the Buccal Aspect

Exercise: Marking the Length of the Crown and the Root

The crown length of 8.5 mm and root length of 14.0 mm are measured and marked on the prepared wax block as described in previous chapters (Figure 13.3a–c). Then the division of the crown into equal thirds is done with junctional lines marked on the wax block (Figure 13.3d).

Exercise: Marking the Mesiodistal Dimensions

Mesiodistal diameter of the crown, which is the bulk dimension of 7.0 mm is marked at the occlusal edge (3.5 mm on either side of the midline; Figure 13.3e). Then, the mesiodistal diameter of the crown at the cervix of 5 mm (2.5 mm on either side of the midline) is marked at the cervix (Figure 13.3f). Then the reference points on both the mesial (Figure 13.3g) and distal sides (Figure 13.3h) are joined to get the dimension of the crown, within which the crown needs to be carved from the buccal aspect [4].

Exercise: Marking the Outline of the Crown and Carving Excess Wax

Within the dimension of the crown obtained on the buccal surface, the outline of the crown is carved, with the features of the crown previously mentioned (Figure 13.3i). The wax outside the outline of the crown is considered as the excess wax which is indicated in blue colour (Figure 13.3j). This excess wax is carved out to get the crown with outline.

Because the concavities are seen above and below the crest of contour on the mesial outline, the curved end of the cutting edge of the carver is used both above and below it and moved in a labiolingual direction (Figure 13.3k–n). The chunk of the wax at the crest is carved to get a smooth outline (Figure 13.3o). The same steps are repeated on the distal side to get the outline of the crown (Figure 13.3p).

Mesial Aspect

From this aspect the crown is roughly rhomboidal in shape (Figure 13.4a). The tip of the buccal cusp is in line with the long axis of tooth [4]. The crown appears tilted in the lingual direction over the root trunk (Figure 13.4b). The buccal crest of contour is at the cervical third of the crown. The lingual crest of contour approaches the middle third of the

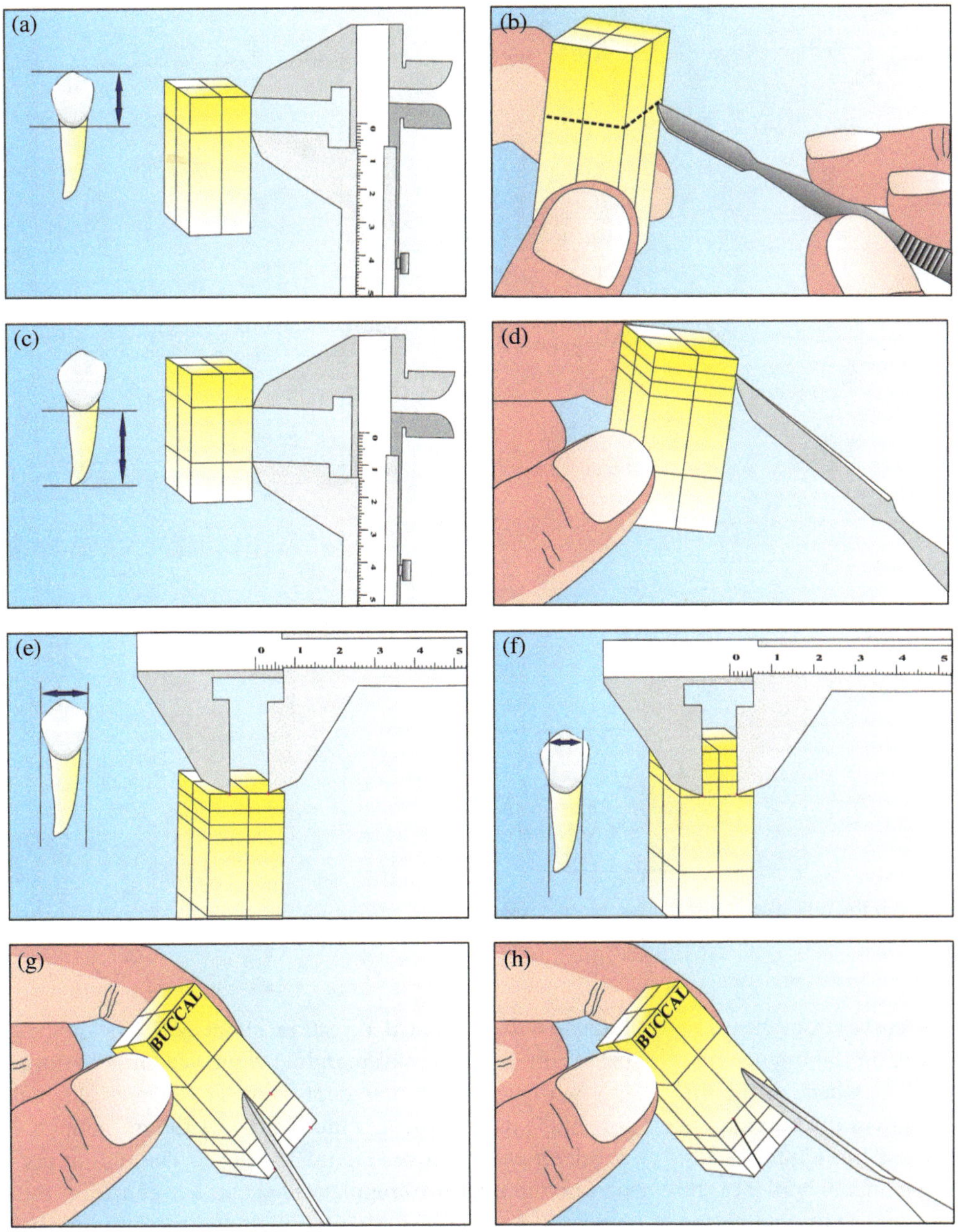

Figure 13.3 (a–h) Measuring and marking the crown dimension and root length on the buccal aspect of the wax.

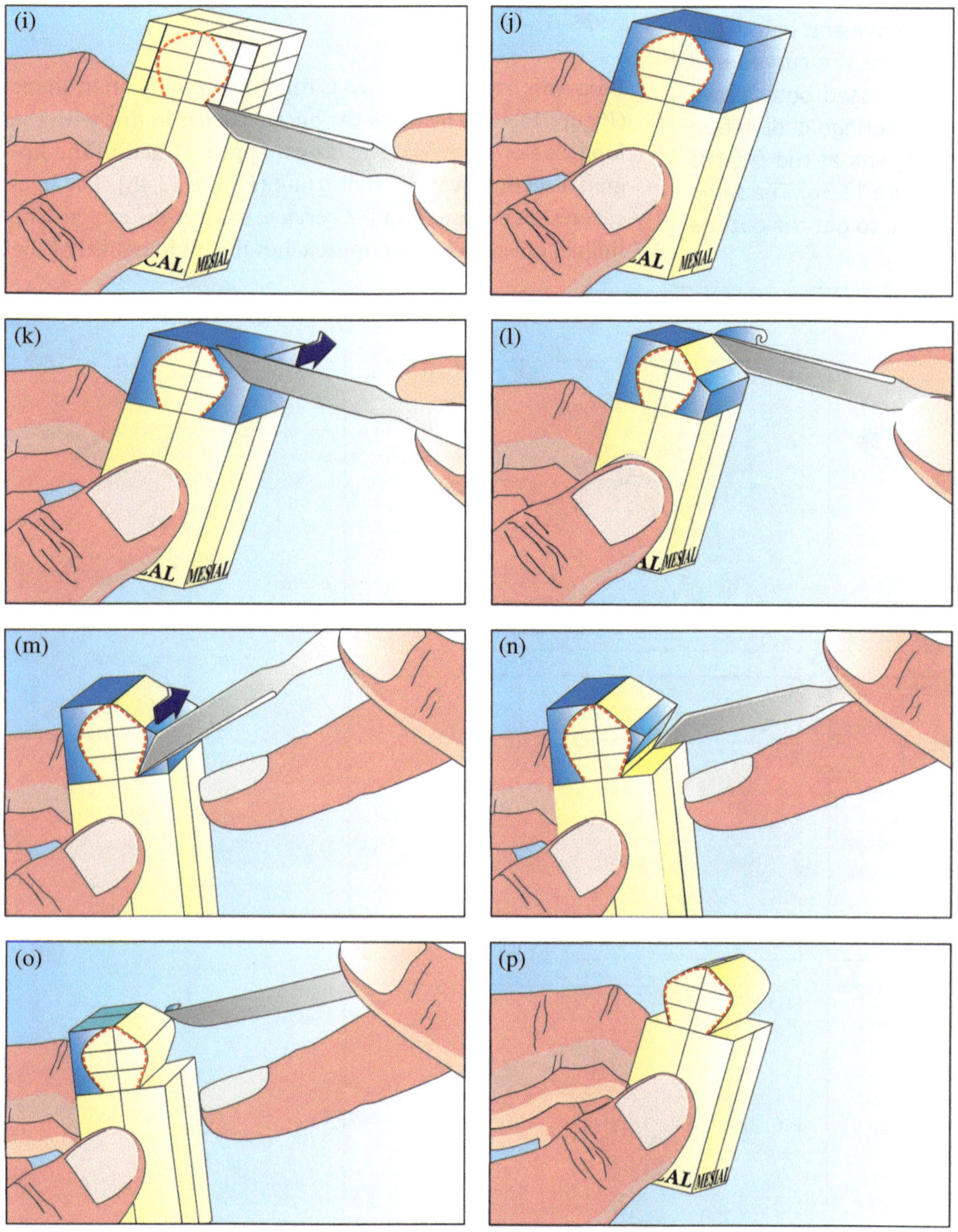

Figure 13.3 (i–p) Carving excess wax from the mesial and distal sides of the crown.

crown length [2]. The buccal outline curves from the cervical line to the cusp tip. The curvature on the lingual cusp ends at the cusp tip (Figure 13.4c). The length of the lingual cusp is about two thirds the length of the buccal cusp from the cervical line to the buccal cusp tip (Figure 13.4d). The lingual cusp tip is in line with the lingual border of the root [4]. The mesial marginal ridge has a sharp inclination lingually in a cervical direction about 45°. The lingual extension of the mesial marginal ridge becomes continuous with developmental depression at the mesiolingual line angle of the crown, which harbours the mesiolingual developmental groove (Figure 13.4e) [3]. The mesial portion of the buccal triangular ridge can be seen from this aspect, the slope of which parallels the mesial marginal

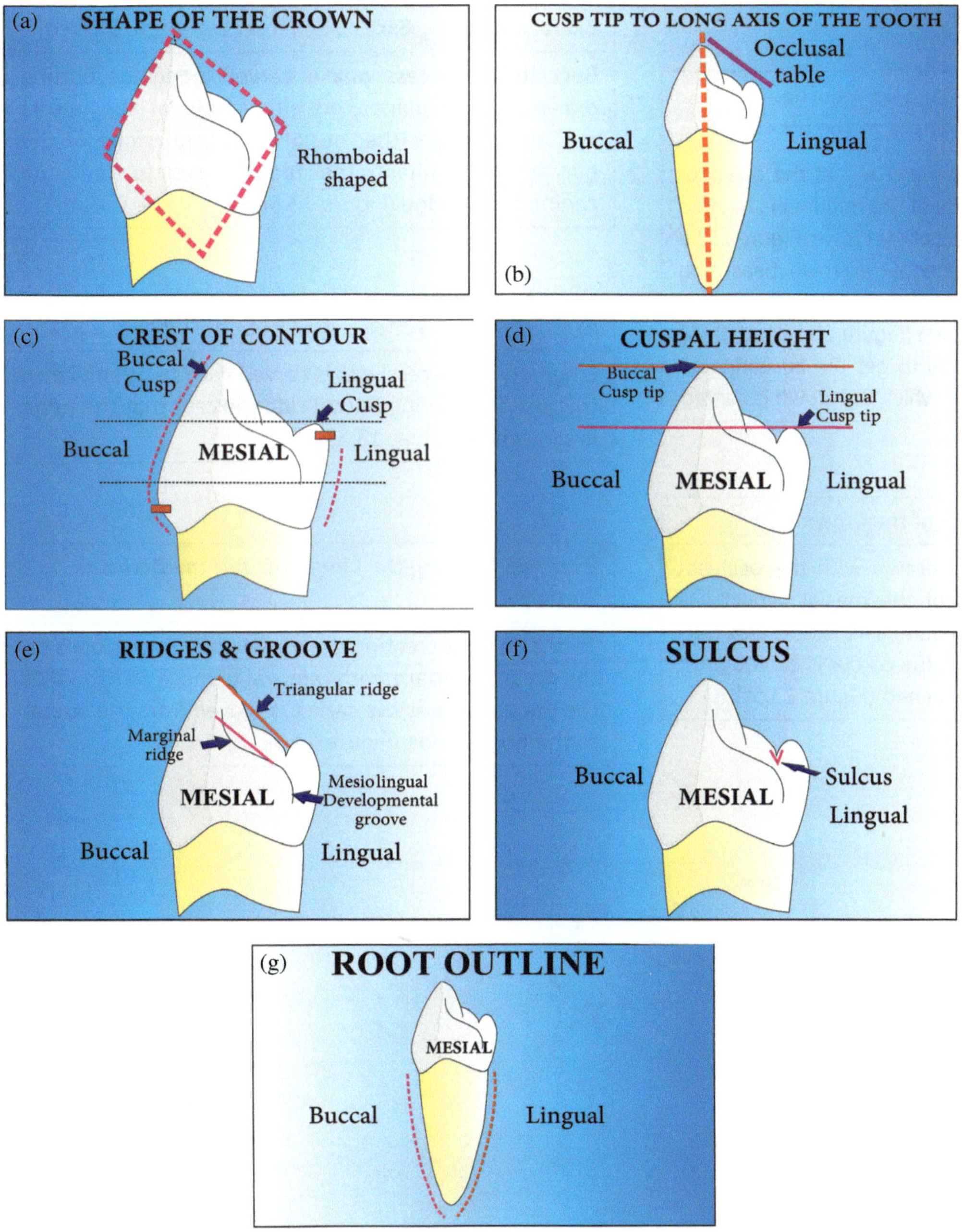

Figure 13.4 (a–g) Description of the permanent mandibular right first premolar from the mesial aspect.

ridge (Figure 13.4e). Convergence of the buccal and lingual cusps creates the sulcus directly above the mesiolingual groove (Figure 13.4f) [4]. Curvature of the cervical line occlusally is 1 mm [5].

The root tapers uniformly from cervix to apex, with the lingual outline being more tapered than the buccal outline (Figure 13.4g) [2].

Carving from the Mesial Aspect

Exercise: Marking the Buccolingual Dimension of the Crown on the Mesial Surface of the Wax Block

The buccolingual diameter of the crown at the cervix of 6.5 mm (3.25 mm on either side of the midline) is marked at the cervix of the mesial aspect of the crown (Figure 13.5a and b). The buccolingual diameter of the crown measuring 7.5 mm (3.75 mm on either side of the midline) is marked at the occlusal edge of the crown (Figure 13.5c and d) [4]. The reference points are joined to get the buccolingual dimension of the crown within which the crown is carved.

Exercise: Marking the Outline of the Crown

The outline of the crown is drawn with the occlusal sloping, and other features of the mesial aspect are drawn on the crown (Figure 13.5e). The excess wax outside the outline, indicated by blue colour is carved until the outline of the crown is reached (Figure 13.5f).

Exercise: Carving Excess Wax from the Bucal Surface

Buccally the excess wax is carved along the outline drawn, in two planes, on either side of the buccal midline to create the mesial and distal slope of the buccal ridge, similar to the steps followed to create the canine labial ridge (Figure 13.5g–i).

Exercise: Carving Excess Wax from the Lingual Surface

Lingually the excess wax is carved with steps similar to that used in carving buccal ridge, except that the ridge is smoothed (Figure 13.5j).

Exercise: Creating the Lingual Tilt of the Occlusal Surface

This is done by creating the mesial and distal slopes on the occlusal surface, with removal of more wax towards the lingual side as the carver is moved from the buccal to the lingual side (Figure 13.5k–n).

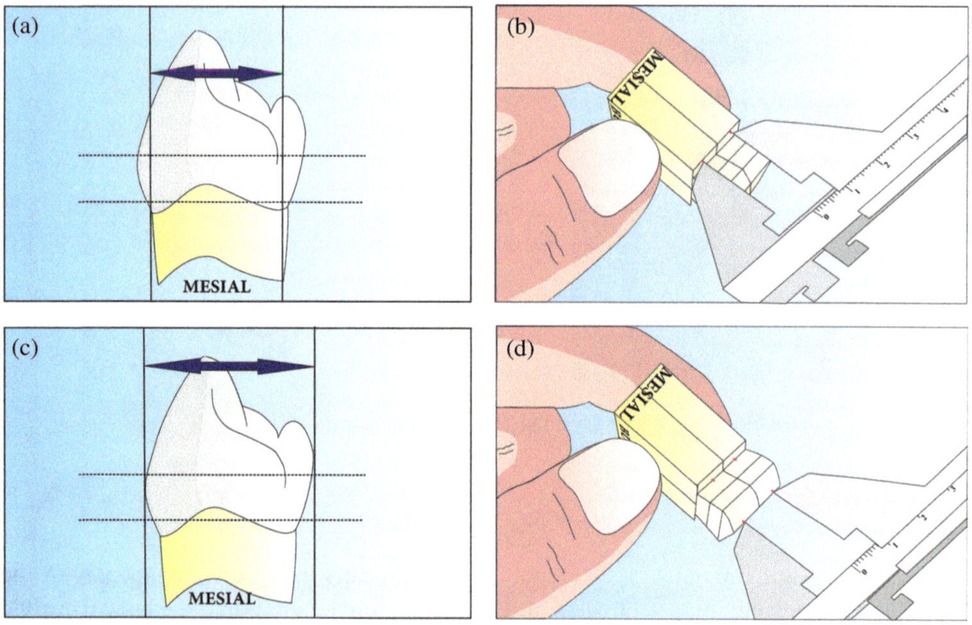

Figure 13.5 (a–d) Measuring and marking the dimension of the crown on the mesial aspect of the wax.

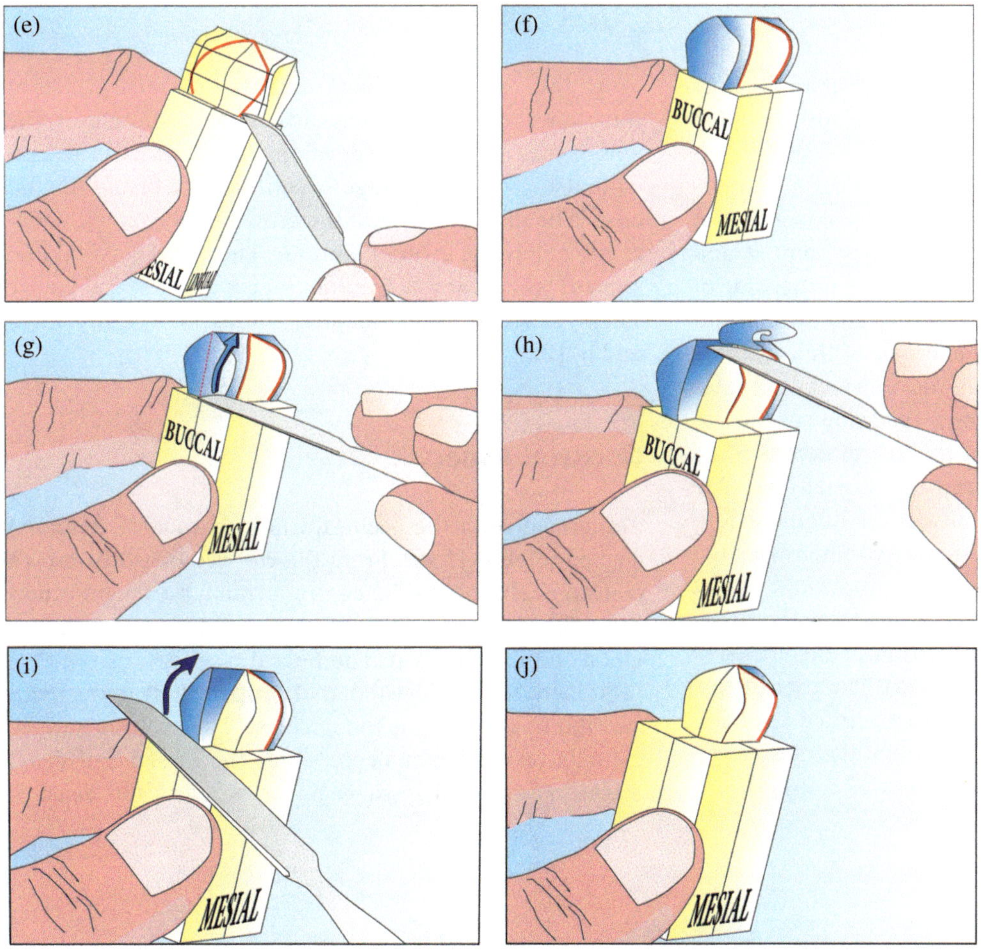

Figure 13.5 (e–j) Drawing the crown outline and carving excess wax from the buccal and lingual surfaces.

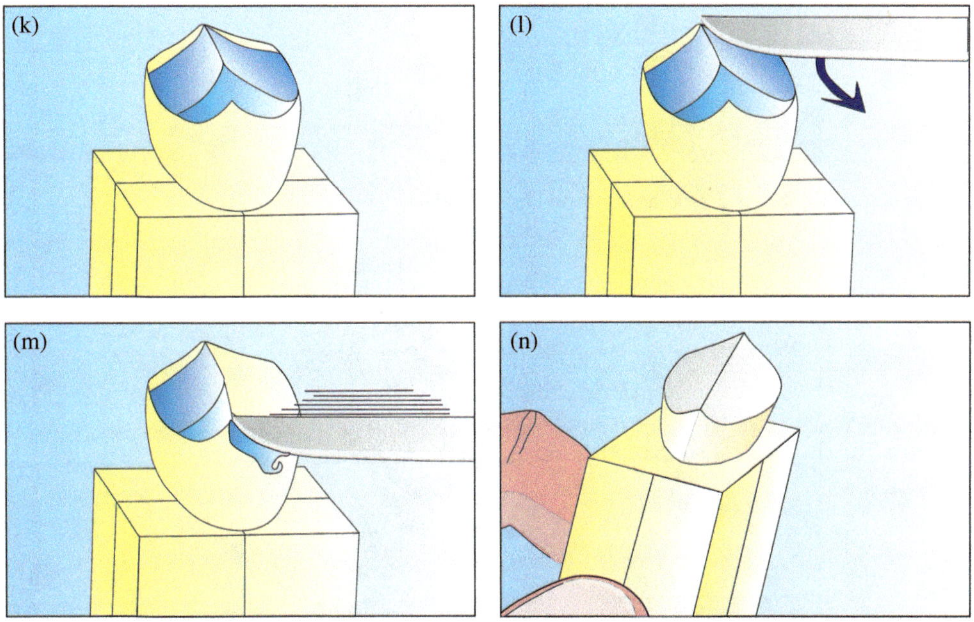

Figure 13.5 (k–n) Creating lingual tilt (45°) of the occlusal surface.

Lingual Aspect

From this aspect, the lingual cusp is shorter than the buccal cusp. Because of this the occlusal table appears tilted lingually towards the cervix and most of the occlusal surface can be seen [5]. The mesial and distal surface tapers lingually. With these features the crown resembles that of the canine [2]. The small lingual cusp is pointed and aligned with the buccal triangular ridge. On either side of the buccal triangular ridge are the mesial and distal triangular fossae. An important characteristic of this aspect is the mesiolingual developmental groove, which separates the mesial marginal ridge and the mesial slope of the lingual cusp [2]. This groove forms the line of demarcation between the mesiobuccal lobe and the lingual lobe. The mesiolingual developmental groove is the lingual extension of the mesial developmental groove that crosses the mesial marginal ridge. The mesial marginal ridge slopes lingually and is placed at a level lower than the distal marginal ridge [3]. The cervical portion of the crown is narrow with concavities (Figure 13.6a). The root of this tooth tapers evenly from the cervix to a pointed apex and also exhibits lingual convergence, so that the mesial and distal sides of the root can be seen (Figure 13.6b) [4].

Distal Aspect

From this aspect, the distal marginal ridge is placed at the higher level and is more nearly at right angles to the axis of the tooth [2]. The developmental groove is absent, so that the marginal ridge is confluent with the lingual cusp. The distal surface of the crown is convex with concavity below the crest of contour. The distal cervical line shows less curvature. The root tapers apically and shows the presence of developmental depression (Figure 13.7a and b) [2].

Occlusal Aspect

The crown from the occlusal aspect is roughly diamond shaped (Figure 13.8a). From the contact areas, the crown converges sharply to the centre forming a triangular outline, with the base at the buccal cusp and apex of the triangle at the lingual cusp. The buccal cusp is larger with a prominent buccal ridge that makes up the bulk of the tooth and the lingual cusp is the smallest. The occlusal surface exhibits two irregular depressions, the mesial and distal fossae. The mesial fossa is linear, whereas the distal is

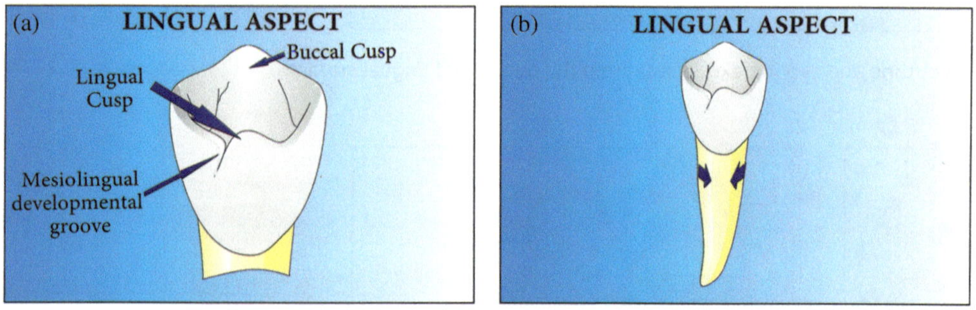

Figure 13.6 (a–b) Description of the mandibular right first premolar from the lingual aspect.

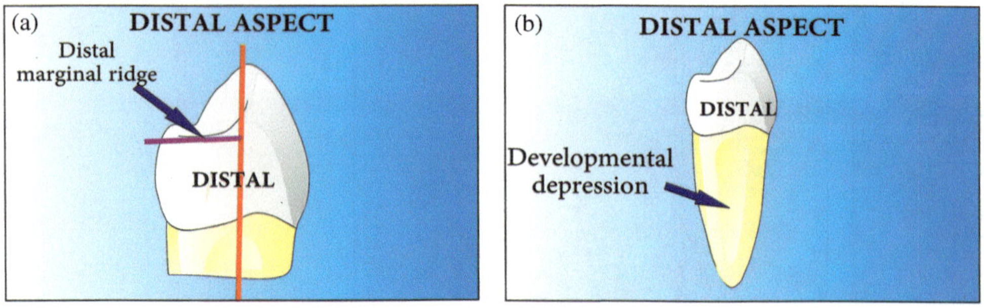

Figure 13.7 (a–b) Description of the mandibular right first premolar from the distal aspect.

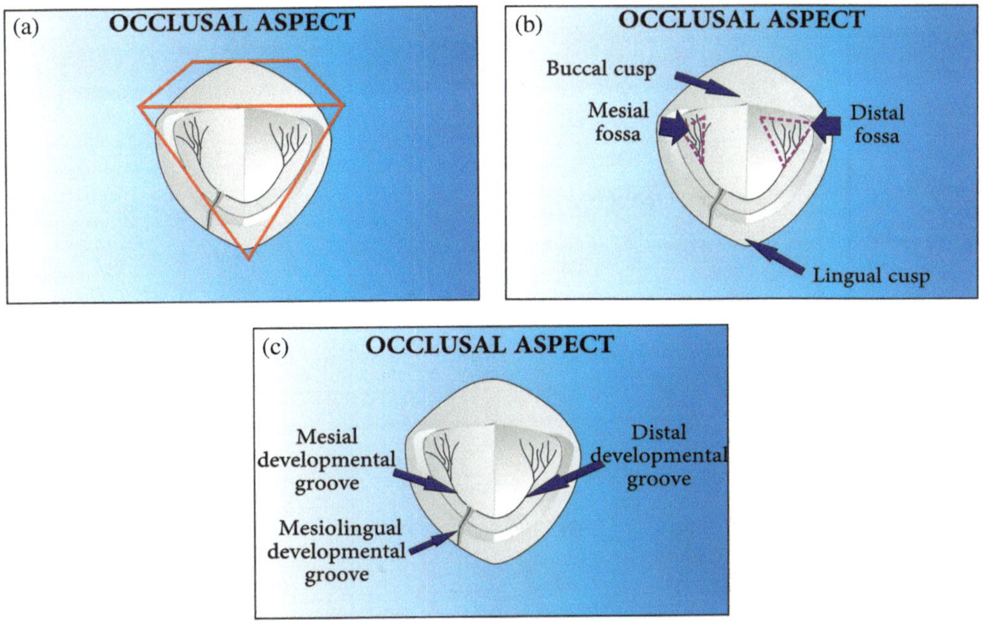

Figure 13.8 (a–c) Description of the mandibular right first premolar from the occlusal aspect.

circular (Figure 13.8b). Marginal ridges are well developed. The most important feature is the mesiolingual developmental depression and groove. The mesial developmental groove extends from the mesial fossa, crosses the marginal ridge mesiolingually, and runs on the mesiolingual surface. Contents of the distal triangular fossa are the distal pit, distal developmental groove, and supplemental groove (Figure 13.8c).

Carving from the Occlusal Aspect

Exercise: Marking the Groove Outline and Carving Fossae

After creating the lingual tilt with the mesial and distal slope, the outline for grooves and fossae is marked (Figure 13.9a and b). The distal fossa is created by moving the carver from one end of the 'V', with the non-cutting end of the carver facing the wax and the tip facing the groove. The carver is moved deep into the wax towards the pit and then the carver is moved out along the other arm of the 'V' (Figure 13.9c and d). The mesial fossa is created in a similar way (Figure 13.9e).

Exercise: Creating the Mesial and Distal Slopes of the Buccal Triangular Ridge and Sulcus

With the non-cutting end facing the wax with an angulation (45°) and the tip of the carver at the distal pit, the carver is moved to the crest of the ridge by pulling it towards the surface (Figure 13.9f and g). Then the carver is pushed deep into the wax while moving towards the mesial pit to complete the triangular ridge (Figure 13.9h and i). The undermined wax along the marginal ridge is carved to create the sulcus with groove (Figure 13.9j and k).

Exercise: Carving the Mesiolingual Developmental Groove

The tip of the carver is moved along the mesial developmental groove crossing the marginal ridge at the mesiolingual line angle, which runs on the surface for short distance (Figure 13.9l–o).

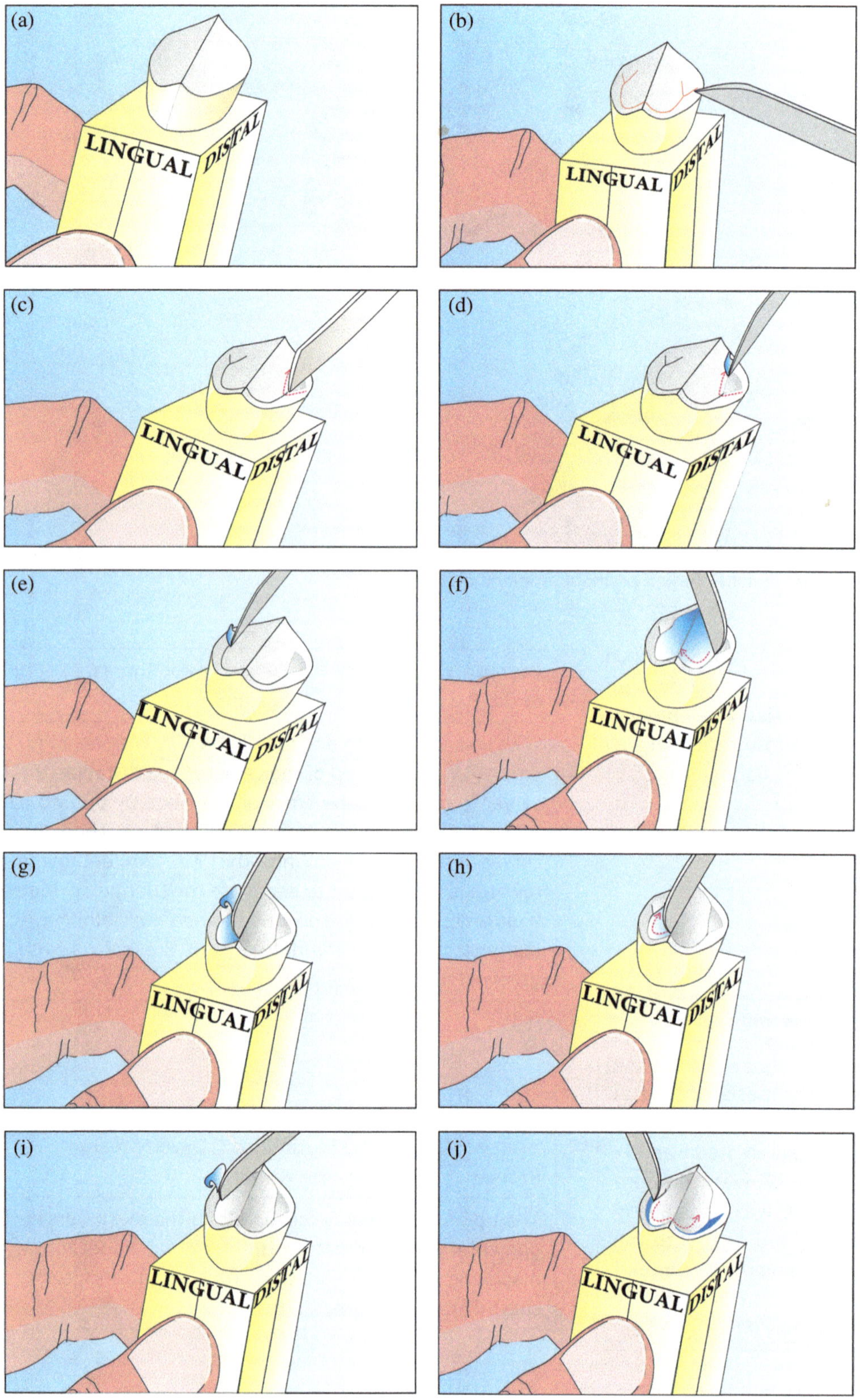

Figure 13.9 (a–o) Step sequence to carve occlusal features of the mandibular right first premolar.

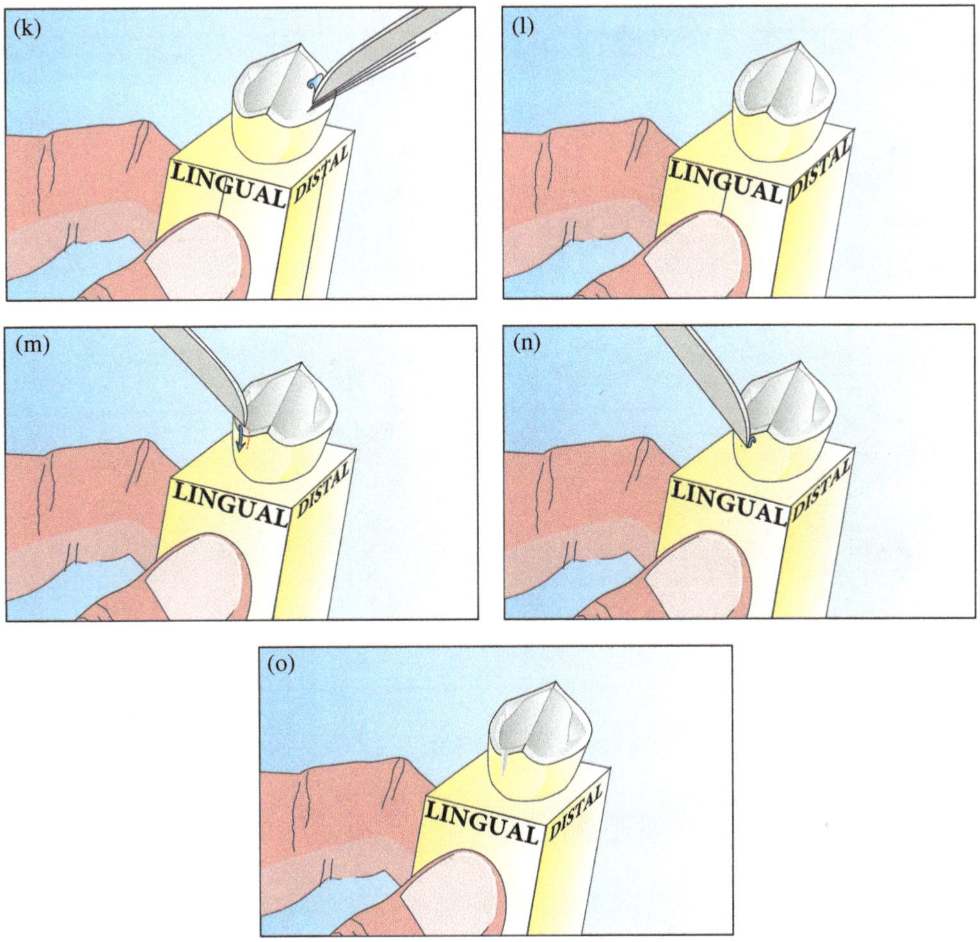

Figure 13.9 (Cont'd) (a–o)

Carving the Root

Exercise: Carving the Root from the Lingual Aspect
The outline of the root with distal curvature at the apex is drawn on either the lingual surface (Figure 13.10a). Then the excess wax indicated in blue colour is carved from both the mesial and distal sides up to the outline of the root (Figure 13.10b–d).

Exercise: Carving the Root from the Mesial Aspect
From the mesial aspect, the buccal and lingual outline of the root is drawn, and excess wax is carved up to the outline (Figure 13.10e–g).

Exercise: Creating the Lingual Convergence of the Root
The lingual convergence is created on the mesial and distal sides (Figure 13.10h and i).

Exercise: Creating Developmental Depression on Root Surfaces
The developmental depression outline is marked on both the mesial and distal surfaces of the root portion (Figure 13.10j). The excess wax within the outline, indicated in blue colour, is carved using the excavating end of the carver. The carver is moved in the cervico-apical direction, shallow near the outer border and deeper near the centre of the outline (Figure 13.10k–m). Finally the cervical line is marked on both the mesial and distal sides.

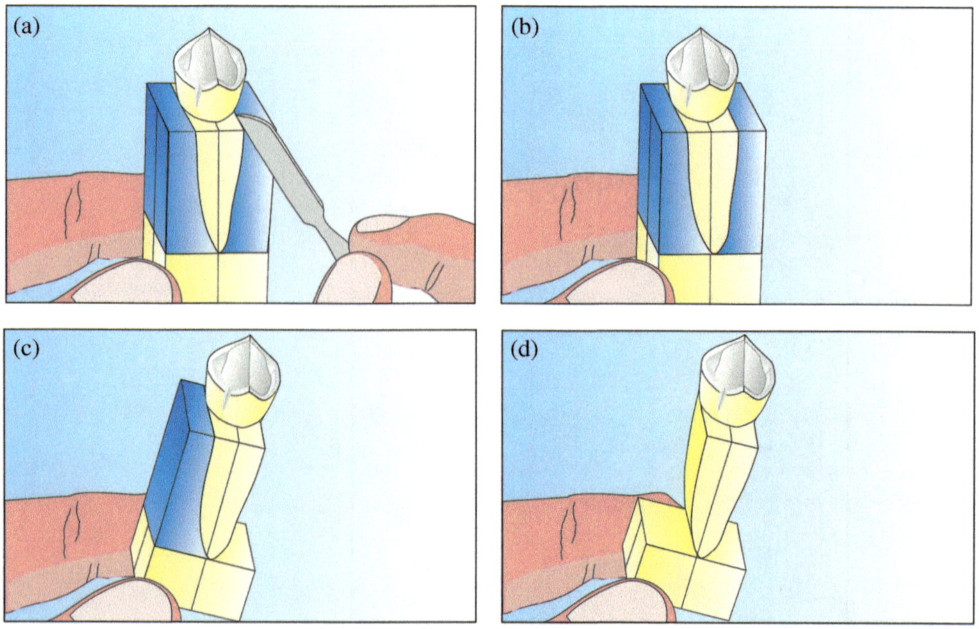

Figure 13.10 (a–d) Carving the root from the lingual aspect.

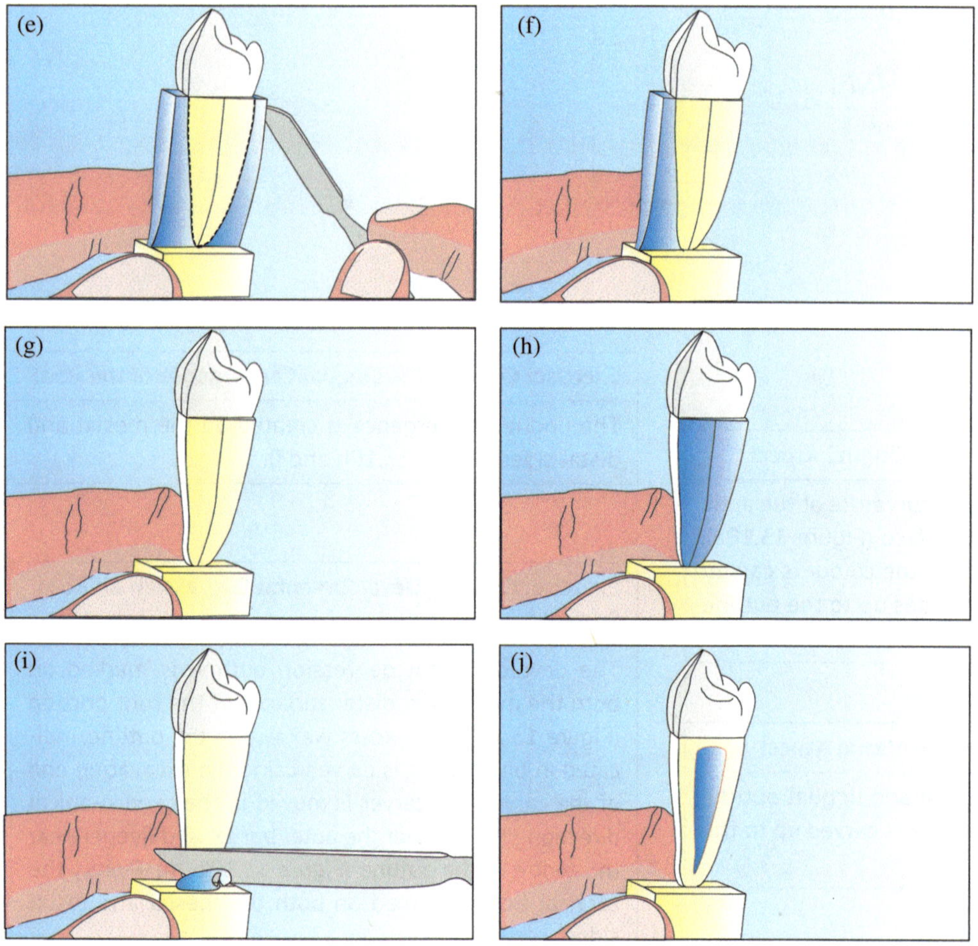

Figure 13.10 (e-j) Carving the root from the mesial aspect.

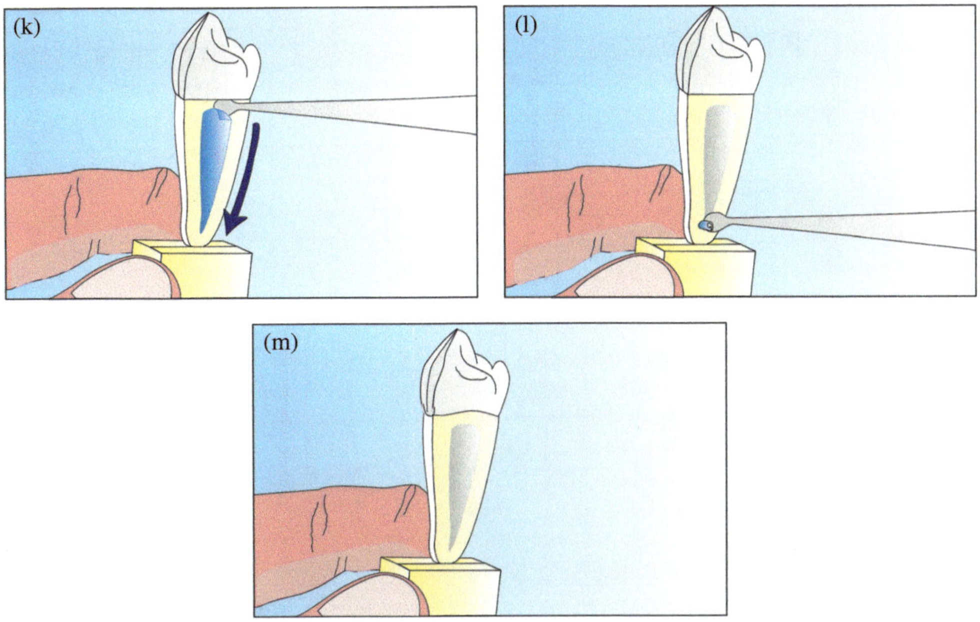

Figure 13.10 (Cont'd) (k–m) Carving the root from the mesial aspect.

References

1 James, L.F., Gerald, E.D., and Thomas, M. (2001). *Concise Dental Anatomy and Morphology*, 44e. Iowa City, IA: University of Iowa College of Dentistry.

2 Rickne, C.S. and Weiss, G. (2012). *Woelfel's Dental Anatomy*, 8e. Philadelphia: Lippincott Williams & Wilkins.

3 Hillson, S. (2012). *Dental Anthropology*, Cambridge University Press, Kindle Edition.

4 Stanley, J.N. and Major, M.A.C. (2010). *Wheeler's Dental Anatomy and Occlusion*, 9e. St. Louis, MO: Saunders Elsevier.

5 Nagaş, I.C., Eğilmez, F., and Kivanç, B.H. (2018). The permanent maxillary and mandibular premolar teeth. In: *Dental Anatomy* (ed. B.H. Kivanç). http://dx.doi.org/10.5772/intechopen.79464 (accessed 23 March 2020).

14

Permanent Mandibular Second Premolar

LEARNING OBJECTIVE

At the end of the chapter, the student should have knowledge of the permanent mandibular second premolar and develop the psychomotor skills for carving and waxing the same.

Permanent Mandibular Right Second Premolar – Three-Cusp Type

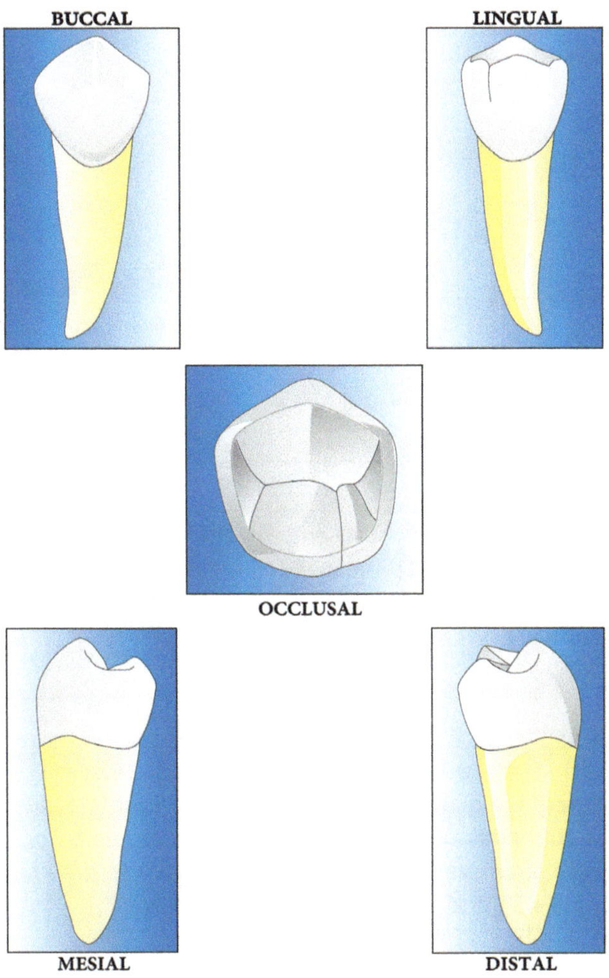

Buccal Aspect

The permanent mandibular second premolar is the fifth tooth from the midline (Figure 14.1). The shape of the cusp is roughly pentagonal (Figure 14.2a). The crown appears shorter and wider. From this aspect, the buccal cusp is less well developed compared to that of the first mandibular premolar, with less angulated mesial and distal cuspal ridges [1, 2]. Slopes of the cuspal ridges meet at an angle of about 130° [2]. The tooth has wider mesial and distal contact areas. The mesial crest of contour is at the junction between the middle and occlusal third. The distal crest of contour is more cervical than the mesial crest (Figure 14.2b and c) [2]. The mesial cuspal ridge is shorter than the distal cuspal ridge (Figure 14.2d [1, 2].

The root is broader mesiodistally and the length almost twice the length of the crown. The root appears gradually tapered with blunted root apex (Figure 14.2e) [2].

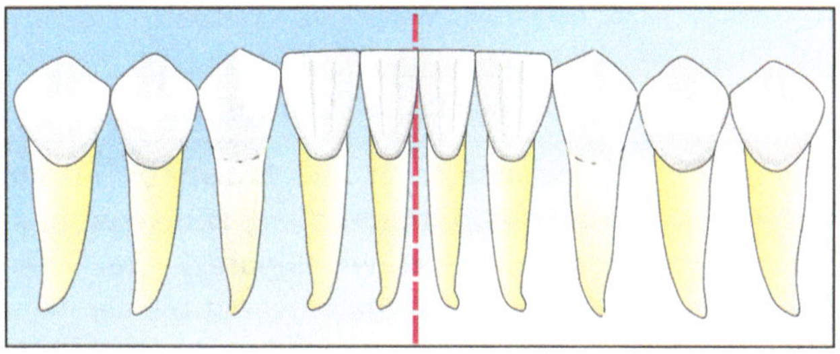

Figure 14.1 Position of the mandibular second premolar in relation to the midsagittal plane.

An Illustrated Atlas of Tooth Carving and Wax-Up Techniques, First Edition. Anil Bangalore Shivappa.

Companion website: www.wiley.com/go/bangalore/toothcarving

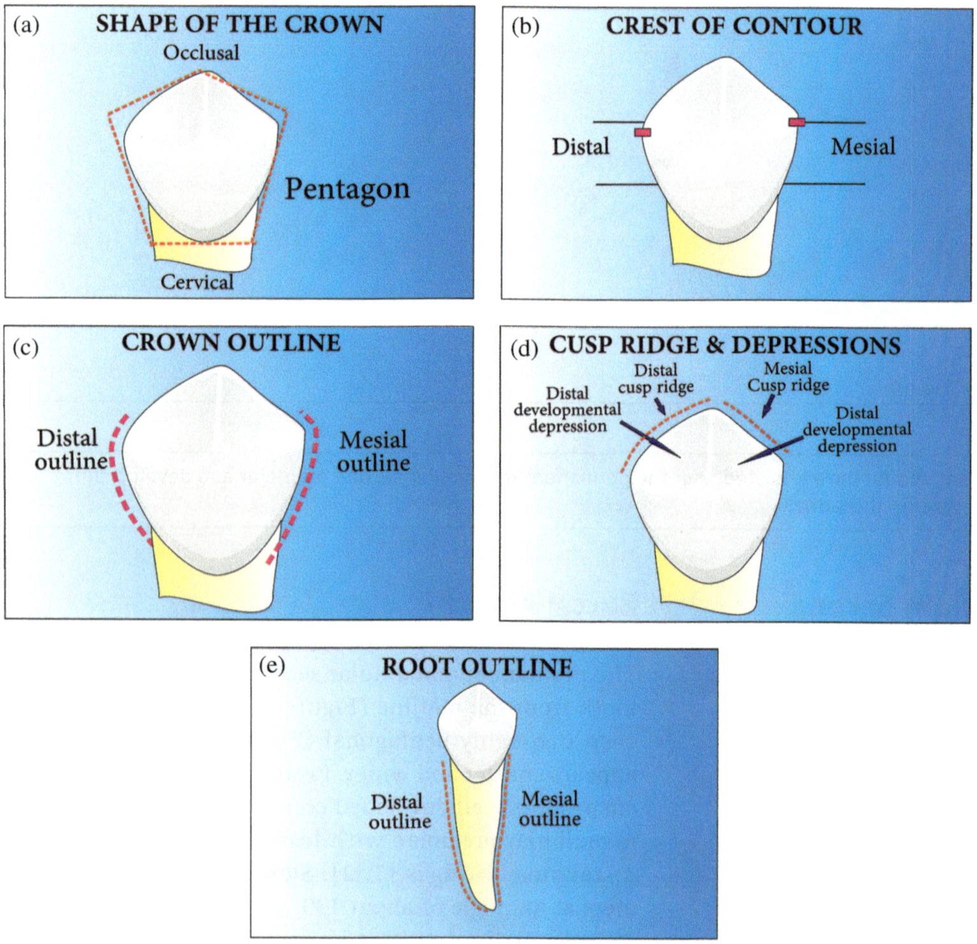

Figure 14.2 (a–e) Descriptive features of the permanent mandibular right second premolar from the buccal aspect.

Carving from the Buccal Aspect

Exercise: Marking Length of the Crown and the Root

After pre-carve preparation of the wax, the length of the crown of 8.0 mm, is marked from the occlusal edge (Figure 14.3a and b). The length of the root of 14.5 mm is marked from the cervical end of the crown length (Figure 14.3c and d) [1]. The marking is extended to other surfaces as well.

Exercise: Marking the Mesiodistal Dimensions

The mesiodistal diameter of the crown of 7.0 mm (3.5 mm on either side of the midline) is marked near the occlusal edge of the crown (Figure 14.3e). Then the mesiodistal diameter of the crown at the cervix of 5.0 mm (2.5 mm on either side of the midline) is marked at the cervix of the crown (Figure 14.3f) [1]. The reference markings are then joined on the mesial and distal sides of the crown to get the dimension of the crown, where the outline of the crown is drawn (Figure 14.3g and h).

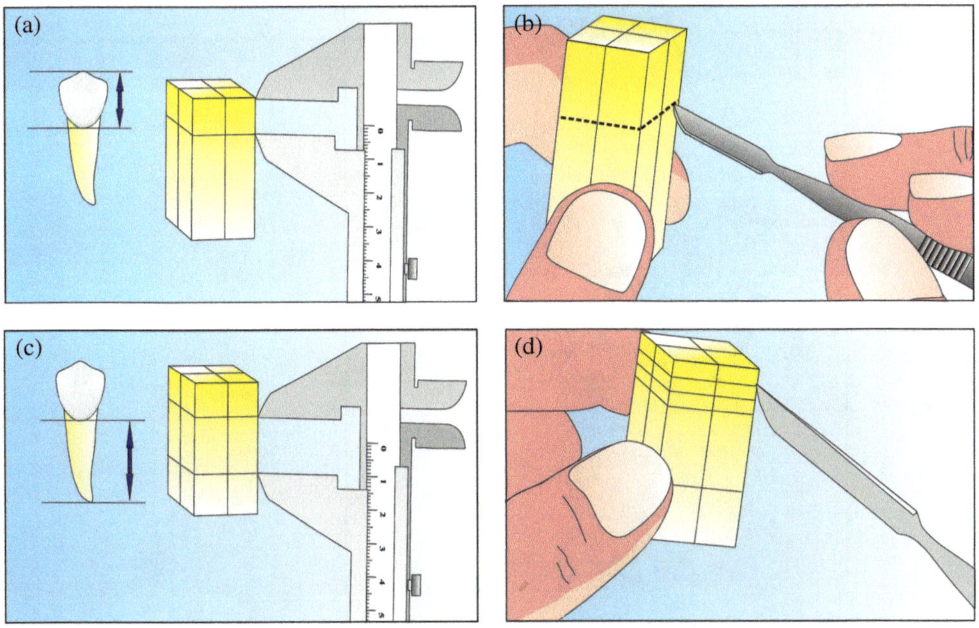

Figure 14.3 (a–d) Marking the crown and root length of the mandibular right second premolar on the wax block.

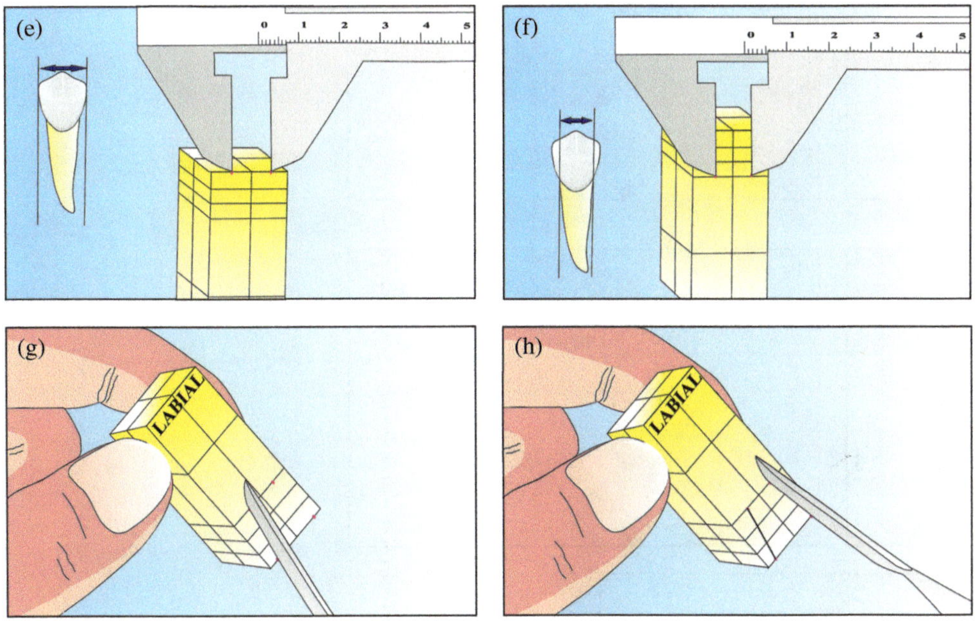

Figure 14.3 (e–h) Marking the mesiodistal dimension of the crown on the wax block.

Exercise: Marking the Outline of the Crown and Carving Excess Wax

Within the dimension of the crown, the outline is drawn, with the features of the crown from the buccal aspect mentioned (Figure 14.4a). The excess wax indicated in blue colour is carved up to the outline (Figure 14.4b). The wax at the mesial cuspal ridges and the mesial side of the crown is carved using the curved part of the cutting edge of the carver moved in a labiolingual direction from the surface until the outline is reached (Figure 14.4c–g). The excess wax is carved out from the distal cuspal ridge and distal side in the steps mentioned previously (Figure 14.4h and i).

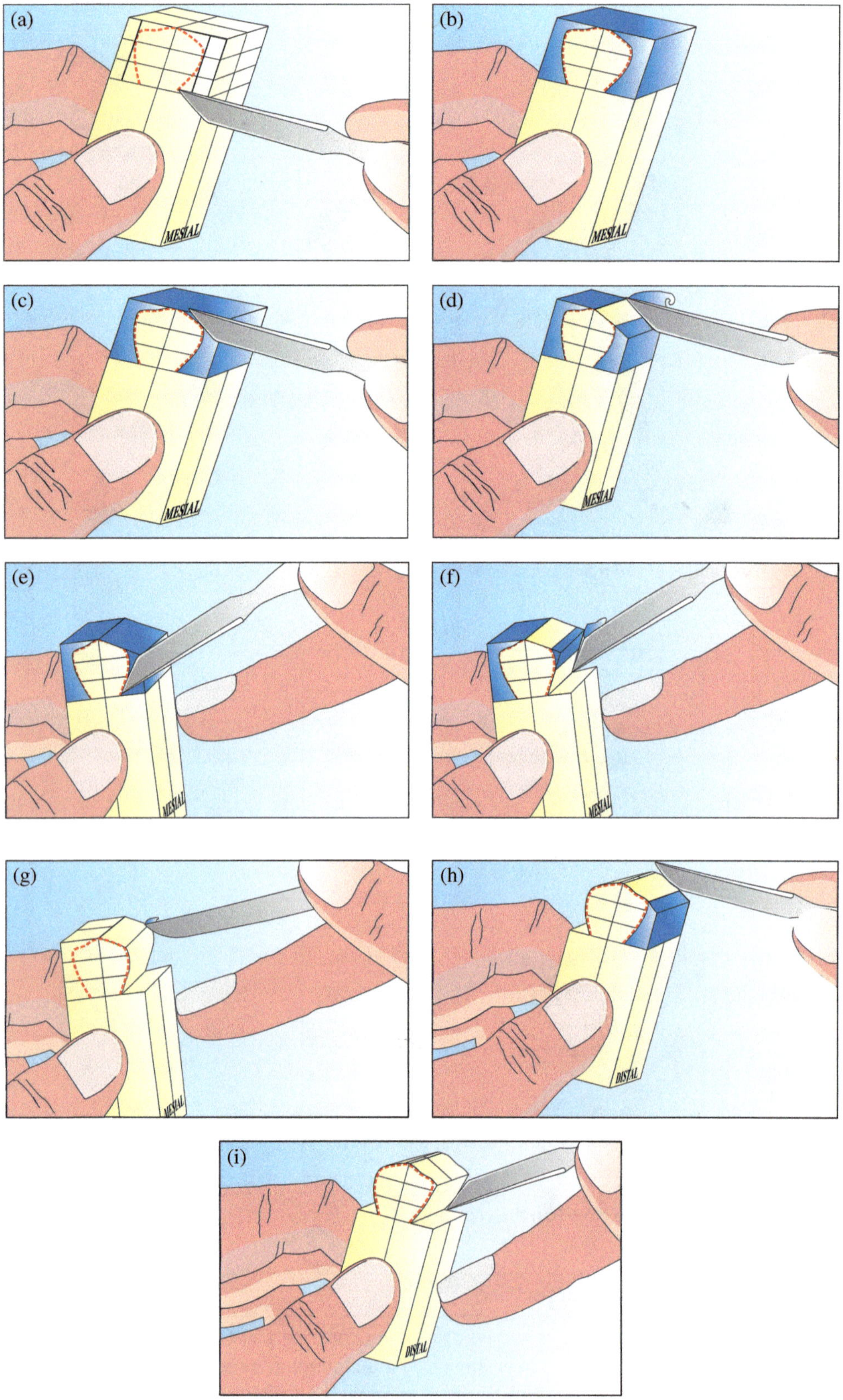

Figure 14.4 (a–i) Marking the crown outline on the buccal aspect of wax and carving the excess wax.

Mesial Aspect

From this aspect, the tooth is rhomboidal in shape and wider buccolingually (Figure 14.5a) [2]. The crown tilts lingually but less compared to the tilt of the mandibular first premolar (Figure 14.5b). The lingual inclination of the occlusal surface is 30° when compared to that of the first premolar which is 45° [4]. The tip of the buccal cusp is slightly buccally placed to the long axis of the tooth, at the junction of the buccal and middle third [1, 2]. The buccal crest of contour is at the junction of the cervical and middle thirds. The lingual crest of contour is slightly above the middle of the middle third. The buccal surface is flat above the crest of contour (Figure 14.5c) [2]. The lingual cusps are well developed and tips of the cusps are placed more occlusally compared to the first premolar. The mesial marginal ridge is placed at a higher level than that of the distal marginal ridge, so less of the

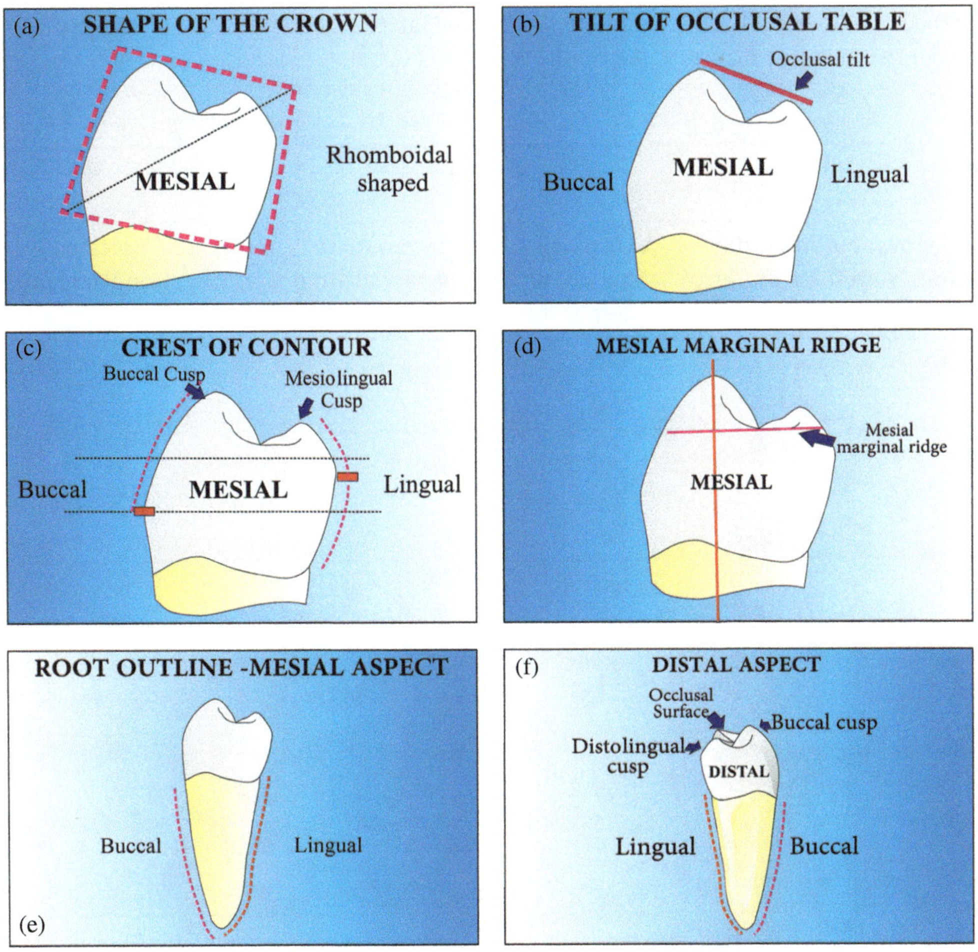

Figure 14.5 (a–f) Description of the permanent mandibular right second premolar crown from the mesial and distal aspect.

occlusal surface is seen from this aspect. The mesial marginal ridge is perpendicular to the long axis of the tooth and is straight (Figure 14.5d) [2–4].

The root tapers slightly in the cervical and middle third abruptly in the apical third and ends in a blunt apex. The root surface appears smooth and convex. Developmental depressions are not seen on the root surface (Figure 14.5e) [2, 3].

Distal Aspect

The tooth from this aspect is similar to that of the mesial aspect. The distal marginal ridge is placed more cervically, so that most of the occlusal surface can be seen. The distal marginal ridge is more concave. A part of the mesiolingual cusps can be seen. The developmental depressions can be seen on the distal surface of the root (Figure 14.5f) [2, 3].

Carving from the Mesial Aspect

Exercise: Marking the Buccolingual Dimension of the Crown on the Mesial Surface of the Wax Block

The buccolingual diameter of the crown at the cervix of 7.0 mm (3.5 mm on either side of the midline) is marked at the cervix (Figure 14.6a and b). Then, labiolingual diameter of the crown of 8.0 mm (4.0 mm on either side of the midline) is marked at the occlusal edge of the crown (Figure 14.6c and d) [1].

Exercise: Marking the Outline of the Crown

After marking the dimension, the crown outline is drawn on the mesial side of the wax block, with the features of the mesial aspect mentioned earlier (Figure 14.6e). The wax outside the crown outline is excess wax indicated in blue colour and is carved from the buccal and lingual sides to the outline of the crown (Figure 14.6f)

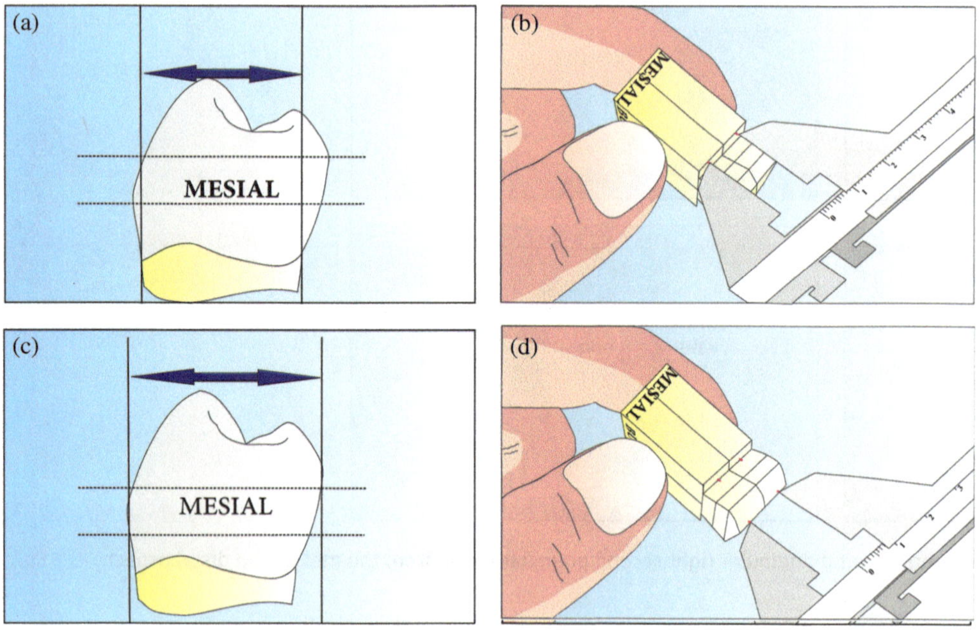

Figure 14.6 (a–d) Measuring and marking the dimension of the crown on the mesial aspect.

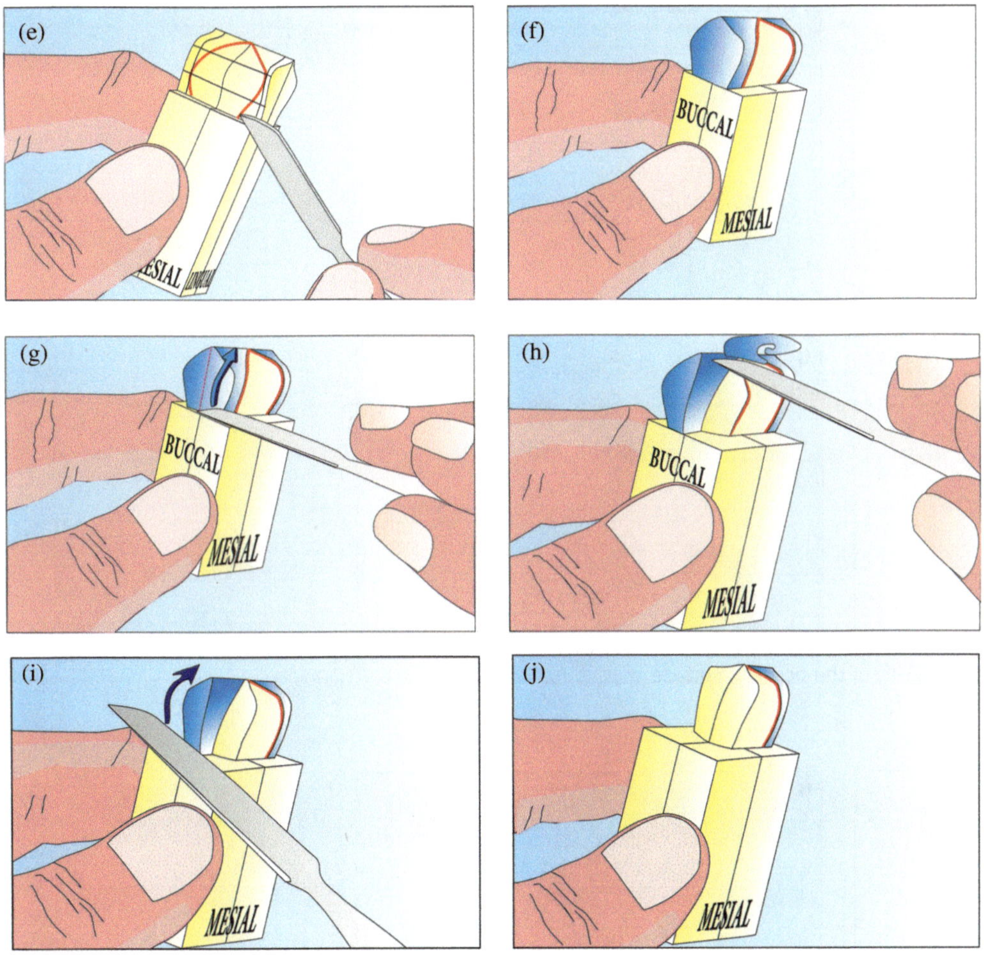

Figure 14.6 (e–j) Drawing the crown outline (mesial aspect) and carving excess wax from the buccal surface.

Exercise: Carving on the Buccal Surface
Excess wax on the buccal surface is carved in two planes, on either side of the buccal midline to create the mesial and distal slope of the buccal ridge (Figure 14.6g–j).

Exercise: Creating the Lingual Sloping of the Occlusal Surface
The lingual sloping of the occlusal table is created by moving the carver on the mesial and distal slopes of the occlusal surface in such a way that more of the wax is carved on the lingual side while moving the carver in labiolingual direction on each slope (Figure 14.6k–p).

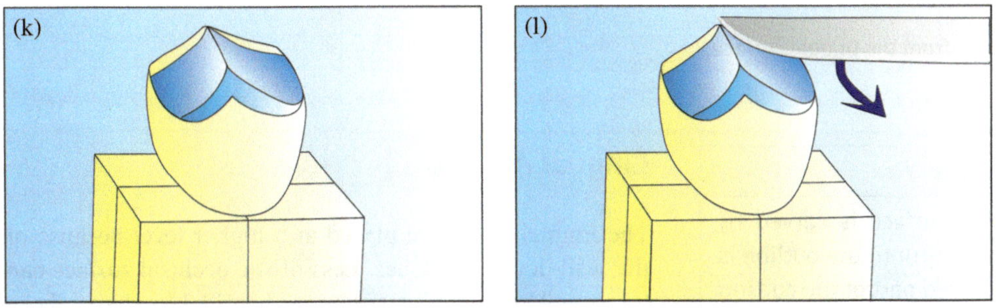

Figure 14.6 (k and l) Creating lingual tilt (30°) of the occlusal surface.

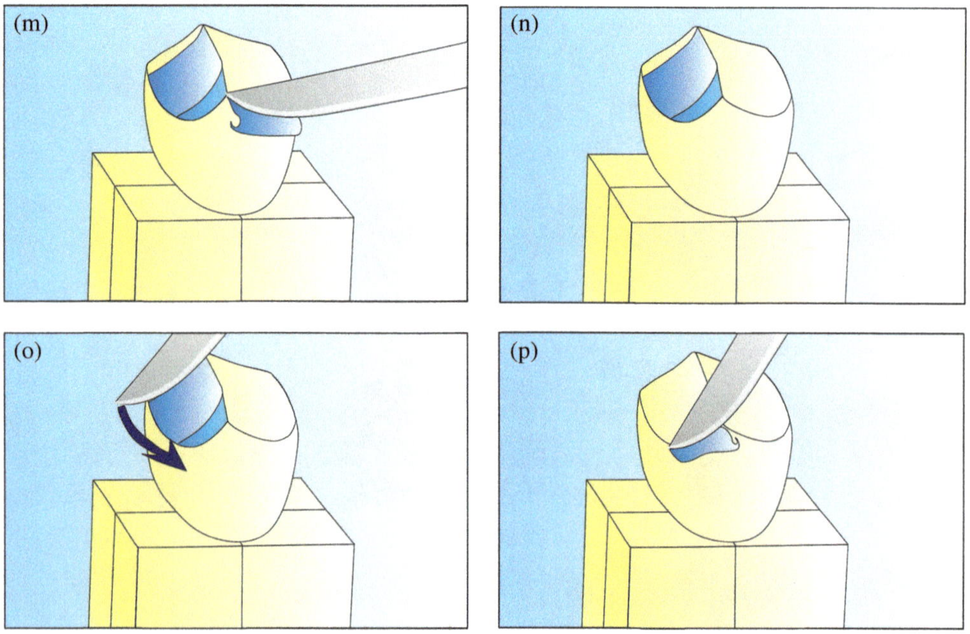

Figure 14.6 (m–p) Creating lingual tilt (30°) of the occlusal surface.

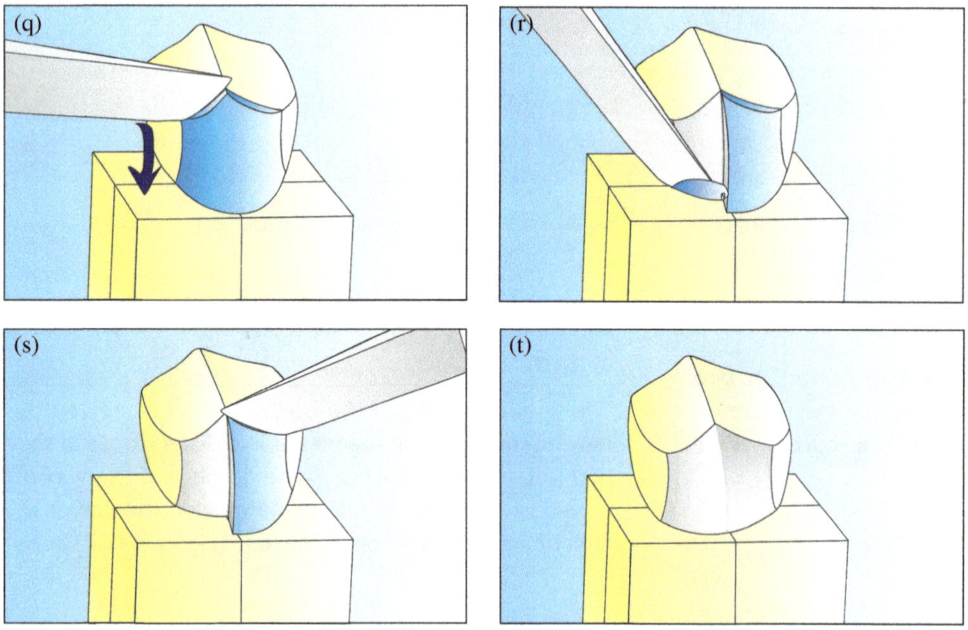

Figure 14.6 (q–t) Carving excess wax from the lingual surface.

Exercise: Carving the Lingual Excess Wax

Excess wax on the lingual side surface is carved by moving the carver occluso-cervically until the outline is reached (Figure 14.6q–t). The curved part of the cutting edge of the carver is used, to carve wax in this step.

Lingual Aspect

The lingual cusps are placed at a higher level because of the well-developed lobes. Less of the occlusal surface can be seen. The lingual surface is spheroidal in shape above the cervical constriction [1–3].

In case of the three-cusp type, the crown is wider mesiodistally, compared to that of the two-cusp type where the crown becomes narrower mesiodistally. In the three-cusp type, two cusps are seen from this aspect. They are mesiolingual and distolingual cusp. The lingual groove is seen in between the cusps that runs for a shorter distance. The mesiolingual cusp is wider and placed at a higher level than the distolingual cusp (Figure 14.7a). In the two-cusp type, only one lingual cusp is seen without any presence of developmental grooves (Figure 14.7b) [2, 3].

The root from this aspect appears wider compared to another single rooted tooth. The width is less than that of the buccal root width. Less of the mesial and distal surfaces can be seen (Figure 14.7c) [2, 3, 5].

Occlusal Aspect

The outline of the two-cusp type second premolar is round or ovoid, broader buccally than lingually. The three-cusp type premolar appears as a square from the occlusal view because the lingual part of the crown is broader owing to the presence of two cusps on the lingual half [1–5].

The three-cusp type is the most common type seen. It has one buccal and two lingual cups. Cusps in the descending order are the buccal cusp, mesiolingual cusp, and distolingual cusp. The buccal cusp is larger than the other two. Lingually the mesiolingual cusp is larger and wider than the distolingual. Triangular ridges of the cusps are well formed and separated by deep developmental grooves. The developmental grooves unite to form a 'Y' pattern on the occlusal surface. The three-cusp type has three fossae and pits. The three fossae are the mesial fossa, the distal fossa and the central fossa. The corresponding pits are harboured within these fossae. Grooves on the occlusal surface are the mesial groove, distal groove, and lingual groove. The mesial groove runs mesiobuccally from the central pit to the mesial fossa and ends in the mesial pit. The distal groove runs in a distobuccal direction from the central pit, whereas the lingual groove runs lingually towards the lingual surface, crosses the lingual cuspal ridges, and ends at a distance on the lingual surface. Supplemental grooves are more often seen radiating from the main groove (Figure 14.8a and b) [1–5].

The two-cusp type is seen less frequently. In this type, the lingual cusp is smaller than the buccal cusp. The buccal triangular ridge joins the lingual triangular ridge to form the transverse ridge. Based on the alignment of the central groove, there are two patterns in the two-cusp type.

The central groove runs from the distal fossa to mesial fossa in a straight manner that combines with the grooves in the mesial and distal fossa to form the 'H' type (Figure 14.8c). In a similar way, the central groove curves towards the lingual side to form the 'U' type (Figure 14.8d) [2, 3, 5].

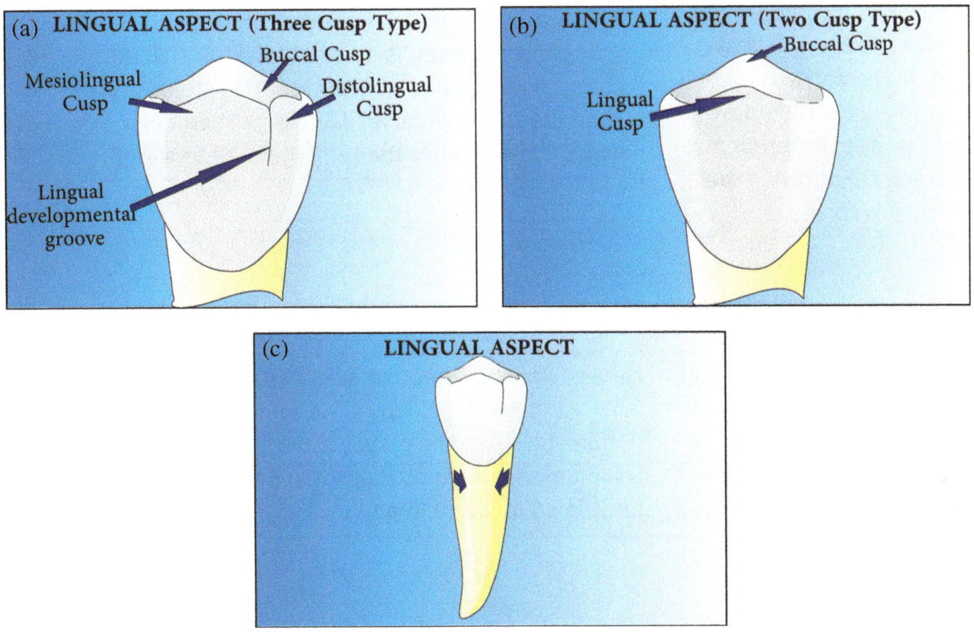

Figure 14.7 (a–c): Description of the permanent mandibular right second premolar from the lingual aspect.

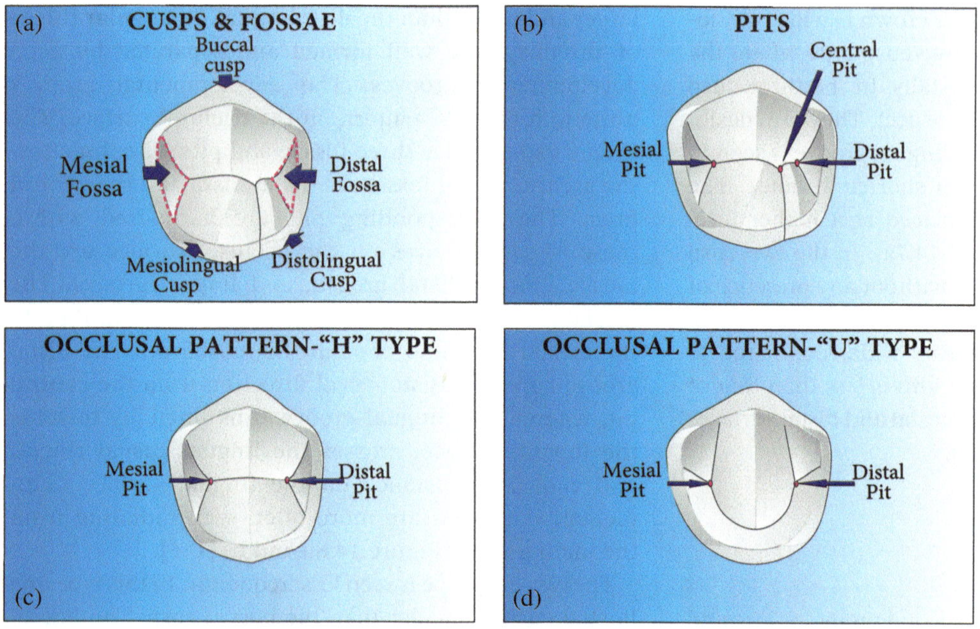

Figure 14.8 (a–d) Description of the permanent mandibular right second premolar from the occlusal aspect.

Carving from the Occlusal Aspect

Exercise: Carving the Mesial and Distal Triangular Fossae

The 'Y' pattern outline of the grooves for the three-cusp type is drawn on the occlusal surface of the wax (Figure 14.9a). The distal fossa is carved by moving the carver from the terminal end of the lingual groove of the distal fossa and moved in a 'V' pattern. With the non-cutting end of the carver facing the wax and the tip at the groove, the carver is pushed deep into the wax at an angle until the pit (mid-part of the 'V') is reached. Then from the pit, the carver is pulled along the buccal groove of the distal fossa (the other end of the 'V') to its terminal to complete the fossa (Figure 14.9b and c). Following the aforementioned steps, the mesial fossa is carved.

Exercise: Carving the Buccal Cusp

Starting from the distal pit, with the back (non-cutting end) of the carver facing occlusal wax, the buccal cusp is carved by directing the carver from the distal pit along the distobuccal groove and part of the mesiobuccal groove until the buccal triangular ridge is reached. During this step, the carver is pulled out from the pit to the surface (Figure 14.9d and e).

Then the carver is moved towards the mesial pit along the mesiobuccal groove. In this step, the pressure is applied on the carver so it is pushed deep into the wax until it reaches the pit (Figure 14.9f and g).

Exercise: Carving the Distolingual Cusp

The carving is started from the distal pit (Figure 14.9h). With the back of the carver at the lingual groove of distal fossa and the tip of the carver facing the distal pit, the carver is run along the distobuccal groove, pulled up on to the surface to form the ridge. From the ridge, the carver is pushed into the wax with application of pressure, to progress deep as it ends at the central pit (Figure 14.9i–k). The carver is then moved from the central pit along the lingual groove to complete the triangular ridge (Figure 14.9l and m).

Exercise: Carving the Mesiolingual Cusp

With the tip of the carver at the central pit and the back of the carver at the lingual groove, the carver is moved along the mesiobuccal groove pulling towards the surface to create the distal slope and ridge (Figure 14.9n). With the application of pressure, the carver is moved into the wax to the mesial pit to complete the mesial slope (Figure 14.9o and p).

Carving the Root

Exercise: Carving the Root from the Lingual Aspect

With the root outline, described earlier, the mesiodistal outline of the root is drawn with the features described and the excess wax is then carved on the mesial and distal side (Figure 14.10a–d).

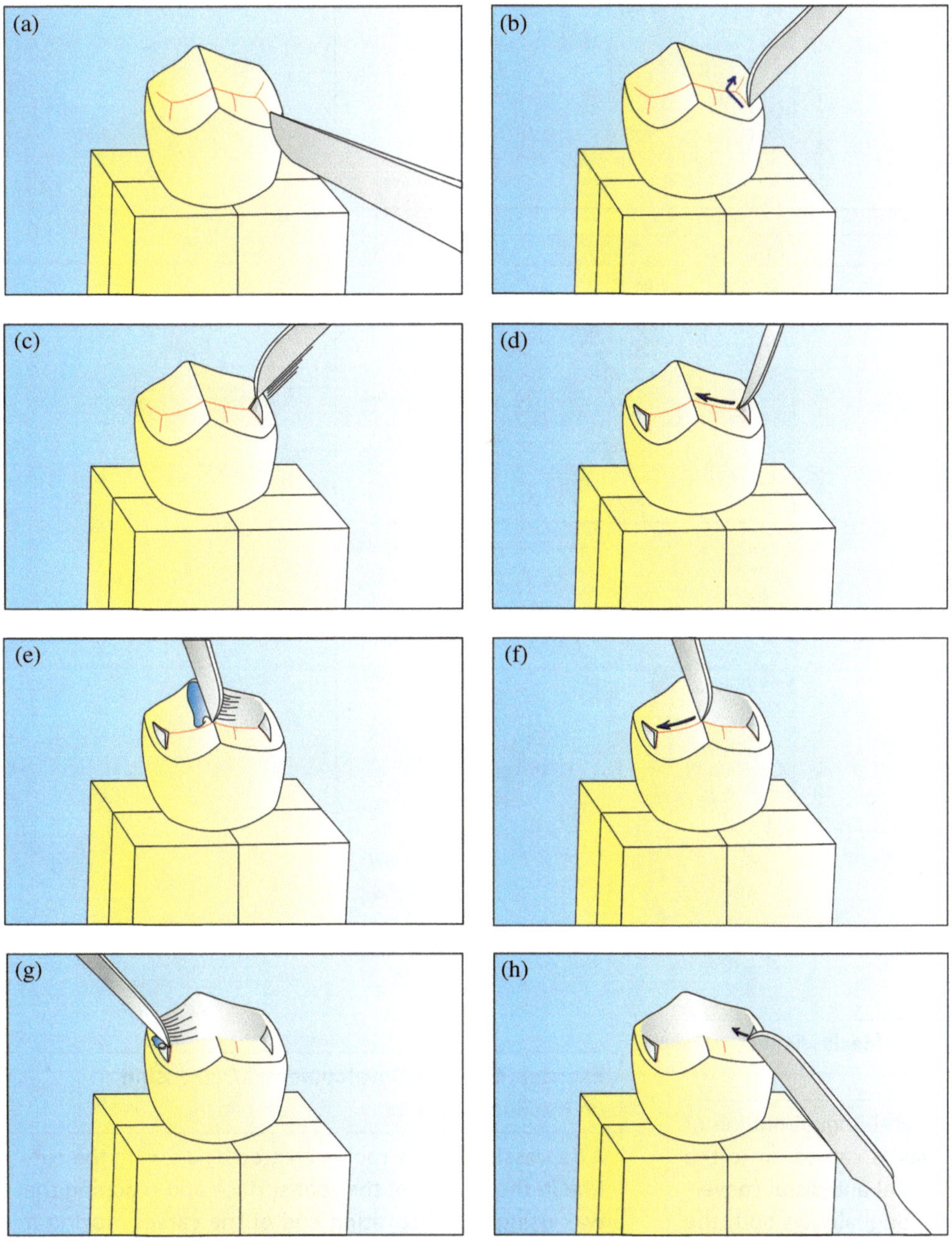

Figure 14.9 (a–p) Step sequence to carve occlusal features of the permanent mandibular right second premolar.

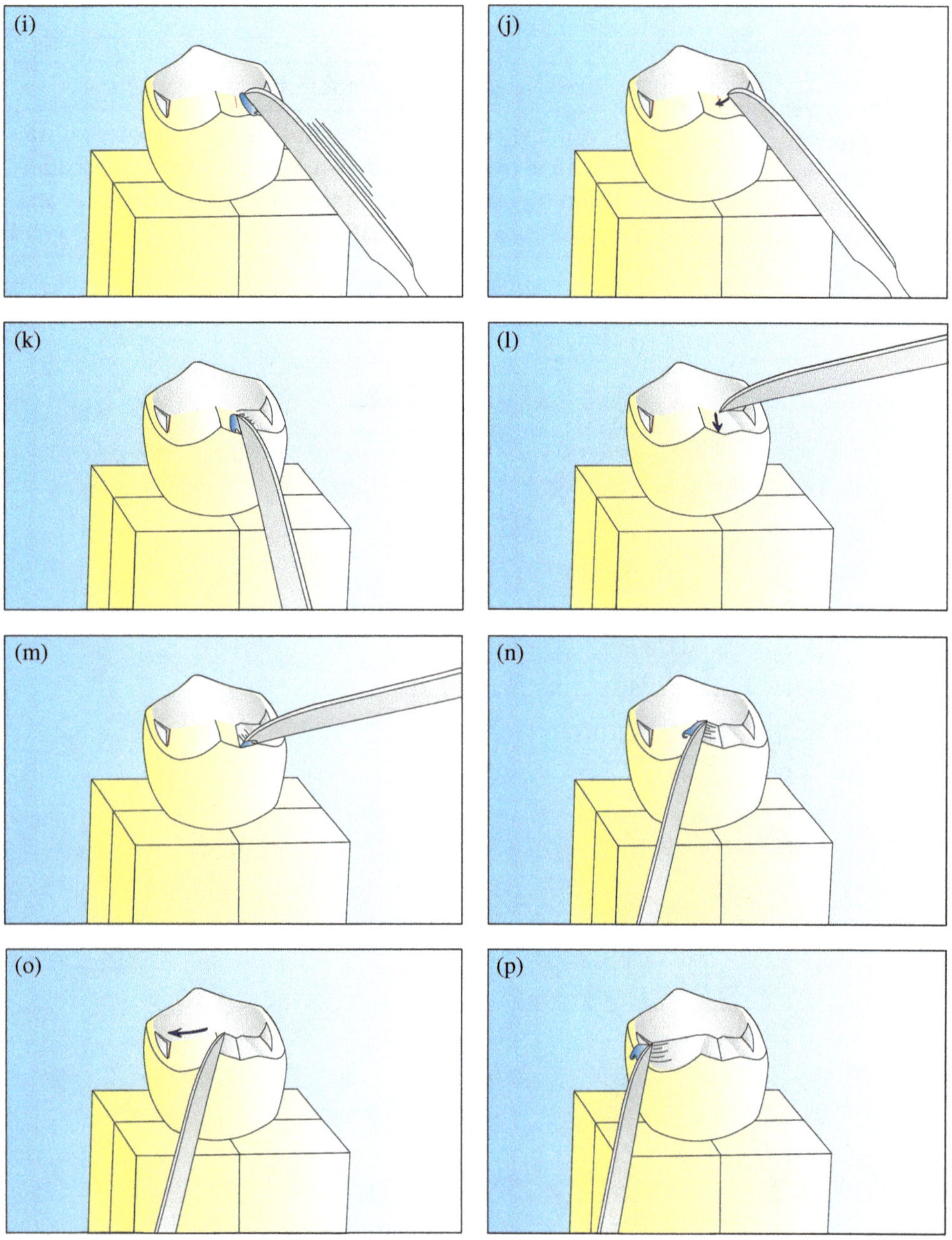

Figure 14.9 (Cont'd) (a–p)

Exercise: Carving the Root from the Mesial Aspect with Lingual Convergence

On the mesial aspect, the buccal and lingual outline of the root is drawn, and excess wax is carved up to the outline (Figure 14.10e–g). The mesial and distal convergence is created by carving wax lingually on both the mesial and distal surfaces (Figure 14.10h and i).

Exercise: Creating Developmental Depression on the Root Surfaces

A depression on the root is created by drawing the outline in the middle of the root surface and scooping the wax using the excavating end of the carver, moving it cervico-apically (Figure 14.10j–m).

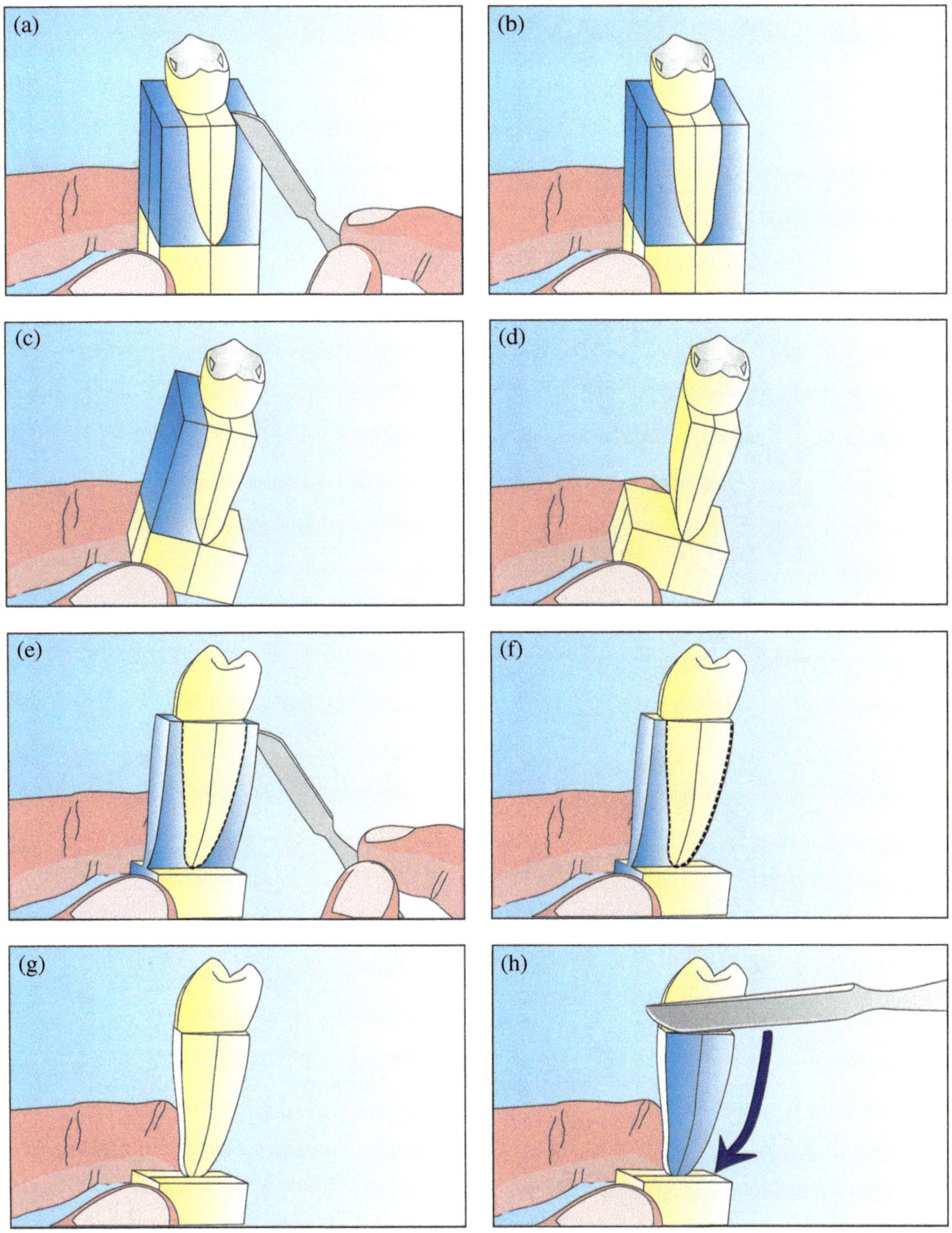

Figure 14.10 (a–m) Carving the root from the lingual and mesial aspect.

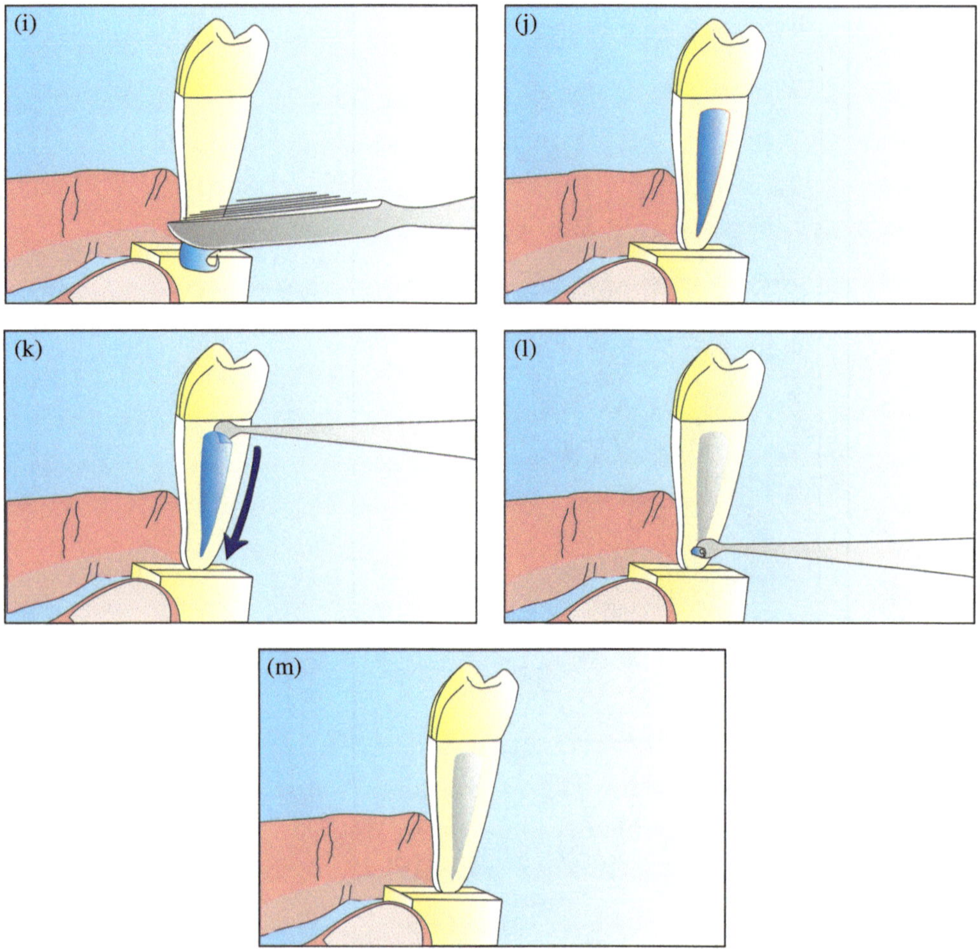

Figure 14.10 (Cont'd) (a–m)

References

1 Stanley, J.N. and Major, M.A.C. (2010). *Wheeler's Dental Anatomy and Oocclusion*, 9e. St. Louis, MO: Saunders Elsevier.

2 Rickne, C.S. and Weiss, G. (2012). *Woelfel's Dental Anatomy*, 8e. Philadelphia: Lippincott Williams & Wilkins.

3 James, L.F., Gerald, E.D., and Thomas, M.S. (2001). *Concise Dental Anatomy and Morphology*, 4e. Iowa City, IA: University of Iowa College of Dentistry.

4 Geoffrey, C.V.B. (1983). *Dental Morphology. An Iillustrated Guide*, 2e. Philadelphia: Wright Elsevier.

5 Nagaş I. C., Eğilmez F., and Kivanç B. H. (2018). The permanent maxillary and mandibular premolar teeth. In: *Dental Anatomy* (ed. B. H. Kivanç). http://dx.doi.org/10.5772/intechopen.79464 (accessed 23 March 2020).

15

Permanent Maxillary First Molar

LEARNING OBJECTIVE
At the end of the chapter, the student should have knowledge of the permanent maxillary first molar and develop the psychomotor skills for carving and waxing the same.

Permanent Maxillary Right First Molar

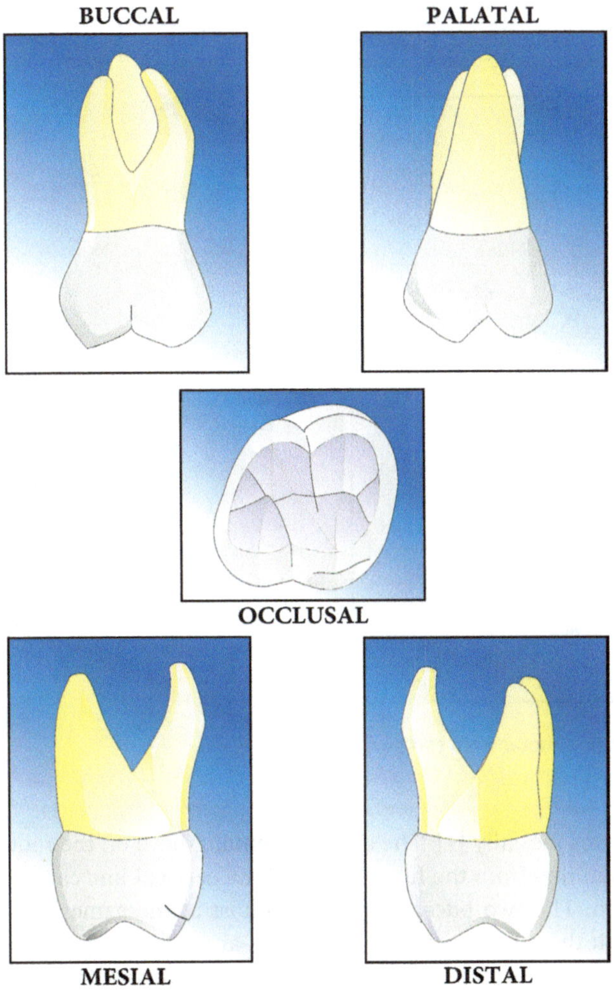

Buccal Aspect

Permanent maxillary first molar is the sixth tooth from the midsagittal plane (Figure 15.1). The crown is roughly trapezoidal in shape with the cervical being the smallest of the uneven sides (Figure 15.2a) [1]. With the tooth held in crown down position, the crest of contour on the mesial outline is at the junction of the middle and occlusal third. The distal crest of contour is placed cervically in the middle third of the crown (Figure 15.2b) [2]. The mesial outline is straight from the cervical line to the crest of contour. From the crest, the outline becomes continuous with mesial slope of the mesiobuccal cusp. The distal outline is concave from the cervix to the crest of contour and convex from the crest of contour to the distobuccal cusp (Figure 15.2c) [1].

Cusps seen from this aspect are mesiobuccal and distobuccal cusps. A part of the mesiopalatal cusp can be seen from this aspect. The mesiobuccal cusp is wider and taller than the distobuccal cusp. The crown appears to taper distally because of the variation in height of the cusp (Figure 15.2d) [2, 3]. The distobuccal cusp is sharper than the mesiobuccal cusp because the mesial slope of the distobuccal cusp meets the distal slope of the same at a right angle. Whereas the mesial slope of the mesiobuccal cusp meets the distal slope of the same at obtuse angle (Figure 15.2e). The buccal developmental groove divides the two buccal cusps and terminates in the middle third of the crown [2]. The cervical line is convex with the convexity towards the roots. Three of the roots seen from this aspect are mesiobuccal, distobuccal, and palatal.

An Illustrated Atlas of Tooth Carving and Wax-Up Techniques, First Edition. Anil Bangalore Shivappa.

Companion website: www.wiley.com/go/bangalore/toothcarving

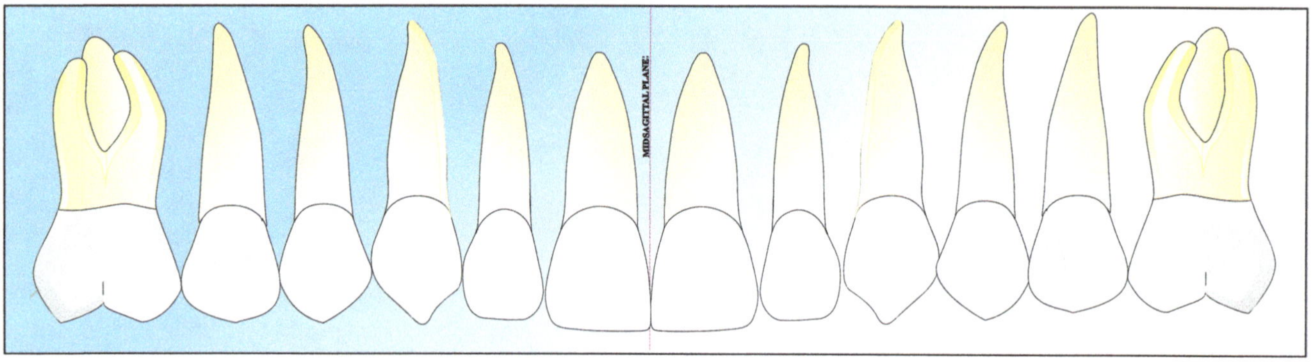

Figure 15.1 Position of the maxillary first molar in relation to the midsagittal plane.

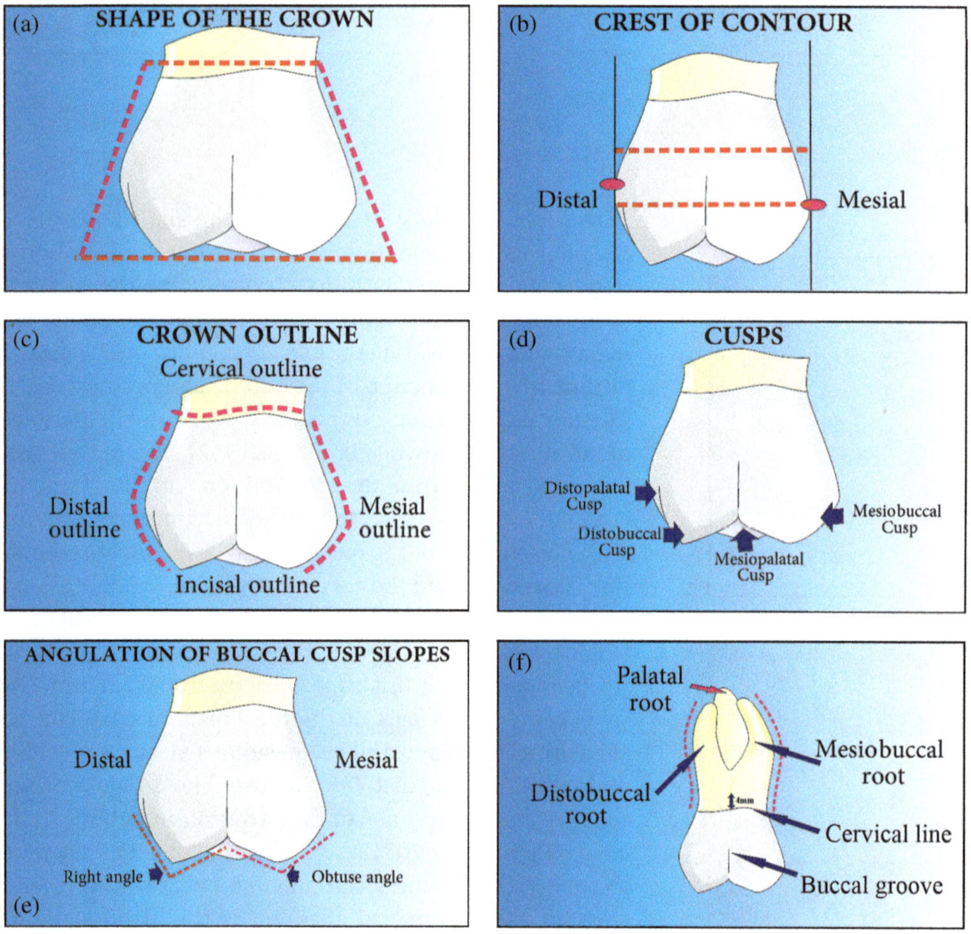

Figure 15.2 (a–f) Descriptive features of the permanent maxillary right first molar from the buccal aspect.

The tooth has longer and well-developed root trunk, with furcation starting near the junction of middle and cervical third. The mesiobuccal root exhibits distal curvature at the midway between the root furcation and the apex. The extent of curvature is such that the apex of the root is placed distal to the buccal groove [2]. The distal root is curves mesially [1]. The developmental groove on the root extending from the furcation until the cervical line can be seen. The two buccal roots are almost at the same level with the palatal root at higher level about 1 mm than the buccal roots. The buccal roots are well confined within the mesiodistal diameter of the crown (Figure 15.2f) [1].

Carving from the Buccal Aspect

Exercise: Marking the Length of the Crown and the Root

The length of the crown measuring 7.5 mm is marked from the occlusal edge of the wax block (Figure 15.3a). This length of the crown is extended onto the other sides of the wax block (Figure 15.3b). The length for the buccal roots measuring 12 mm is marked on the buccal surface of the wax block from the cervical end of the crown length. In the similar way, the length for the palatal root of 13 mm is marked on the palatal surface of the root (Figure 15.3c) [1].

Exercise: Marking the Dimension of the Crown on the Buccal Surface of the Wax Block

The buccal surface is now divided into three equal parts (Figure 15.3d). The mesiodistal diameter of the crown of 10 mm (5 mm marked on either side of the midline) is marked at the occlusal edge of the buccal surface of wax block (Figure 15.3e). Then the mesiodistal diameter of the crown at cervix of 8 mm (4 mm on either side of the midline) is marked at the cervical end of the crown (Figure 15.3f) [1].

Exercise: Marking the Outline of the Crown on the Buccal Surface of the Wax Block

The mesial and distal outline of the crown is drawn on the mesial and distal side of the midline with the features already mentioned (Figure 15.3g).

Exercise: Carving the Excess Wax from the Buccal Aspect of the Wax Block

After marking the outline of the crown, the wax outside this outline is considered as excess or unwanted wax (indicated in blue colour) that needs to be carved (Figure 15.3h). The bulk of the excess wax cervical to the crest of contour on the mesial side is carved with the anterior part of the cutting edge of the carver moved in buccopalatal direction. Then using the non-cutting end (back of the carver) the surface is made smooth (Figure 15.3i). The remaining wax at the occlusal third (above the crest of contour) is then carved using the anterior part of the cutting edge of the carver, moved in a buccopalatal direction (Figure 15.3j and k). In a similar way, the excess wax is carved on the distal side (Figure 15.3l).

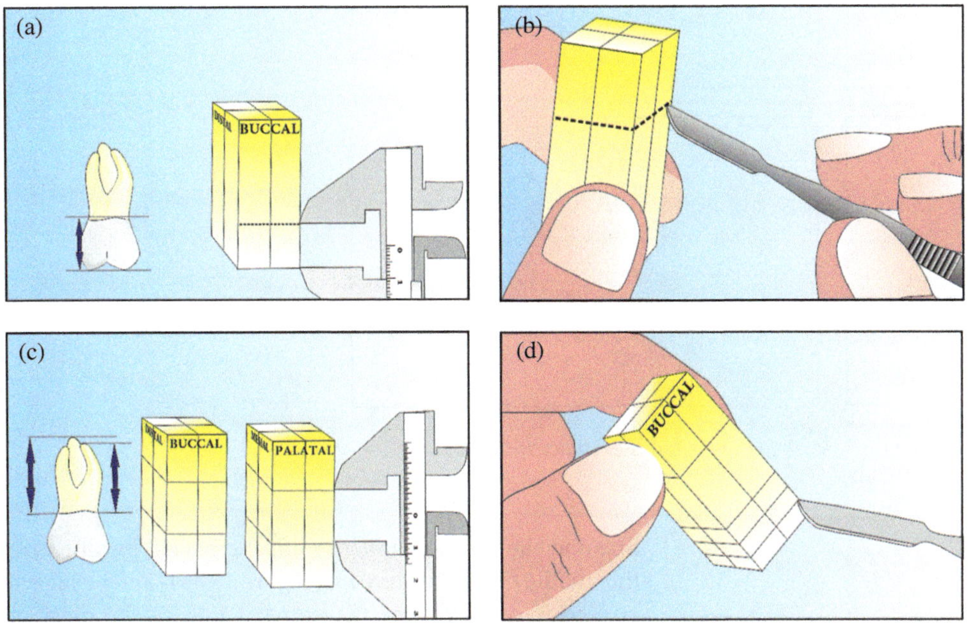

Figure 15.3 (a–h) Measuring and marking the crown dimension and root length on the buccal aspect of the wax block

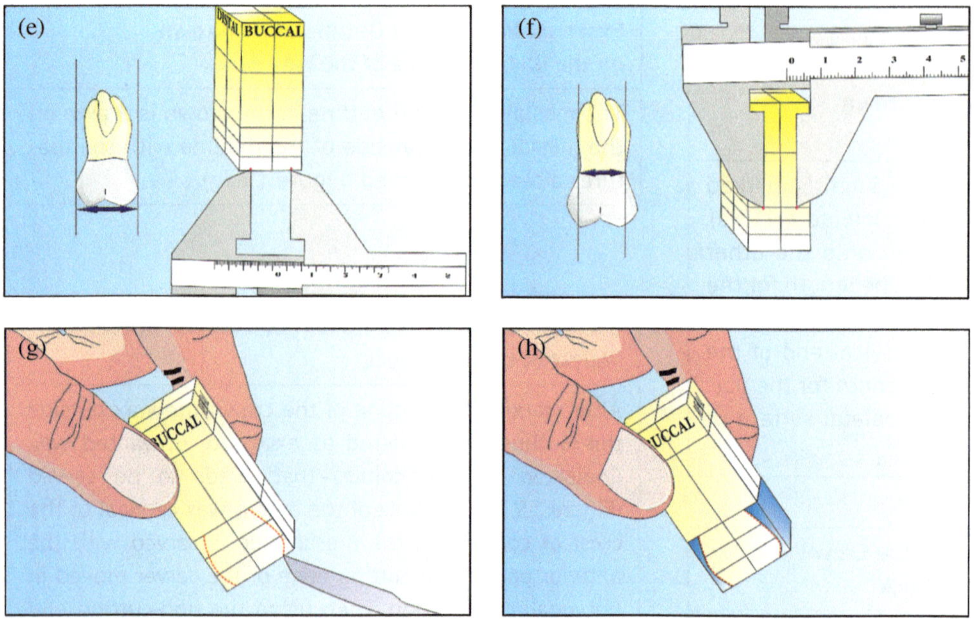

Figure 15.3 (Cont'd) (a–h).

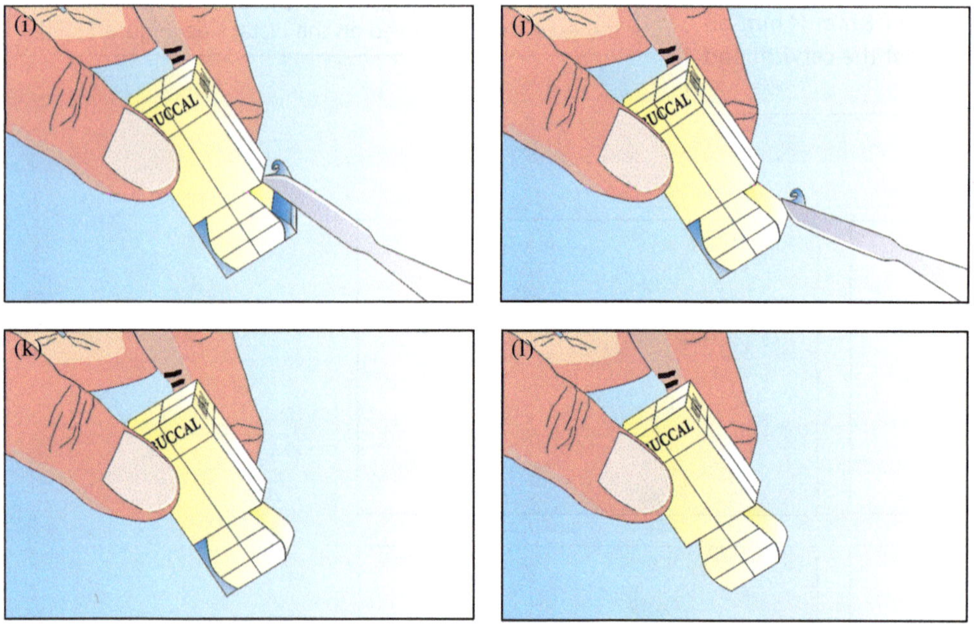

Figure 15.3 (i–l) Carving excess wax from the mesial and distal sides of the crown.

Mesial Aspect

The crown appears broader buccopalatally and shorter cervico-occlusally. The crest of curvature on the buccal outline is at the cervical third more towards the cervical line and the crest of curvature on the palatal outline is at the middle third of the crown (Figure 15.4a) [2]. The buccal outline is convex from the cervical line to the crest of contour and from there it becomes slightly concave on the middle and occlusal third and then convex at the cusp tip

(Figure 15.4b). The palatal outline appears semicircular and the outline dips inward at the cusp of Carabelli (Figure 15.4c) [1]. The cusps seen from this aspect are mesiobuccal, mesiopalatal, and the cusp of Carabelli. The mesial marginal ridge is irregular dipping cervically about one fifth of the crown length. The cervical line is also irregular, curving occlusally. Numerous marginal ridge grooves and enamel projections (tubercle) are seen on the mesial marginal ridge rather than the distal (Figure 15.4d) [2].

The mesiobuccal root is broad and flat. Its width is about two thirds the buccopalatal diameter of the crown at the cervix. The buccal outline of the root extends upward and outward from the crown, ending at the blunt apex. The apex of the mesiobuccal root is in line with the mesiobuccal cusp tip. The palatal outline of the mesiobuccal root is relatively straight from the bluntly rounded apex down to the bifurcation with the palatal root [2]. The level of the bifurcation is a little closer to the cervical line than is found between the roots buccally [1].

The palatal root is longer than the mesial root but is narrower from this aspect. It flares out palatally from the cervical line and it curves buccally at its middle third portion. The root appears more pointed towards the end than does the mesiobuccal root (Figure 15.4e) [1, 2].

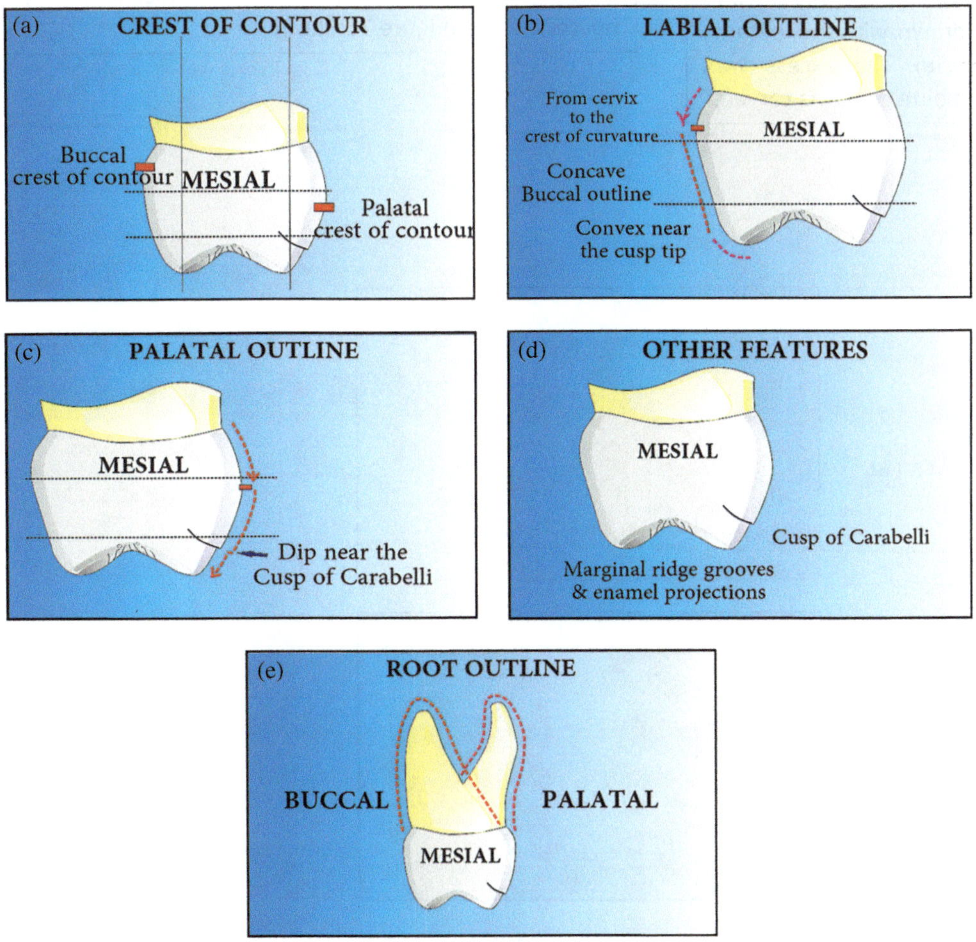

Figure 15.4 (a–e) Descriptive features of the permanent maxillary right first molar tooth from the mesial aspect.

Carving from the Mesial Aspect

Exercise: Marking the Dimension of the Crown on the Mesial Surface of the Wax Block

The buccopalatal diameter of the crown at the cervix of 10mm (5mm on either side of the midline) is marked at the cervix of mesial surface of the wax block (Figure 15.5a and b). Then the buccopalatal diameter of the crown about 11mm (5.5mm on either side of the midline) is marked at the occlusal edge of the crown (Figure 15.5c and d) [1].

Exercise: Marking the Outline on the Mesial Aspect of the Wax Block

Within the outer dimension marked, the buccal and palatal outline of the crown is drawn, with the features mentioned earlier (Figure 15.5e). The excess wax outside the outline, indicated in blue colour, is carved.

Exercise: Carving Excess Wax from the Palatal Surface

The wax cervical to the crest of contour on the palatal side is carved with the cutting edge of the carver facing the wax and the carver moved in a mesiodistal direction until the outline is reached (Figure 15.5f and g). The excess wax occlusal to the crest of contour is carved to get the smooth palatal outline (Figure 15.5h–j).

Exercise: Carving Excess Wax from the Buccal Surface

In a similar way to the carving of the palatal surface, excess wax is carved from the buccal surface to get the buccal outline (Figure 15.5k).

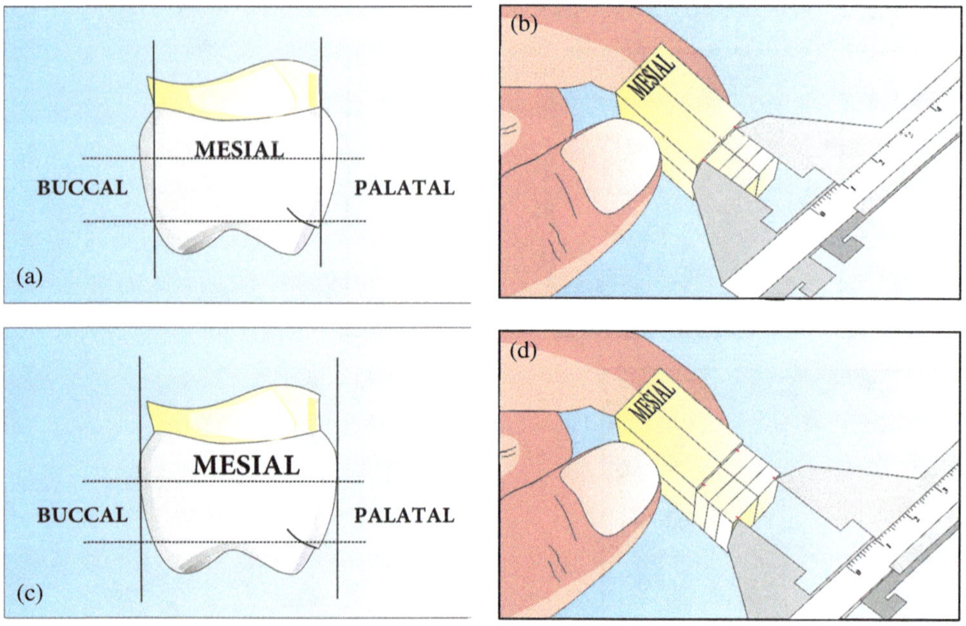

Figure 15.5 (a–d) Measuring and marking the dimension of the crown on the mesial aspect of the wax.

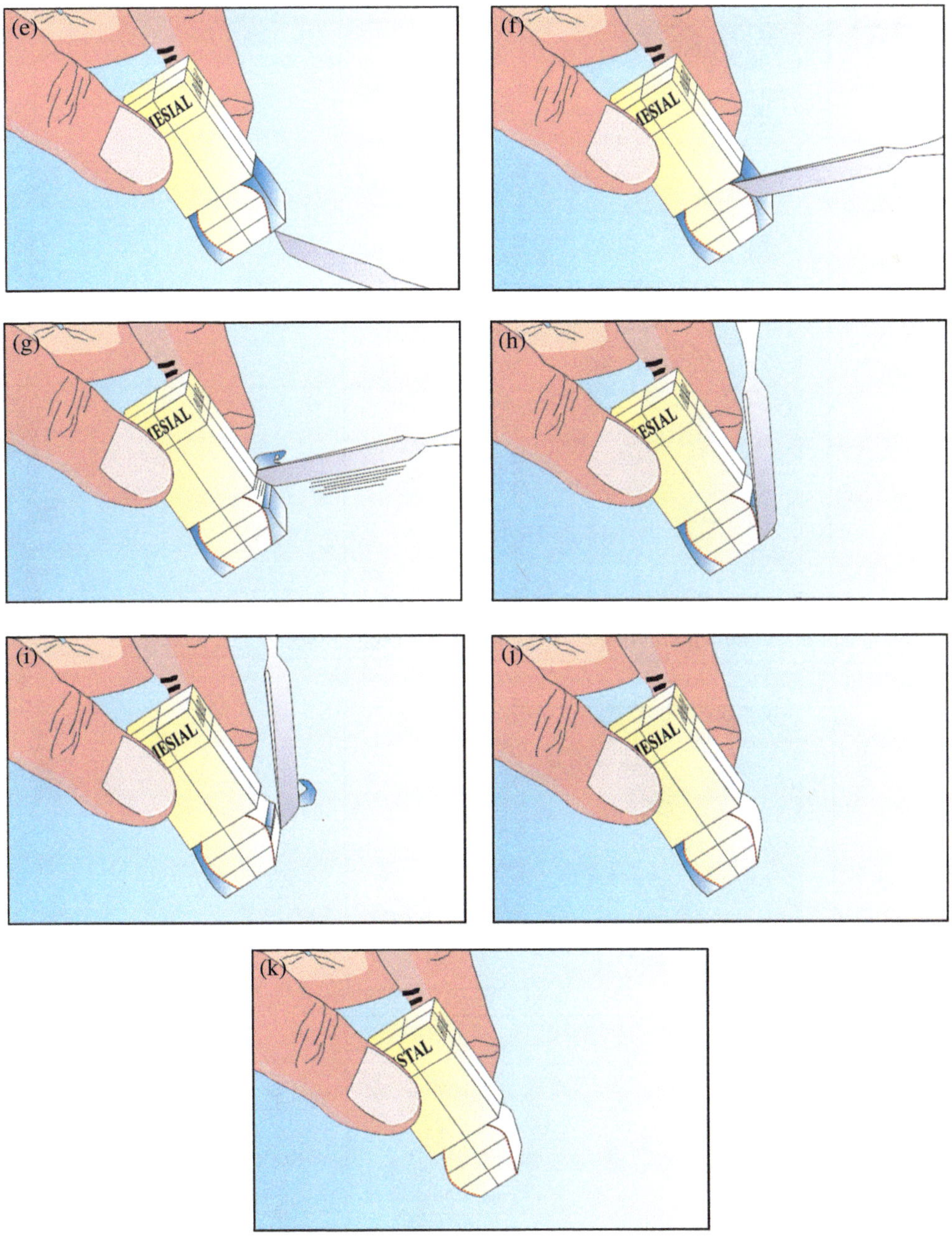

Figure 15.5 (e–k) Drawing the crown outline and carving excess wax from the palatal and buccal surface.

Distal Aspect

The outline from the distal aspect is similar to that of the mesial outline (Figure 15.6a). Because the crown tapers distally, most of the buccal and palatal surfaces can be seen due to the narrow buccopalatal dimension of the distal surface compared to the mesial surface (Figure 15.6b) [1]. All four major cusps can be seen, because the height of the distal cups is less than that of the mesial side [2]. The distal marginal ridge is more concave than mesial, so that the triangular ridges can be seen from this aspect (Figure 15.6c and d) [2].

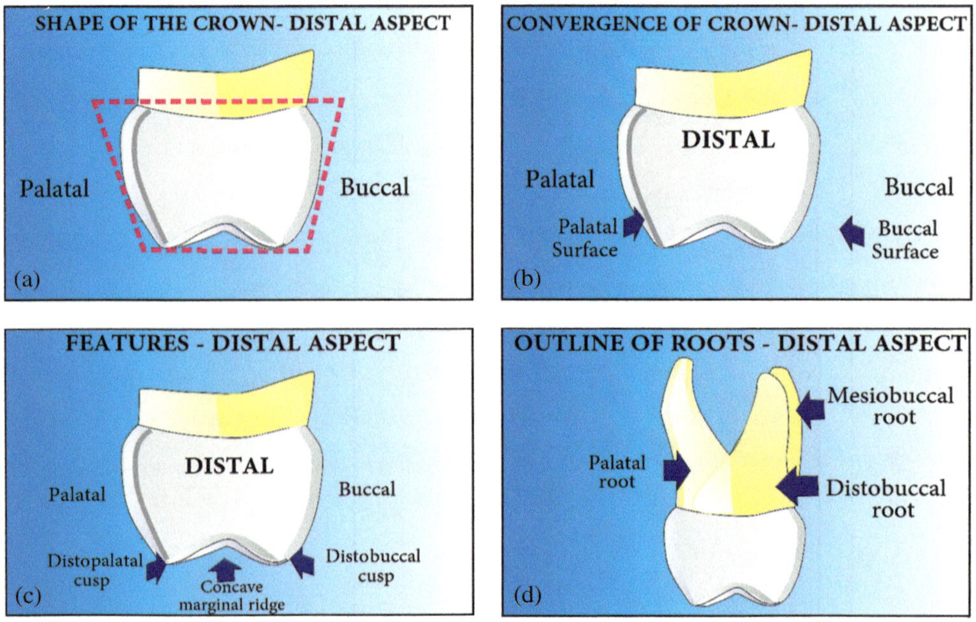

Figure 15.6 (a–d) Description of the permanent maxillary right first molar crown from the distal aspect.

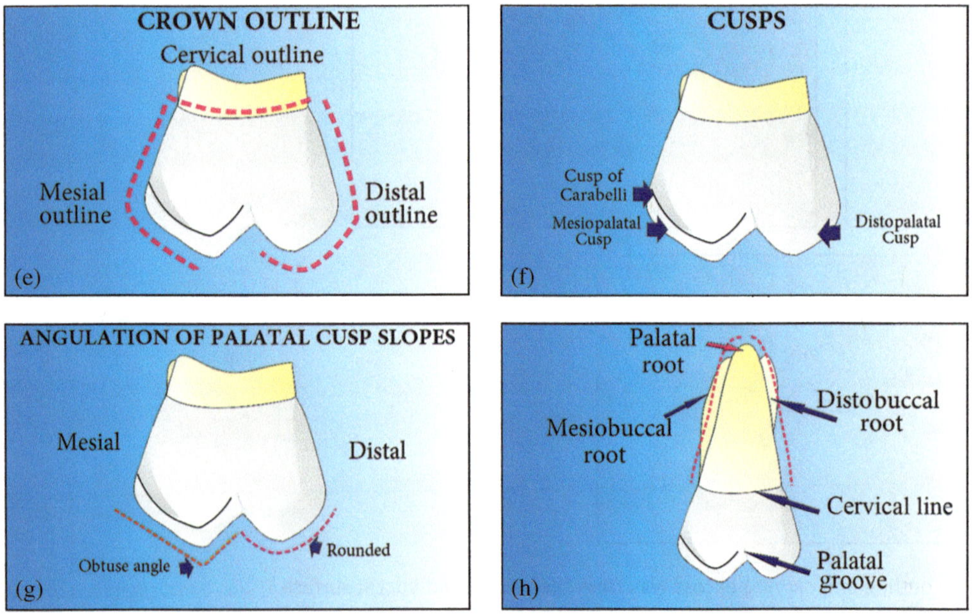

Figure 15.6 (e–h) Description of the permanent maxillary right first molar from the palatal aspect.

Palatal Aspect

The outline of the crown is opposite to that of the buccal aspect. Little buccopalatal convergence towards the palatal surface can be seen (Figure 15.6e) [1]. Only two major cusps can be seen from this aspect: mesiopalatal and distopalatal cusps. The minor cusp is the cusp of Carabelli (Figure 15.6f) [2]. The mesiopalatal cusp is the largest and tallest among the major cusps. Its cuspal ridges form an obtuse angle. The distal cusp is rounded. The mesiodistal width of the mesiopalatal cusp is about three fifths the width of the crown. That of the distopalatal cusp is about two fifths the mesiodistal width of the crown [1]. The cusp of Carabelli is seen on the palatal surface of the mesiopalatal cusp. It is considered a nonfunctional cusp as it is 2 mm shorter than the mesiopalatal cusp tip [2]. An irregular groove outlining this cusp starts at the mesiopalatal line angle that runs towards the cusp tip then turns down at an obtuse angle towards the palatal groove (Figure 15.6g). Roots seen from this aspect are the palatal root and parts of the buccal roots. The palatal root is long and conical in shape and ends in rounded apex [1]. A depression on the palatal root surface can be seen (Figure 15.6h) [2].

Occlusal Aspect

The occlusal outline is roughly rhomboidal in shape with the mesial side wider than the distal and the palatal side wider than the buccal (Figure 15.7a) [1, 2, 4]. The acute line angles of the crown are mesiobuccal and distopalatal; the obtuse line angles are mesiopalatal and distobuccal [1, 2]. It may also appear rectangular and squarish [3]. There are four major cusps and one minor cusp. The minor cusp is the cusp of Carabelli (tuberculum Carabelli), placed at the mesiopalatal line angle of the mesiopalatal cusp [4]. The cusp of Carabelli is also referred to as fifth lobe, fifth cusp, supplemental cusp, accessory cusp, and mesiopalatal prominence [3]. The size of the major cusps in descending order is the mesiopalatal cusp (largest cusp) followed by mesiobuccal, distobuccal, and distopalatal (Figure 15.7b) [2, 3, 5]. The distopalatal cusp is the smallest and more rounded. Of the four major cusps, the mesiopalatal cusp has two triangular ridges: the mesial triangular ridge and the distal cuspal ridge. The remaining three major cusps have their own individual triangular ridges that run from cusp tip to the centre of the crown. The triangular ridge of the mesiobuccal cusp unites with the mesial triangular ridge of the mesiopalatal cusp to form the transverse ridge (Figure 15.7c). The distal cuspal ridge of the mesiopalatal cusp runs obliquely to join the triangular ridge of the distobuccal to form the oblique ridge. The oblique ridge is also known as the 'enamel bridge'. The height of the oblique ridge is reduced at the centre about same height as the marginal ridges (Figure 15.7d) [2].

The occlusal surface has two major and two minor fossae. The major fossae are the central fossa (or fovea centralis) and the distal fossa. The central fossa is mesial to the oblique ridge and is triangular in shape, whereas the distal

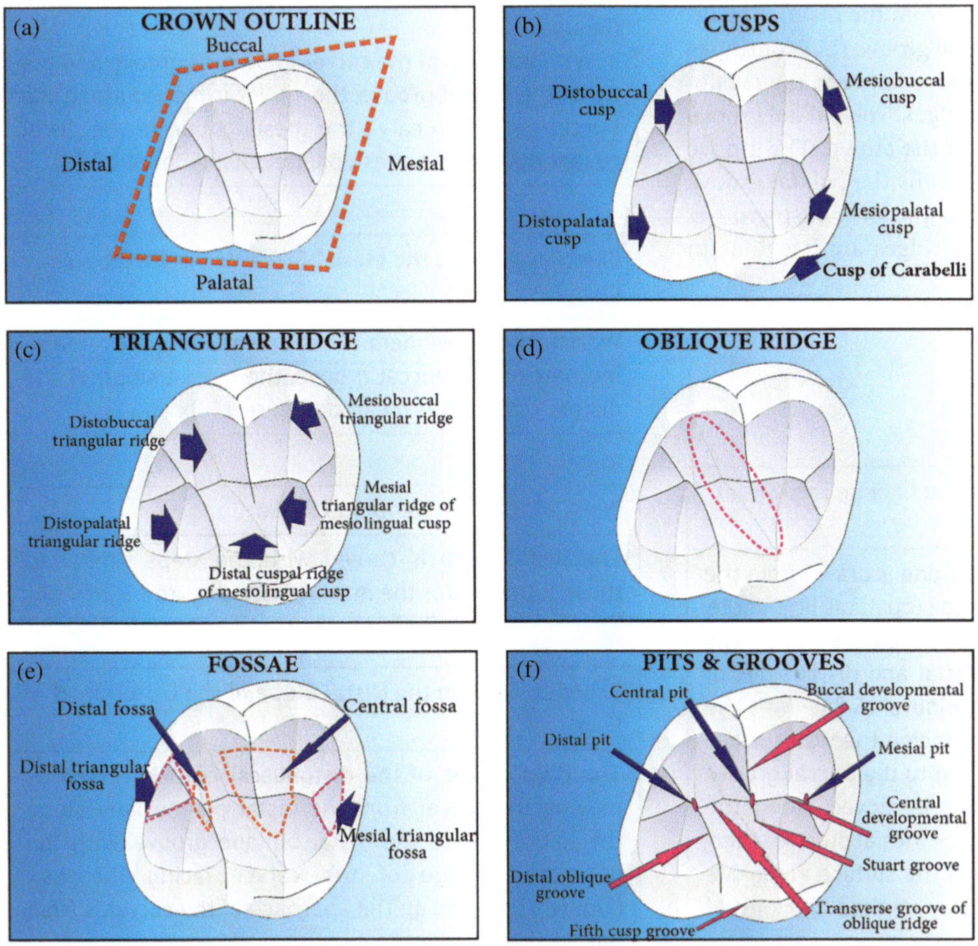

Figure 15.7 (a–f) Description of the permanent maxillary right first molar crown from the occlusal aspect.

fossa is distal to the oblique ridge and is linear. The two minor fossae are the mesial triangular fossa and the distal triangular fossa (Figure 15.7e) [5].

The central fossa is a concave area bounded mesially by the crests of the triangular ridges of the mesiobuccal and the mesiopalatal cusps, buccally by the distal slope of the mesiobuccal cusp and the mesial slope of the distobuccal cusp, and distally by the oblique ridge crest [1, 2]. Contents of the central fossa are the developmental grooves, the supplemental grooves, and the central developmental pit (Figure 15.7e). The developmental grooves radiate forming the central pit. The developmental groove which runs buccally from the central pit is the buccal developmental groove that continues between the buccal cusps over the buccal surface. The developmental groove radiating mesially from the central pit is the central developmental groove which terminates in the mesial triangular fossa. The supplemental grooves arise as branches of the central developmental groove. Also present is the transverse groove of the oblique ridge running distally from the central pit crossing the oblique ridge and ending in the distal pit. The groove arising in the distal fossa from the distal pit running palatally is the distal oblique groove that continues as the palatal developmental groove between the mesiopalatal and distopalatal cuspal ridges. The palatal groove is located exactly at the centre of the crown. The groove bordering the cusp of Carebelli joins the palatal groove at its terminus. This is known as the fifth cusp groove. The mesial and distal marginal ridges are irregular in shape (Figure 15.7f) [2].

Carving from the Occlusal Aspect

Exercise: Marking the Grooves and Carving the Mesial Triangular Fossa

A line representing the oblique ridge is drawn from the mesiopalatal line angle to the distopalatal line angle. With the occlusal features mentioned previously, the grooves are marked on the mesial and distal sides of the oblique ridge line drawn (Figure 15.8a). With the non-cutting edge of the carver facing the wax surface and the tip of the carver pointing to the buccal groove of the mesial fossa, the carver is moved along the groove, deep into the wax until the mesial pit is reached. The carver is then pulled out to the surface along the palatal groove of the fossa to complete the mesial fossa (Figure 15.8b–d).

Exercise: Carving the Triangular Ridge of the Mesio-buccal Cusp

With the non-cutting edge of the carver facing the wax surface and the tip of the carver at the pit, the carver is pulled towards the surface (Figure 15.8e). Then the carver is pushed into the wax by application of pressure to carve the distal slope, with formation of the triangular ridge of the mesiobuccal cusp (Figure 15.8f). The carver is then moved buccally along the buccal groove (Figure 15.8g).

Exercise: Carving the Mesial Triangular Ridge of the Mesiopalatal Cusp

With the tip of the carver in the mesial pit and the back of the carver facing the wax, the carver is moved towards the surface up to the ridge to complete mesial slope (Figure 15.8h and i). Then the carver is pushed into the wax to create the distal slope of the mesial triangular ridge of the mesiopalatal cusp. This distal slope ends by forming a groove called Stuart's groove (Figure 15.8j).

With the back of the carver in Stuart's groove and the tip at the buccal groove, the carver is moved along the buccal groove to carve the mesial slope of the distal cuspal ridge of the mesiopalatal cusp (Figure 15.8k).

Exercise: Carving the Mesial Slope of the Distobuccal Cusp

With further movement of the carver along the remaining part of the buccal groove, the mesial slope of the distobuccal cusp is created (Figure 15.8k and l).

Exercise: Carving the Distal Fossa

The distal fossa is carved with the steps similar to those followed for the mesial fossa (Figure 15.8m–o).

Exercise: Carving the Distal Slope of the Distobuccal Cusp

The distal slope of the distobuccal cusp is carved by moving the carver from the distal pit mesially along the initial half of the distal oblique groove, with the non-cutting edge of the carver facing the wax (Figure 15.8p and q). The approach of the carver is from buccal side.

Exercise: Carving the Distal and Mesial Slope of the Distopalatal Cusp

The distal and mesial slopes of the distopalatal cusps are created by moving the tip of the carver along the whole length of the distal oblique groove, with the non-cutting edge facing the distopalatal part of the occlusal surface of wax (Figure 15.8r–u). The approach of the carver is from the palatal side.

Exercise: Carving the Distal Slope of the Distal Cuspal Ridge of the Mesiopalatal Cusp

With the non-cutting edge on the distal half of the transverse oblique groove, the tip of the carver is moved along the palatal half of the distal oblique groove to create the distal slope of the distal cuspal ridge of the mesiopalatal cusp (Figure 15.8v–x).

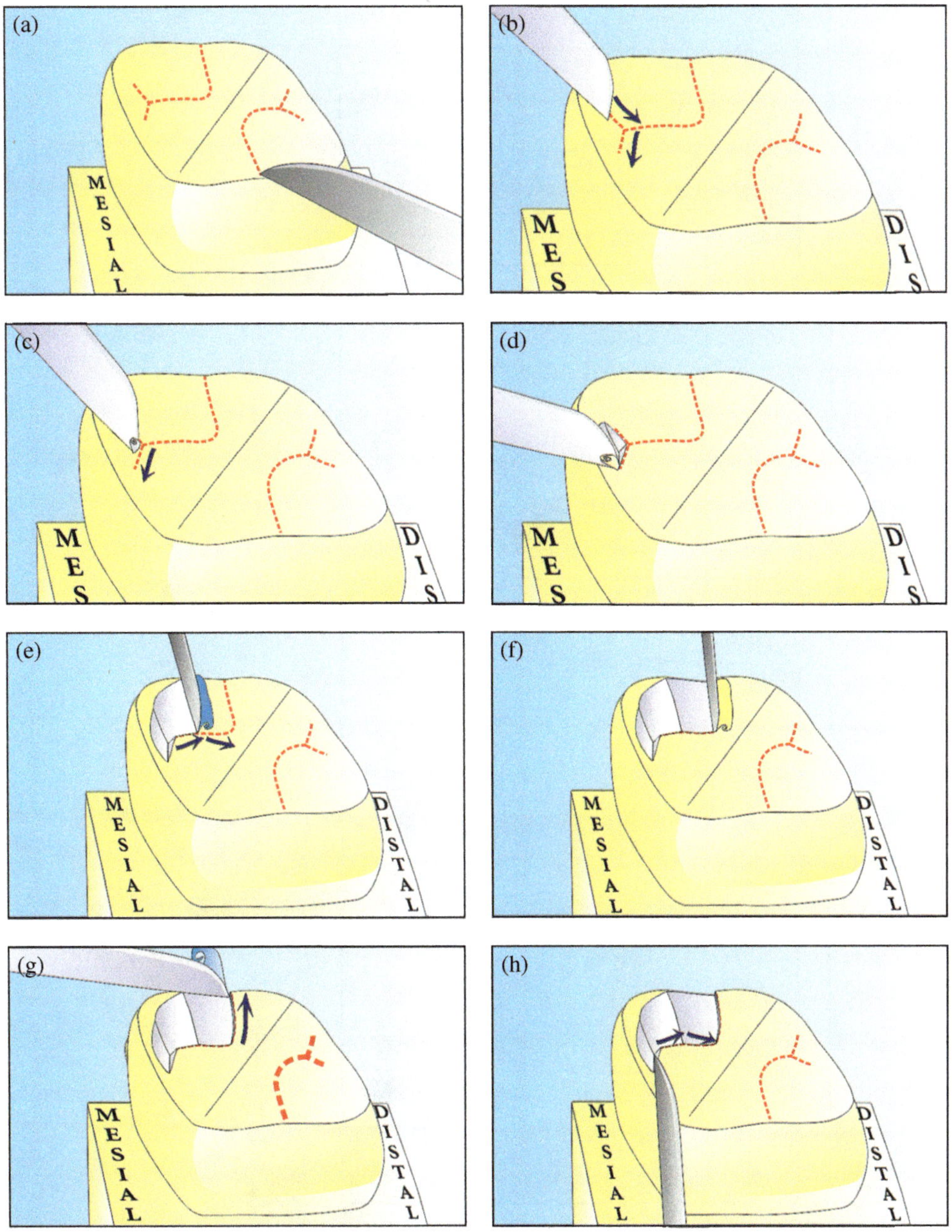

Figure 15.8 (a–x) Carving occlusal features (cusps, their ridges, fossae, and grooves) of the permanent maxillary right first molar.

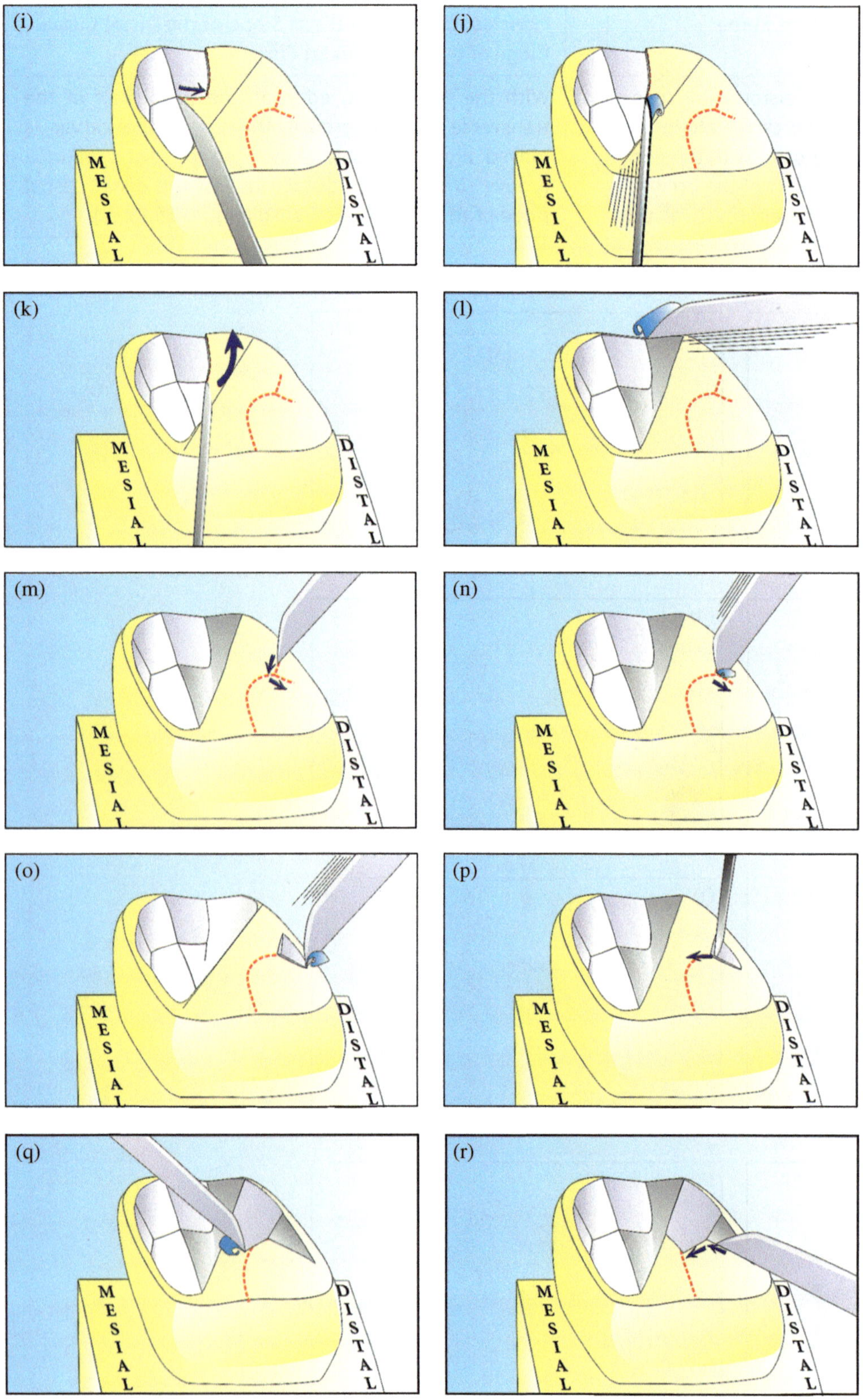

Figure 15.8 (Cont'd) (a–x)

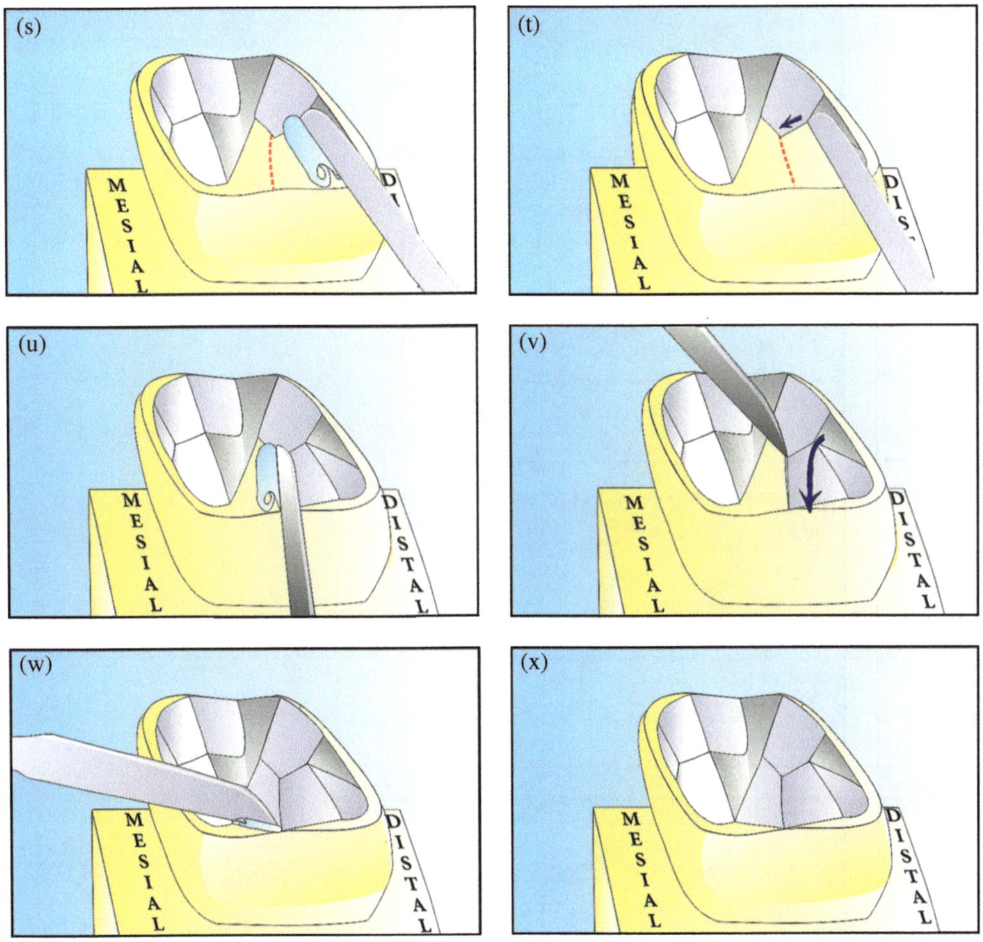

Figure 15.8 (Cont'd) (a–x)

Exercise: Creating the Slopes of the Marginal Ridges

Using the curved part of the cutting edge, the outer slopes of the marginal ridges are created on the mesial and distal sides (Figure 15.9a and b).

Exercise: Creating the Ridges on the Buccal and Palatal Surfaces of Each Cusp

Using the curved anterior part of the carver, the slopes are created on either side of the midline of each cusp (Figure 15.9c). The slopes should be carved from the crest of contour. The mesial slope on the palatal surface of the mesiopalatal cusp is carved starting from the crest of contour at the middle third of the crown and the carver is moved occlusally at an angle (Figure 15.9d and e). The distal slope is also carved in the similar way to obtain the ridge (Figure 15.9f). The ridges of the remaining cusps are carved in a similar way (Figure 15.9g–i).

Exercise: Carving the Cusp of Carabelli

The outline of the cusp of Carabelli is drawn starting at the mesiopalatal line angle, moved towards the tip of the mesiopalatal cusp, forming an obtuse angle that ends at the palatal groove. This outline is placed 2 mm from the occlusal surface, cervically (Figure 15.9j). Then with the non-cutting edge of the carver facing the surface of the mesiopalatal cusp, the carver is moved along the outline from the mesiopalatal line angle towards the palatal groove (Figure 15.9k and l).

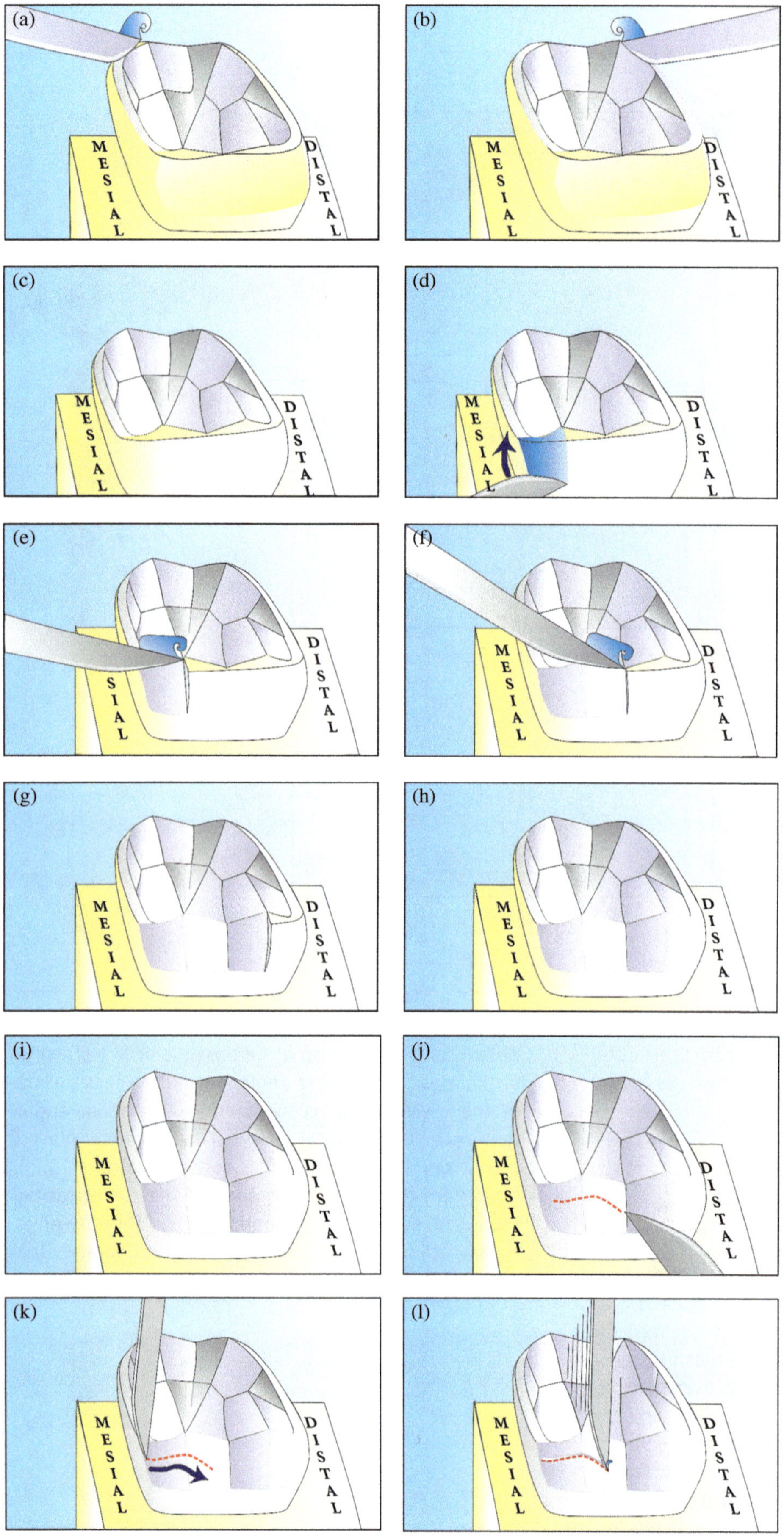

Figure 15.9 (a–l) Carving marginal ridges, ridges on buccal and palatal surfaces, and the cusp of Carabelli on the crown of the maxillary right first molar.

Root Carving

Exercise: Carving the Roots from the Buccal Aspect

The outlines of the buccal roots are drawn on the root portion of the buccal surface of wax with their features mentioned earlier (Figure 15.10a and b). The excess wax outside the outline on the mesial and distal sides needs to be carved (Figure 15.10c). The concave part of the mesial root is carved using the convex anterior part of the carver (Figure 15.10c and d). For the convex parts of the root, the non-cutting part (back) of the carver is used. The carver is run in the buccopalatal direction until the outline of the root is reached (Figure 15.10e and f). The furcal part of the excess wax is carved out using the anterior cutting edge of the carver, run along the inner outline of the buccal roots (Figure 15.10g–i). The excess wax is then carved (Figure 15.10j and k).

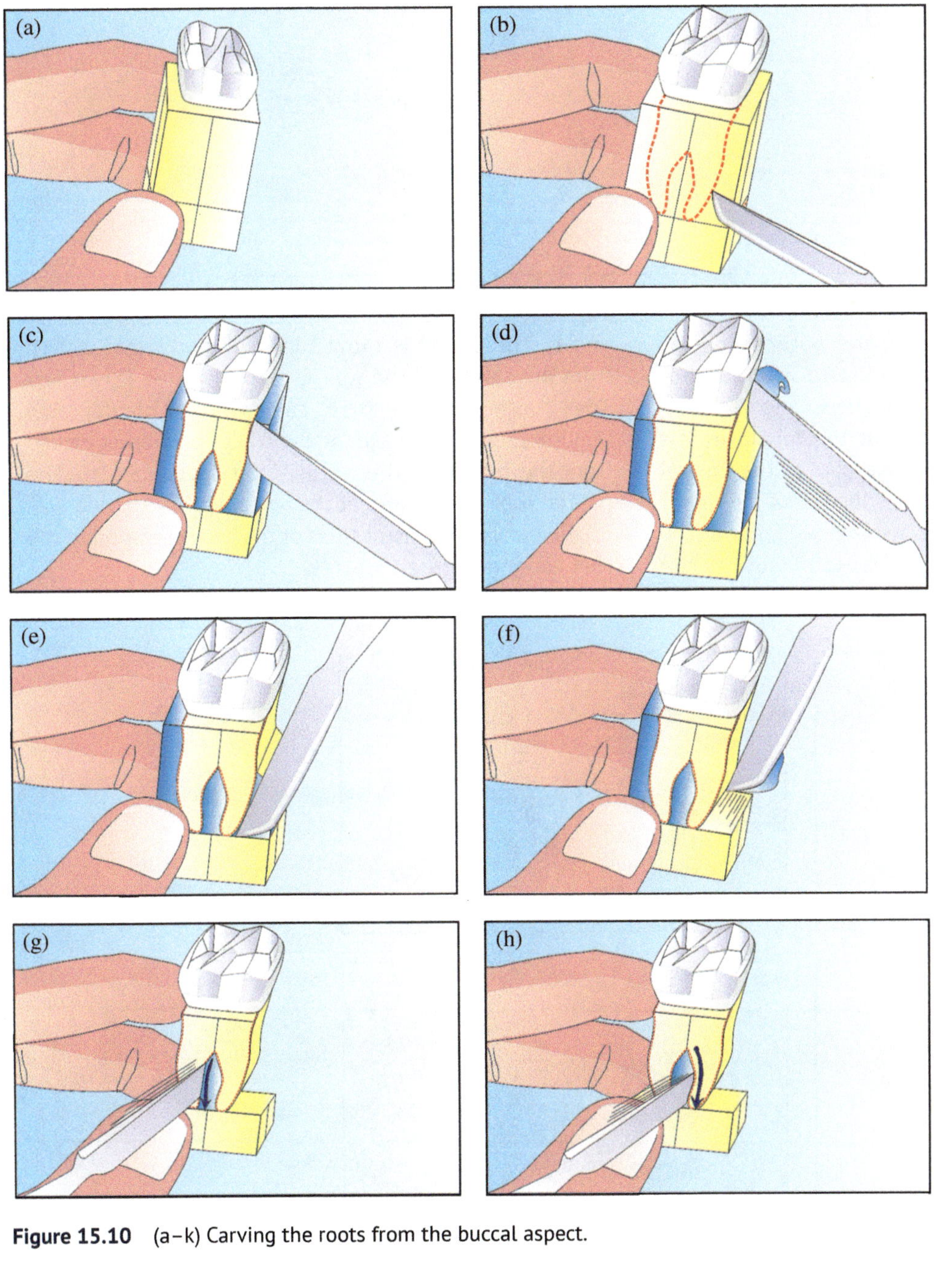

Figure 15.10 (a–k) Carving the roots from the buccal aspect.

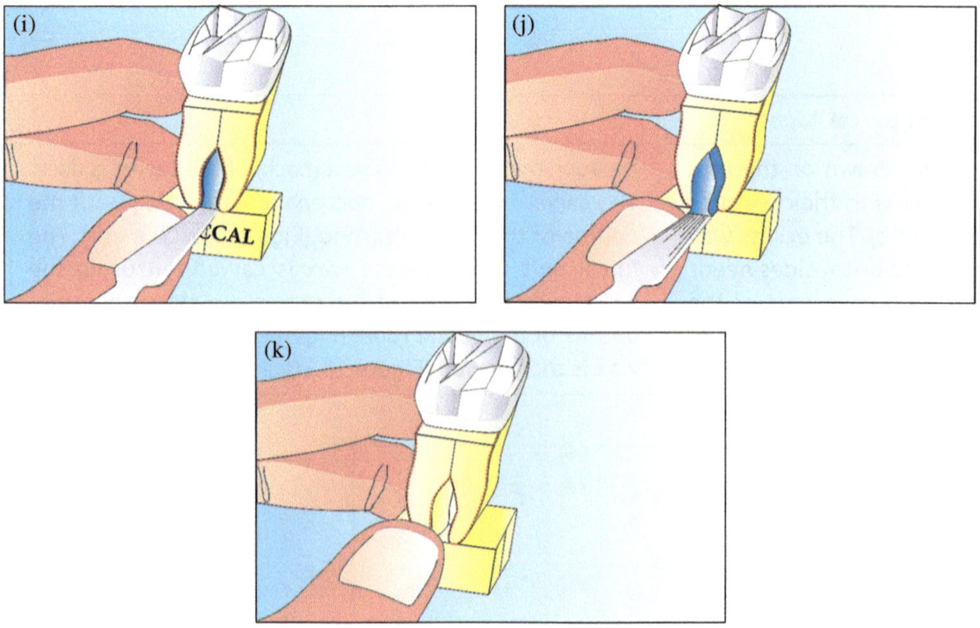

Figure 15.10 (Cont'd) (a–k)

Exercise: Carving the Roots from the Proximal (Mesial) Aspect

On the mesial side of the root, the outlines of the mesiobuccal and palatal roots are drawn with features mentioned earlier (Figure 15.11a). The excess wax outside the outline of the root and at the furcal area is carved (Figure 15.11b). The concave part of the palatal root is carved using the convex anterior part of the carver (Figure 15.11c and d). For the convex part of the root, the non-cutting part (back) of the carver is used (Figure 15.11e and f). The carver is moved in a mesiodistal direction from the surface of the wax, until the outline is reached. The buccal root is then carved in a similar way (Figure 15.11g). The wax at the furcal portion is carved from the mesial to the distal side (Figure 15.11h). The palatal root is narrowed at the apical half by carving wax on the mesial and distal sides of the root to complete the root carving (Figure 15.11i–k).

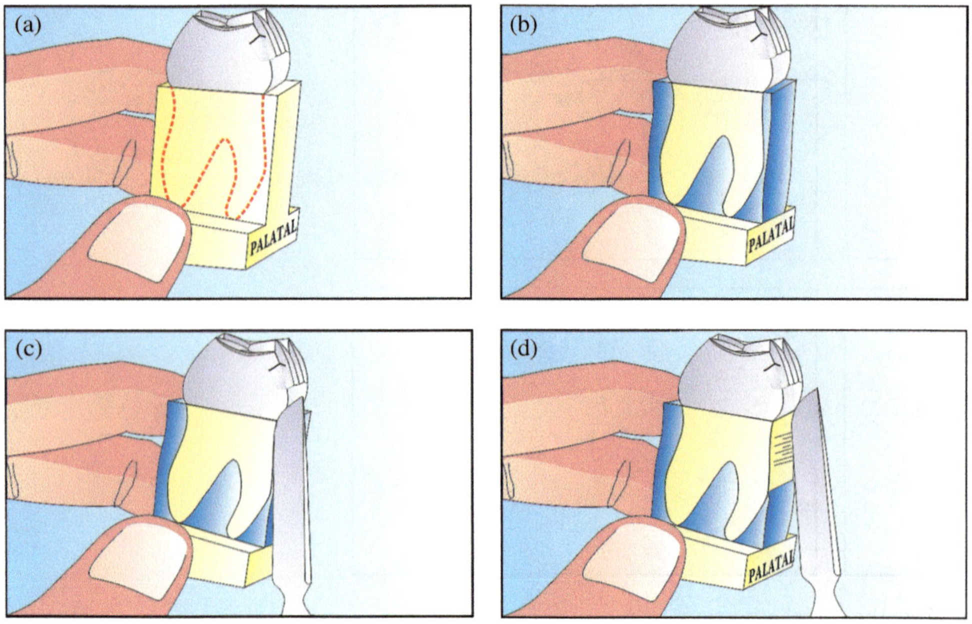

Figure 15.11 (a–k) Carving the roots from the mesial aspect.

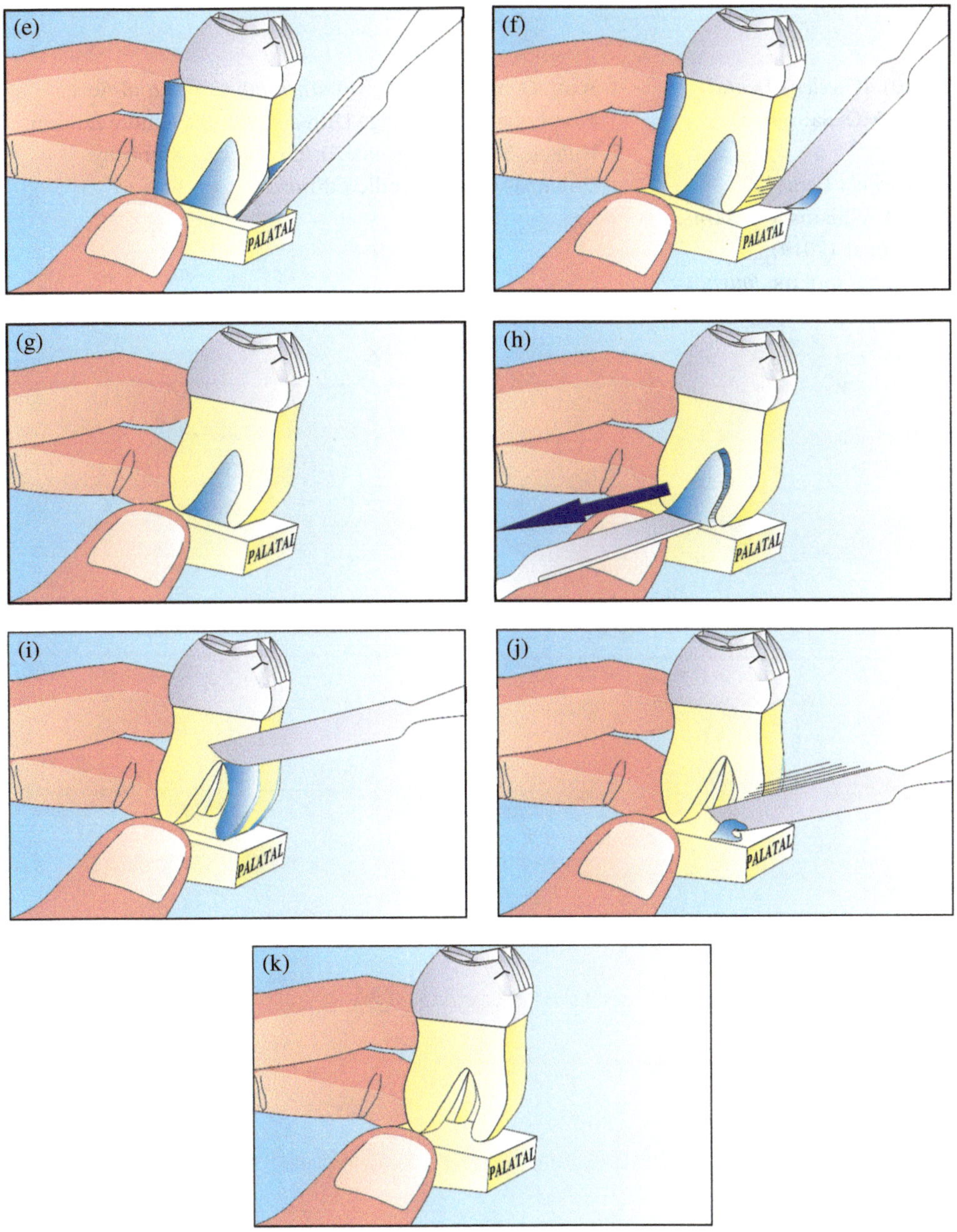

Figure 15.11 (Cont'd) (a–k)

Exercise Drawing the Cervical Line
The cervical line is drawn using the tip of the carver at the junction of the crown and root, with the curvature of the line facing the occlusal surface. The curvature on the mesial surface is 1 mm and on the distal surface is 0 mm [1].

References

1 Stanley, J.N. and Major, M.A.C. (2010). *Wheeler's Dental Anatomy and Occlusion*, 9e. St. Louis, MO: Saunders Elsevier.

2 Rickne, C.S. and Weiss, G. (2012). *Woelfel's Dental Anatomy*, 8e. Philadelphia: Lippincott Williams & Wilkins.

3 Luis, E.G., Gabriely, F., Marcelo, B.C. et al. (2019). Morphological differences between upper molars. *Journal of Morphological Sciences* 36: 303–308.

4 Scott, G. and Richard. *Human Tooth Crown and Root Morphology*. Cambridge University Press. Kindle Edition.

5 Hillson, S. (2012). *Dental Anthropology*. Cambridge University Press. Kindle Edition.

16

Permanent Maxillary Second Molar

LEARNING OBJECTIVE
At the end of the chapter, student should have knowledge of the permanent maxillary second molar and develop the psychomotor skills for carving and waxing the same.

Permanent Maxillary Right Second Molar

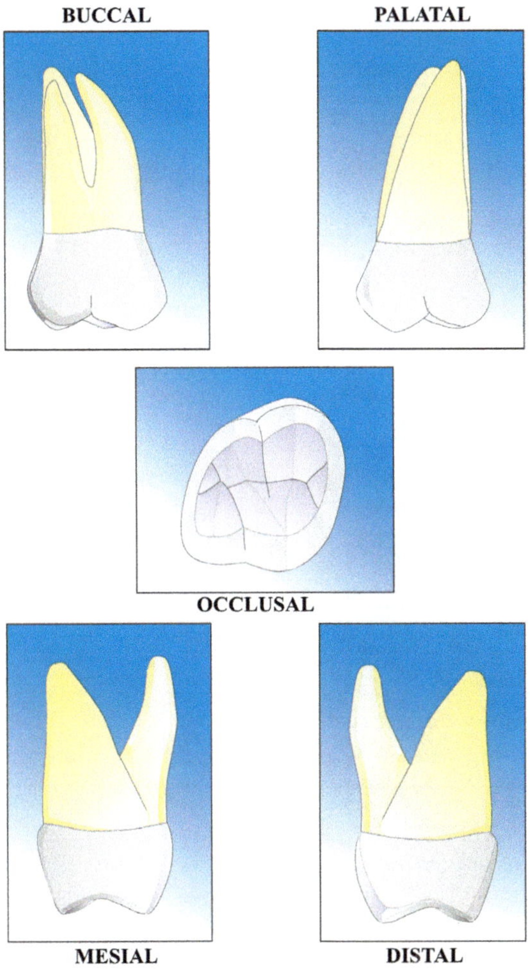

Buccal Aspect

The permanent maxillary second molar is the seventh tooth from the midsagittal plane (Figure 16.1). From this aspect, the crown is similar to that of the first molar except the crown is short and narrow [1]. The crown appears inclined cervically on the distal side because of the smaller and narrower distobuccal cusp [2]. This allows part of the distal marginal ridge and distopalatal cusp to be seen (Figure 16.2a and b) [1]. The buccal groove between the mesiobuccal and distobuccal cusps is shorter and ends in a pit [2]. The roots are shorter, inclined distally, and less spread out (Figure 16.2c) [3]. The mesiobuccal root apex is in line with the buccal groove (Figure 16.2d) [1].

Carving from the Buccal Aspect

Exercise: Marking the Crown and Root Length on the Wax Block
The length of the crown measuring 7.0 mm is marked on the buccal surface of the wax from the occlusal edge (Figure 16.3a). The marking is then extended onto other surfaces (Figure 16.3b). The length of the root of 11 mm is marked on the buccal surface. The root length of the palatal root (12 mm) is marked on the palatal surface of the wax block (Figure 16.3c) [1]. Then the reference points of measurement of the roots are joined on the mesial and distal surfaces of the wax.

An Illustrated Atlas of Tooth Carving and Wax-Up Techniques, First Edition. Anil Bangalore Shivappa.

Companion website: www.wiley.com/go/bangalore/toothcarving

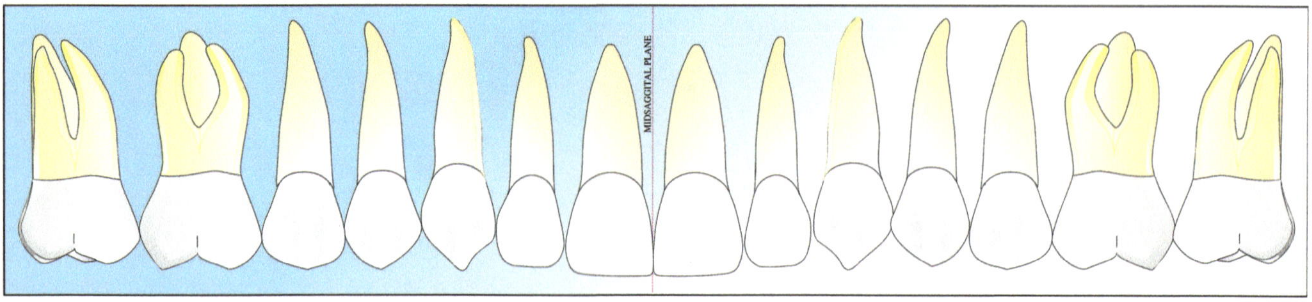

Figure 16.1 Position of the permanent maxillary second molars in relation to the midsagittal plane.

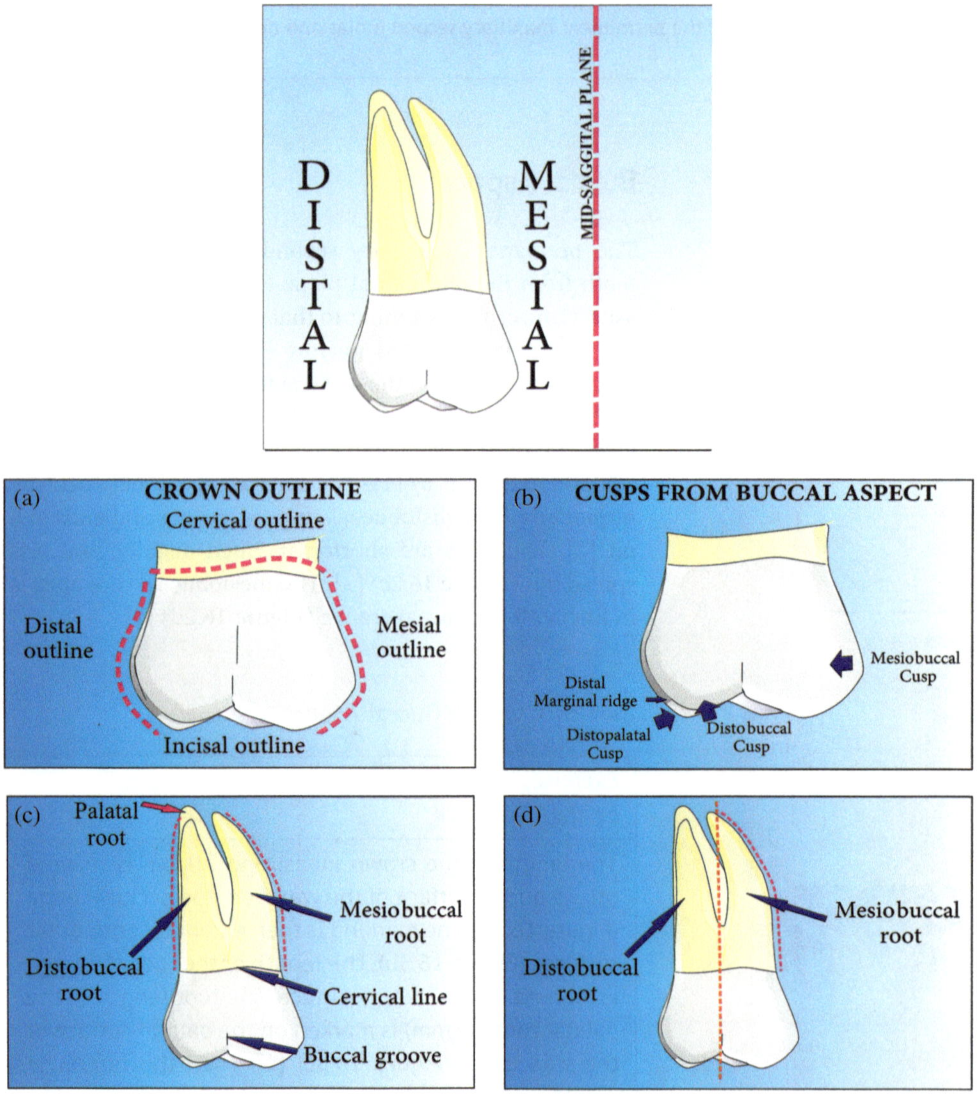

Figure 16.2 (a–d) Descriptive features of the permanent maxillary right second molar from the labial aspect.

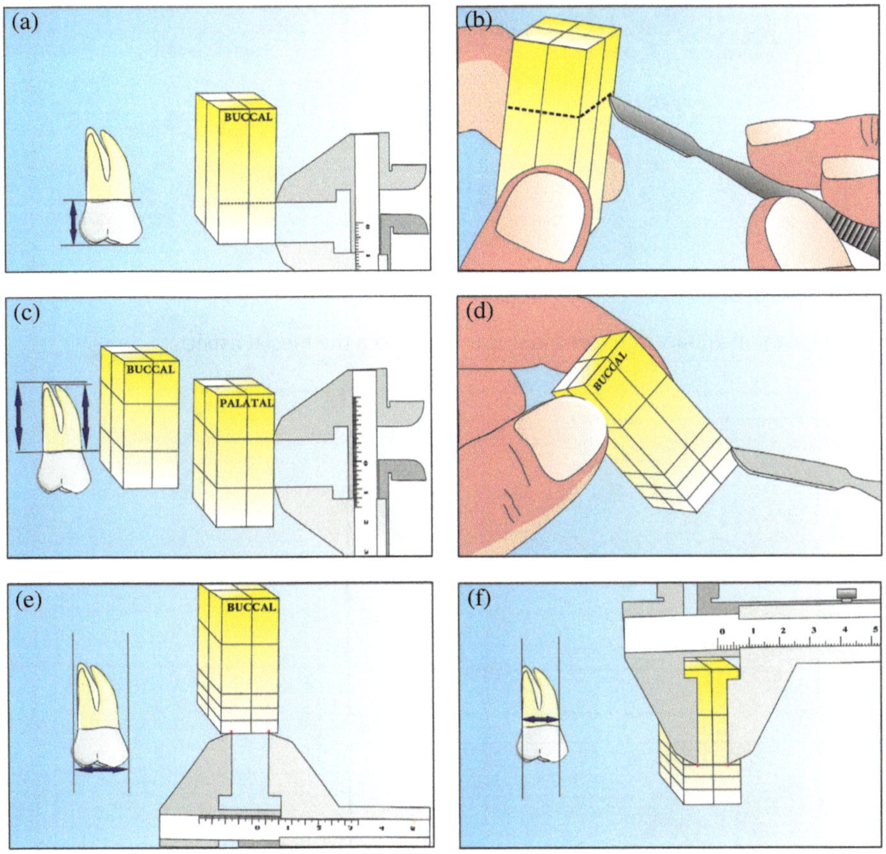

Figure 16.3 (a–f) Measuring and marking the crown dimension and root length on the buccal aspect.

Exercise: Marking the Mesiodistal Dimension on the Buccal Surface

The mesiodistal diameter of the crown of 9.0 mm (4.5 mm on either side of the midline) is marked on the occlusal edge of the buccal surface of the wax block (Figure 16.3e). Then the mesiodistal diameter of the crown at the cervix measuring 7.0 mm (3.5 mm on either side of the midline) is marked at the cervical end of the crown measurement (Figure 16.3f) [1].

Exercise: Marking the Outline and Carving on the Mesial and Distal Side

NOTE: The marking and carving sequence is similar to that followed in the maxillary first molar. Students are directed to refer to Chapter 15 for this particular exercise.

Mesial Aspect

The buccopalatal dimension of crown is the same but the crown length is less than that of the first molar (Figure 16.4a). Outlines and the crest of contour are similar to that of the first molars [1]. The mesial surface is flat [2]. The cusp of Carabelli is absent. The roots are confined within the buccopalatal crown outline (Figure 16.4b). The palatal root is straighter than that of the first molar [3].

Carving from the Mesial Aspect

Exercise: Marking the Buccopalatal Dimension on the Mesial Surface

The buccopalatal diameter of the crown at the cervix measuring 10.0 mm (5.0 mm on either side of the midline) is marked at the cervical end of the crown (Figure 16.5a and b). The buccopalatal diameter of the crown of 11.0 mm (5.5 mm on either side of the midline) is marked on the occlusal edge of the buccal surface of the wax block (Figure 16.5c and d) [1].

Exercise: Marking the Outline and Carving on the Buccal and Palatal Sides

NOTE: The marking and carving sequence is similar to that followed for the maxillary first molar. Students are directed to refer to Chapter 15 for this exercise.

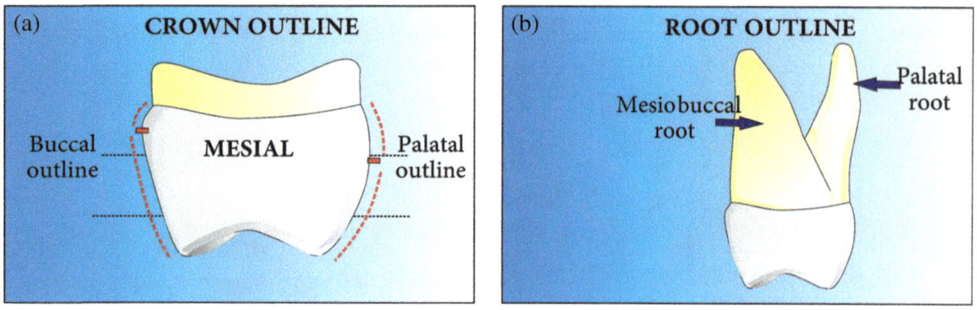

Figure 16.4 (a–b) Descriptive features of the permanent maxillary right second molar tooth from the mesial aspect.

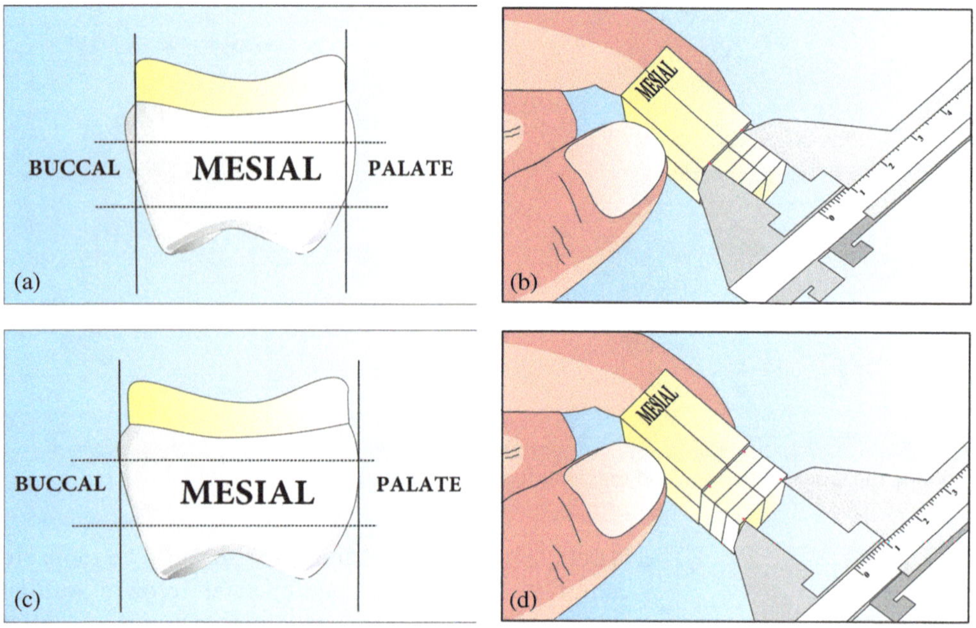

Figure 16.5 (a–d) Measuring and marking the dimension of crown on the mesial aspect of the wax block.

Palatal Aspect

Because of a smaller or nonexistent distopalatal cusp, the crown appears narrower from this aspect. Both the mesiopalatal and distopalatal cusps can be seen (Figure 16.6a) [3]. The fifth cusp is not evident [2]. The crown becomes narrower at the cervical third. There are two types of maxillary second molars based on the number of cusps: the four-cusp type and the three-cusp type. In a majority of cases the four-cusp type is seen, whereas the three-cusp type or tricuspid type is seen in a few cases. In the tricuspid only one large palatal cusp is seen from the palatal aspect and the palatal groove is not seen as much [3, 4]. The palatal root is at a higher level and distally tilted at the apex. Less flaring of the buccal roots is noticed (Figure 16.6b) [1–3].

Distal Aspect

The crown appears narrower buccopalatally towards the distal side, so the buccal and palatal surfaces can be seen from this aspect [3]. Also the distobuccal cusp is smaller than that of the first molar (Figure 16.7a) [1]. The distal marginal ridge is more concave and most of the occlusal surface can be seen (Figure 16.7b). In the tricuspid type of second molar, a single large palatal cusp is seen. The cervical line shows less curvature than the mesial side. The dis-

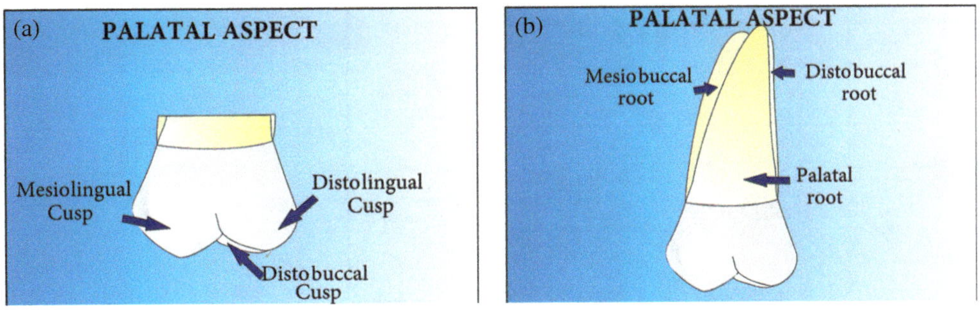

Figure 16.6 (a–b) Description of the permanent maxillary right second molar from the palatal aspect.

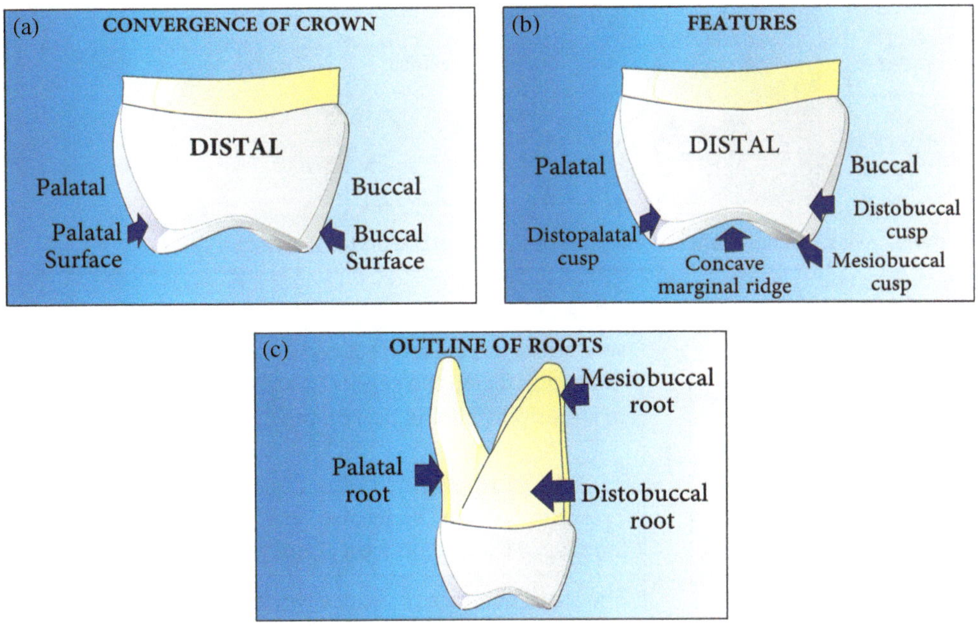

Figure 16.7 (a–c) Description of the permanent maxillary right second molar from the distal aspect.

tobuccal root is shorter and narrower, and therefore the mesiobuccal root can be seen from this aspect. The palatal root shows little curvature compared to that of the first molar (Figure 16.7c) [3].

Occlusal Aspect

From this aspect, the crown is rhomboidal in shape with lesser acute and greater obtuse angle than first molar (Figure 16.8a). The buccopalatal diameter of the crown is the same, but the mesiodistal diameter is less than that of the first molar [1]. There are two types of second maxillary molars, based on the number of cusps. They are the four-cusp (tetracuspid) type and the three-cusp (tricuspid) type [2]. In the tetracuspid type, the cusps in decreasing order of size are mesiopalatal, mesiobuccal, distobuccal, and distopalatal (Figure 16.8b). The buccopalatal length of the crown on the distal part of the crown is less compared to the mesial (Figure 16.8c). The groove pattern in this type resembles an 'H'. In this type the oblique ridge is less frequent, and the height is reduced. In the tricuspid type, the distopalatal cusp is absent [2]. The triangular shape formed by the mesiopalatal, mesiobuccal, and distobuccal cusps is known as the primary cusp triangle [1]. A prominent oblique ridge can be seen in some populations. The groove pattern in this type resembles a 'T', with the distal segment of the letter placed more palatally. Supplemental grooves are often seen (Figure 16.8d) [2].

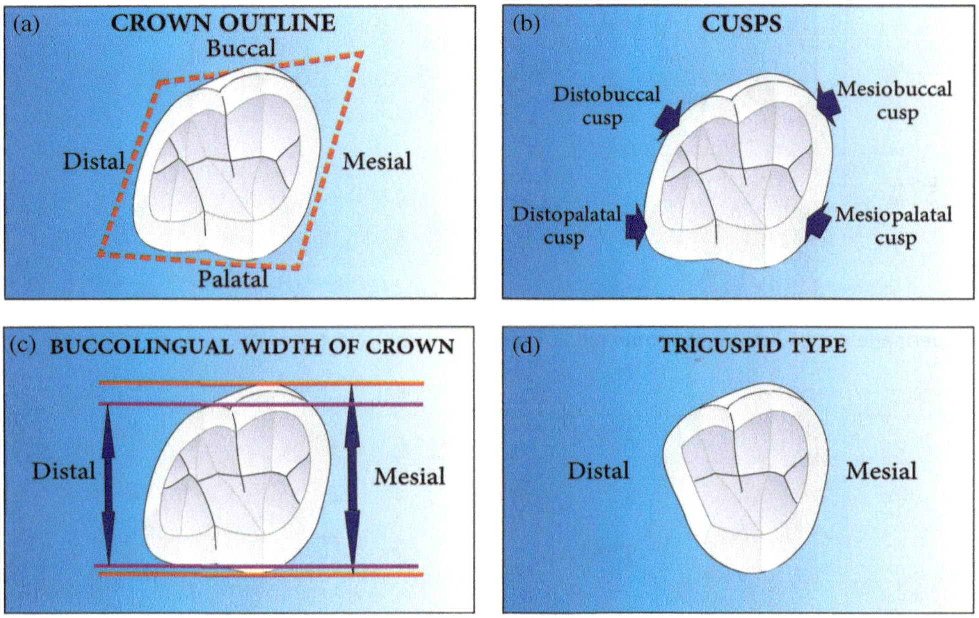

Figure 16.8 (a–d) Description of the permanent maxillary right second molar crown from the occlusal aspect.

Carving from the Occlusal Aspect

Exercise: Carving the Cuspal Ridges, Fossae, and Ridges

Steps for carving the occlusal part of the maxillary second molar crown are similar to that of the maxillary first molar. Students are directed to refer to the occlusal carving section of Chapter 15 for the sequence of steps (Figure 15.8a–x and Figure 15.9a–h).

Exercise: Reducing the Buccopalatal Dimension on the Distal Half of the Crown

Once the crown is carved with features of the maxillary first molar (Figure 16.9a), excess wax is marked on the distal half of the crown to reduce the crown distally (Figure 16.9b). Excess wax is indicated in blue colour.

Exercise: Carving the Excess Wax from the Palatal Surface of the Distopalatal Cusp

The excess wax on the palatal surface of the distopalatal cusp is reduced while maintaining the ridge on the palatal surface of that particular cusp. This is done by carving excess wax while creating mesial and distal slopes (Figure 16.9c–f). The excess wax is carved with the cutting edge of the carver facing the wax and run in an occluso-cervical direction from the occlusal surface to the palatal crest of contour (Figure 16.9c and d). Then the wax below the crest is reduced by placing the back end of the carver facing the cervical part of the wax and moving in a mesiodistal direction on the distopalatal cusp.

Exercise: Carving the Excess Wax from the Buccal Surface of the Distobuccal Cusp

The step sequence to reduce the wax on the buccal surface of the distobuccal cusp is similar to that followed in the previous exercise (Figure 16.9g and h).

Exercise: Carving the Excess Wax from the Distal Surface of the Crown

The excess wax is carved on the distal surface of the crown, with the anterior part of the cutting edge of carver facing the wax and moving in an occluso-cervical direction on the entire distal surface (Figure 16.9i and j).

Carving the Root

The step sequence for carving the root of this (second molar) tooth is similar to that of the maxillary first molar, except for a slight change in the root outline. The root outlines are drawn with their features mentioned earlier in this chapter. Students are directed to the root carving section in Chapter 15.

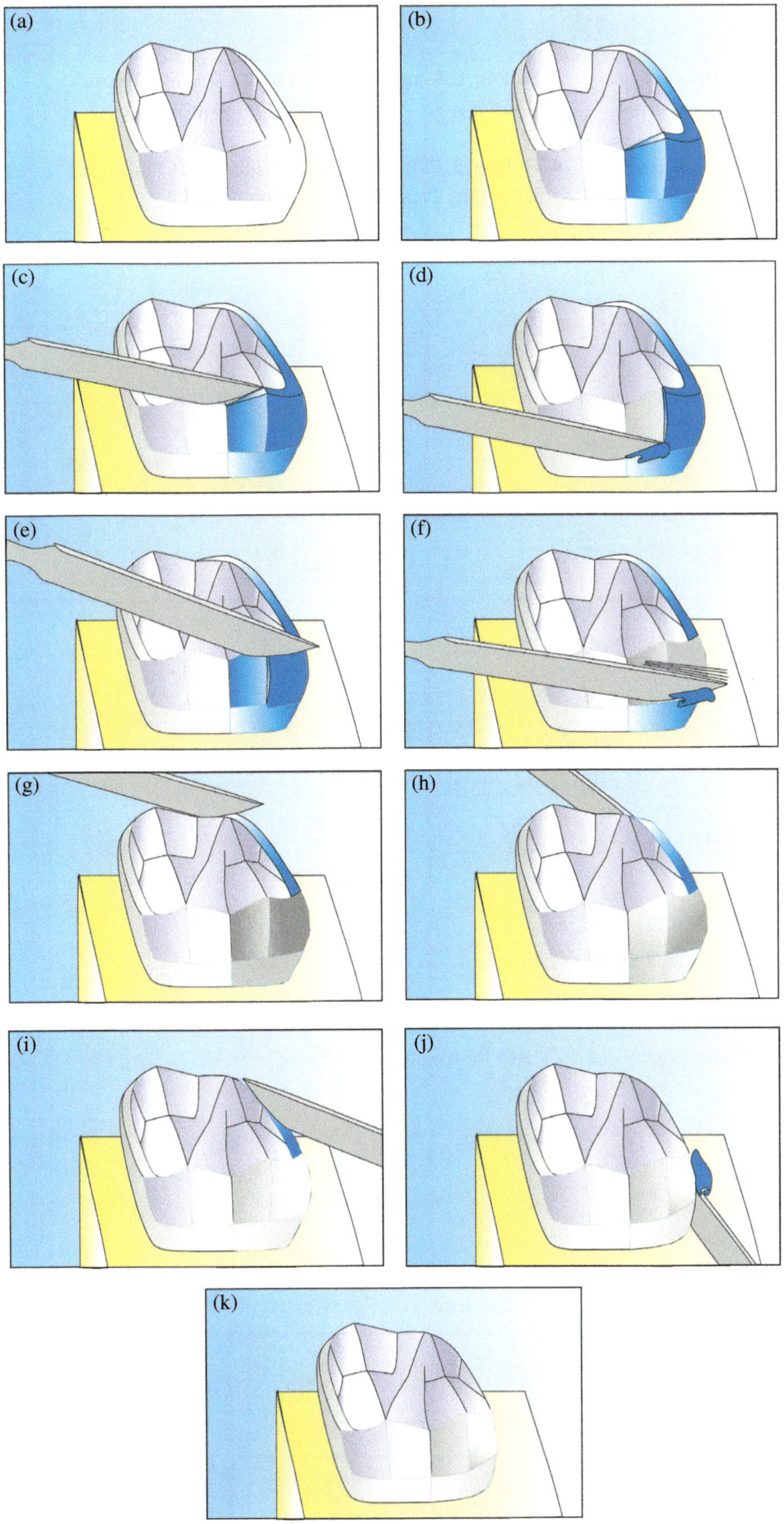

Figure 16.9 (a–k) Creating the distal convergence of buccal and palatal surfaces.

References

1 Stanley, J.N. and Major, M.A.C. (2010). *Wheeler's Dental Anatomy and Occlusion*, 9e. St. Louis, MO: Saunders Elsevier.
2 Luis, E.G., Gabriely, F., Marcelo, B.C. et al. (2019). Morphological differences between upper molars. *Journal of Morphological Sciences* 36: 303–308.
3 Rickne, C.S. and Weiss, G. (2012). *Woelfel's Dental Anatomy*, 8e. Philadelphia: Lippincott Williams & Wilkins.
4 Hillson, S. (2012). *Dental Anthropology*. Cambridge University Press. Kindle Edition.

17

Permanent Mandibular First Molar

LEARNING OBJECTIVE
At the end of the chapter, the student should have knowledge of the permanent mandibular first molar and develop the psychomotor skills for carving and waxing the same.

Permanent Mandibular Right First Molar

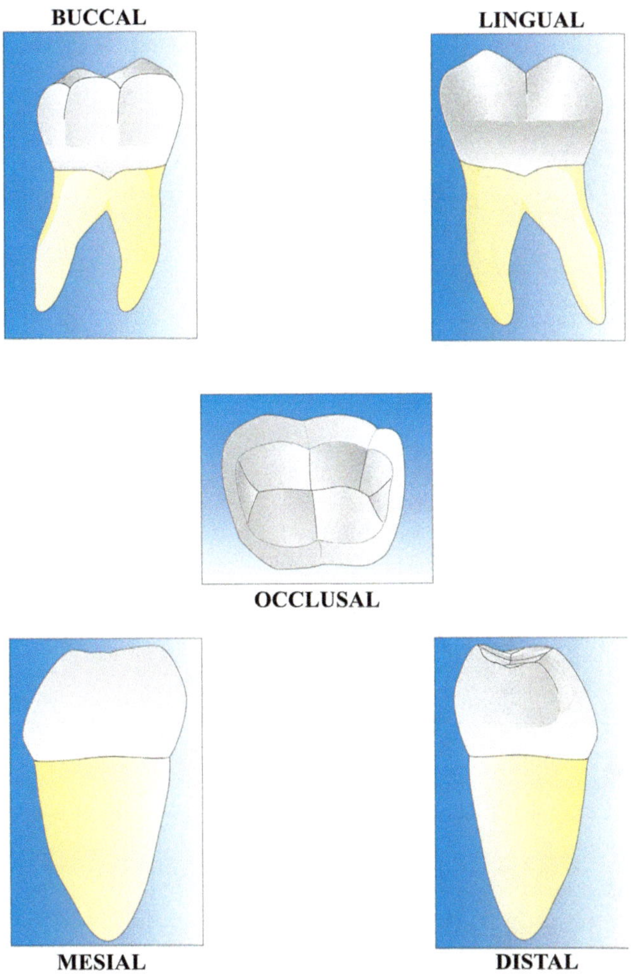

Buccal Aspect

The permanent mandibular right first molar is the sixth tooth from the midline (Figure 17.1). The tooth outline from this aspect appears roughly trapezoidal in shape, with the longer side of the trapezoid represented by the occlusal outline and the shorter by the cervical line (Figure 17.2a) [1–3]. The mesial crest of curvature or mesial contact is at the junction of the occlusal and middle thirds and the distal crest of contour is at the middle of the middle third (Figure 17.2b) [2]. The mesial outline below the contact is concave whereas the distal outline is straight (Figure 17.2c) [1, 3].

From this aspect all five cusps can be seen: two buccal cusps, a part of the distal cusp, and two lingual cusps (Figure 17.2d). Lingual cusps are seen from this aspect due to their higher position [1, 3]. There are two developmental grooves, seen in this aspect. The mesiobuccal developmental groove between the mesiobuccal and distobucal cusps. The distobuccal developmental groove lies between the distobuccal and distal cusps [1–3]. The mesiobuccal groove is shorter than the distobuccal groove, ending exactly at half the length of the crown [1]. The distobuccal groove terminates near the distobuccal line angle at the cervical third or sometimes in the middle third of the crown (Figure 17.2d) [1, 3].

The cuspal ridge of the mesiobuccal and distobuccal cusps has less curvature, with the distal cusp being pointed [2]. The major portion of the buccal surface is formed by the mesiobuccal and distobuccal cusp. The mesiobuccal cusp is the widest cusp, followed by the distobuccal cusp

An Illustrated Atlas of Tooth Carving and Wax-Up Techniques, First Edition. Anil Bangalore Shivappa.

Companion website: www.wiley.com/go/bangalore/toothcarving

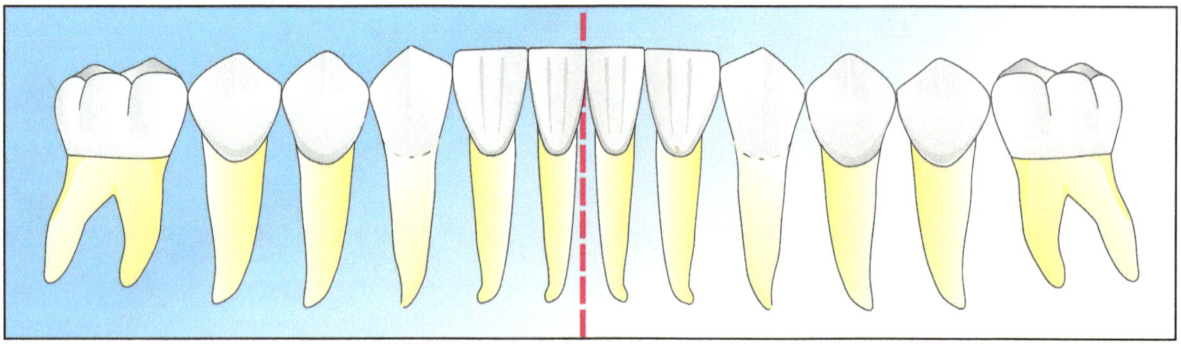

Figure 17.1 Position of the permanent mandibular first molar in relation to the midsagittal plane.

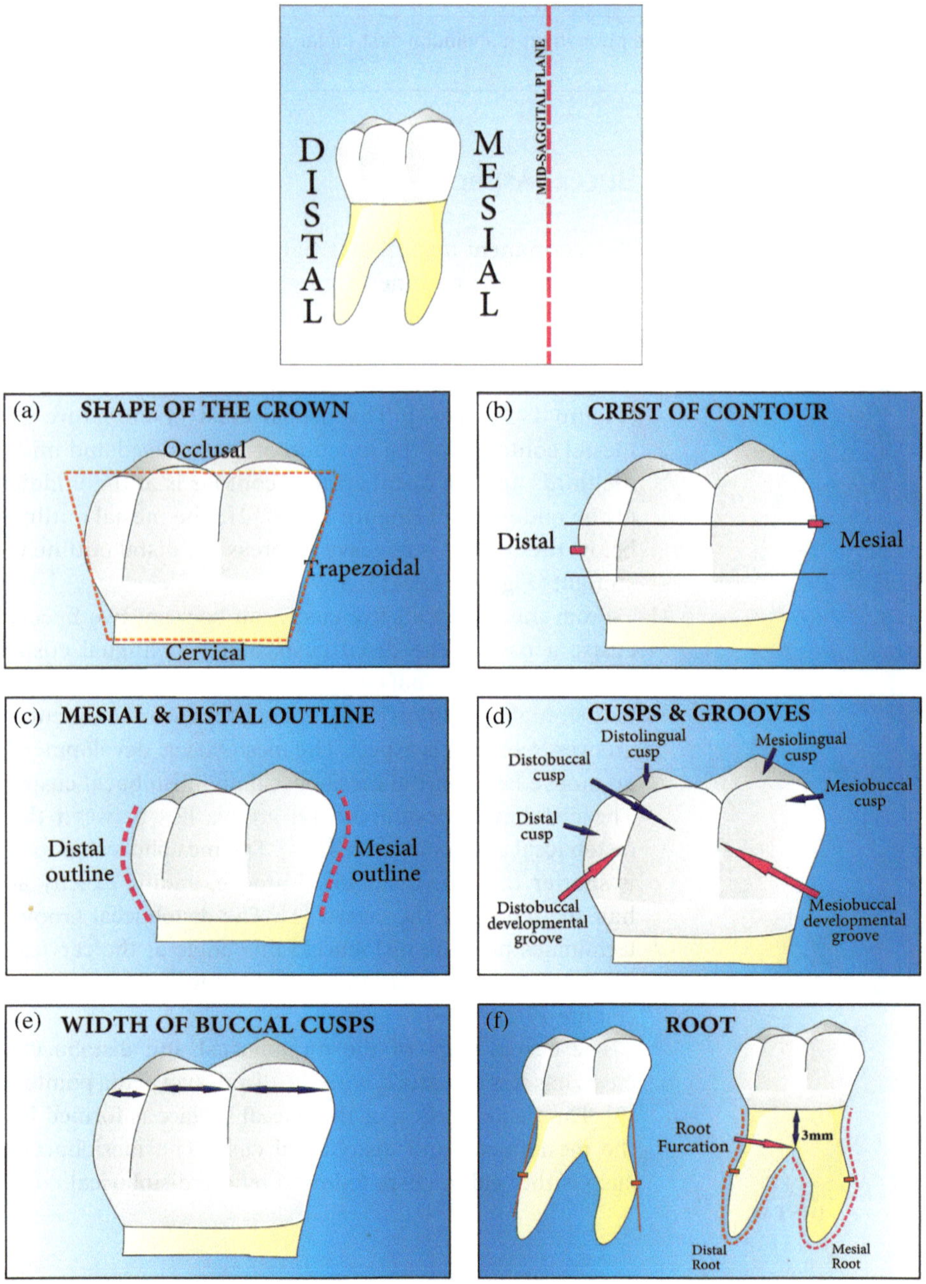

Figure 17.2 (a–f) Descriptive features of permanent mandibular right first molar from the buccal aspect.

and then the distal cusp (Figure 17.2e). The surface of the crown is smooth and convex. The cervical line dips towards the root bifurcation [1–3]. The buccogingival ridge is the prominent mesiobuccal convexity at the cervical third of the buccal surface of crown. This is more commonly seen on the mesial side [4].

The mesial root curves mesially from the cervical line to the mesial crest of curvature. The crest of curvature of the root is in the middle third of the root and mesial to the crown cervix. From this point, the root curves distally to the tapered apex, which is located directly below the mesiobuccal cusp [1].

The distal outline of the mesial root is concave from the bifurcation of the root apex (Figure 17.2f).

The distal root curves distally from the cervix to the root apex. The root curves at its apical third either in mesial or distal direction. The apex of distal root is more pointed than the mesial root and is distal to the distal contact area of the crown (Figure 17.2f) [1, 2]. The root furcation is near the cervical line, starting approximately about 3 mm from the cervical line (Figure 17.2f) [1, 2, 5]. Because of this the root trunk appears shorter than that of the maxillary molar [2, 6].

Lingual Aspect

From this aspect the crown appears narrower [2, 3]. Two lingual cusps and a part of the distal cusp can be seen (Figure 17.3a). Because the lingual cusps are placed at the higher level, the buccal cusps cannot be seen from this aspect [1]. Of the two lingual cusps, the mesolingual cusp is wider and at a higher level than the distolingual cusp (Figure 17.3b) [2, 3]. The two lingual cuspal ridges meet at an obtuse angle [1]. The lingual developmental groove separates the two lingual cusps and extends lingually for a shorter distance to the junction of the occlusal and middle third (Figure 17.3a) [3]. It has the convex mesial outline from the cervix to the marginal ridge. The distal outline is straight above the crest of contour (Figure 17.3c). The mesial crest of contour is at a higher level than the distal crest [1, 3].

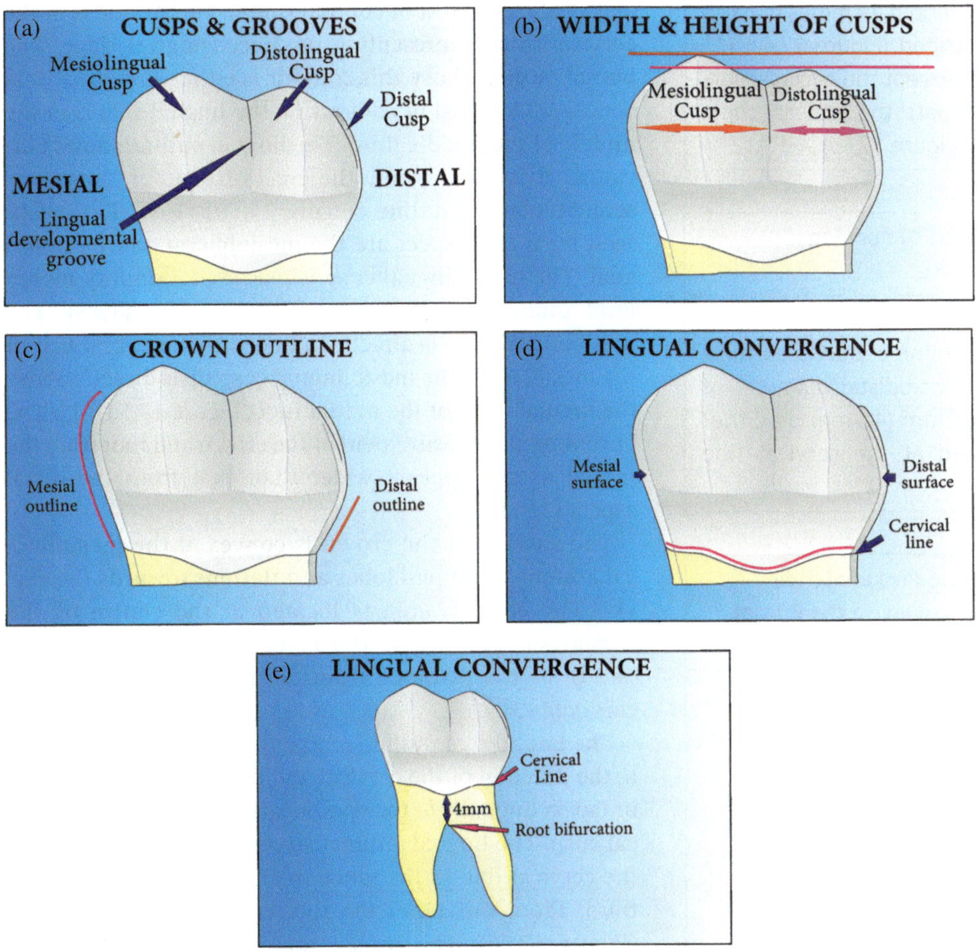

Figure 17.3 (a–e) Description of the permanent mandibular right first molar from the lingual aspect.

The cervical line in this aspect is shorter and is placed at a higher level than that of the buccal [3]. The cervical line dips sharply towards the root bifurcation (Figure 17.3d) [1]. Due to the lingual convergence, the mesial and distal surfaces of the crown and root trunks can be seen from this aspect (Figure 17.3d) [1, 2].

The root trunk appears longer than that of the buccal side and the root appears 1 mm longer than that of the buccal aspect, due to the higher position of the cusps and cervical line from the lingual aspect [1, 2, 6]. Lingually the root bifurcates about 4 mm below the cervical line (Figure 17.3e) [1].

Carving on the Buccal Aspect

Exercise: Marking the Length of the Crown and the Root

After preparation of the wax block by smoothing the surface and drawing the midlines to divide the surfaces into two equal parts, the cervico-occlusal measurement of about 7.5 mm is marked on the buccal surface (Figure 17.4a). The same measurement is also taken on the lingual, mesial, and distal surfaces (Figure 17.4b). In a similar way, the length of root of about 14 mm is marked on the surfaces previously described (Figure 17.4c) [1]. Then each surface of the crown, except the occlusal surface, is divided into three equal part: the occlusal third, middle third, and cervical third (Figure 17.4d).

Exercise: Marking the Mesiodistal Dimension of the Crown on the Buccal Surface

The mesiodistal diameter of the crown about 11 mm (5.5 mm on either side of the midline of buccal surface) is marked (Figure 17.4e). The mesiodistal diameter of the crown at the cervix about 9 mm (4.5 mm on either side of the midline) is marked at the cervical line (Figure 17.4f) [1].

Exercise: Reduction of Wax on the Proximal Side and Marking the Outline of the Crown on the Buccal Surfaces of the Wax Block

After marking the reference points for the dimensions (Figure 17.4g), the points are then joined on the mesial (Figure 17.4h) and distal (Figure 17.4i) sides to get the outer dimension of the crown within which the crown is carved (Figure 17.4j). Excess wax is then carved out on both the mesial and distal surfaces (Figure 17.4k). Then the mesial and distal outline of the crown is drawn with the features described (Figure 17.4l).

Exercise: Carving the Excess Wax from Mesial and Distal Side of Outline

Excess wax outside the mesial outline (Figure 17.4m) is carved in two steps. The wax above the mesial crest of contour is carved with the anterior part of the cutting edge of the carver facing excess wax (Figure 17.4n). The carver is then moved in a buccolingual direction until the outline is reached (Figure 17.4o). Excess wax below the contact, that is, the middle and the cervical third, is carved with the non-cutting end of the carver facing the wax and the tip of the carver at the cervix (Figure 17.4p). The carver is moved in the same direction as mentioned previously (Figure 17.4q). Wax on the distal side is carved out above and below the contact, with the steps mentioned (Figure 17.4r).

Mesial Aspect

The crown appears rhomboidal in shape (Figure 17.5a) [3]. From this aspect two cusps and one root can be seen. The crown appears to tilt lingually in relation to the root axis [1, 3]. The crest of contour on the buccal side is in the cervical third, representing the buccogingival ridge. The buccal outline above this contour is either straight or less concave. The crest of contour on the lingual side is in the middle of the middle third. The lingual outline shows curvature above and below the crest of contour, appearing semicircular in outline (Figure 17.5b) [1–3]. Two cusps seen from this aspect are the mesiobuccal and mesiolingual. The mesiolingual cusp is placed at a slightly higher level than the mesiobuccal (Figure 17.5c) [1, 3]. The mesiobuccal cusp is directly in line with the buccal half of the mesial root. The mesiolingual cusp tip is directly above the lingual third of the mesial root (Figure 17.5d) [1]. The buccolingual measurement of the crown and root from the mesial aspect appears wider than that from the distal aspect [2].

The surface of the crown is convex at the mesiobuccal and mesiolingual lobes and flattens towards the cervix. The contact area is located at the centre of the mesial surface, below the marginal ridge crest about one third the distance from the marginal ridge to the cervix [1–3].

The buccal root outline is straight from the cervical line to the junction of the cervical and middle third and curves or tapers lingually to the apex located below the mesiobuccal cusp. The lingual outline curves buccally directly from the cervical line to the junction of the middle and apical third. From this point the root curves abruptly, bucally (Figure 17.5e). The mesial root is flat and shows the

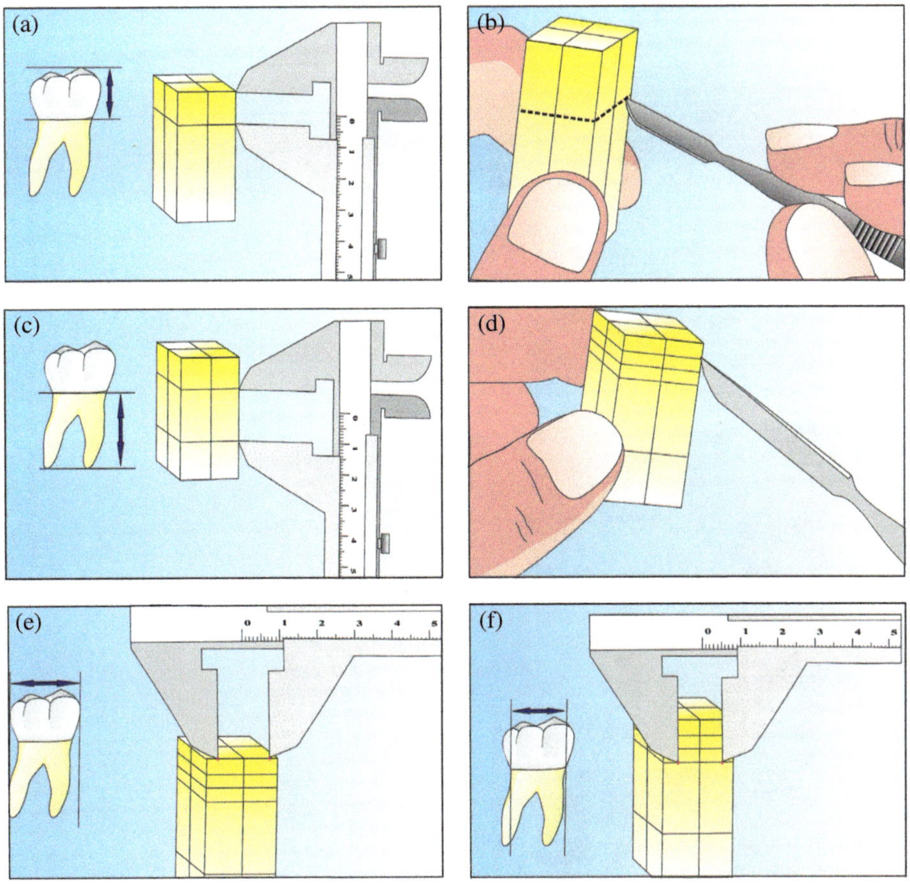

Figure 17.4 (a–f) Measuring and marking the crown dimension and root length on the buccal aspect of the wax block.

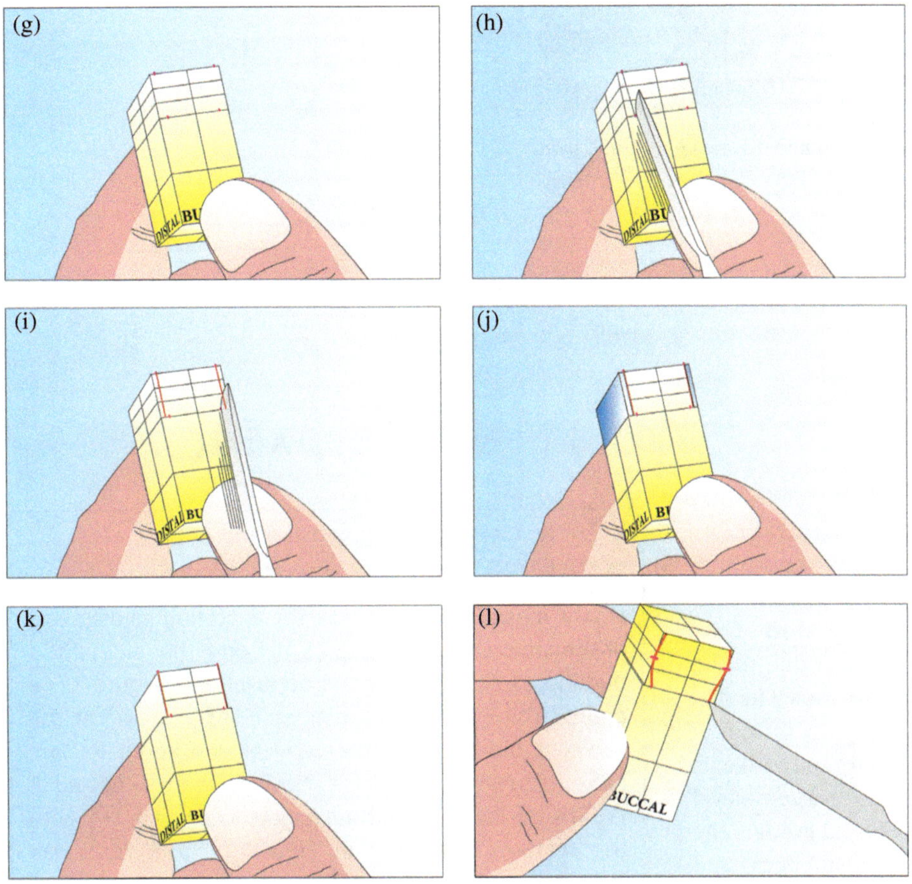

Figure 17.4 (g–l) Marking and carving the dimension and marking outline of the crown from the buccal aspect.

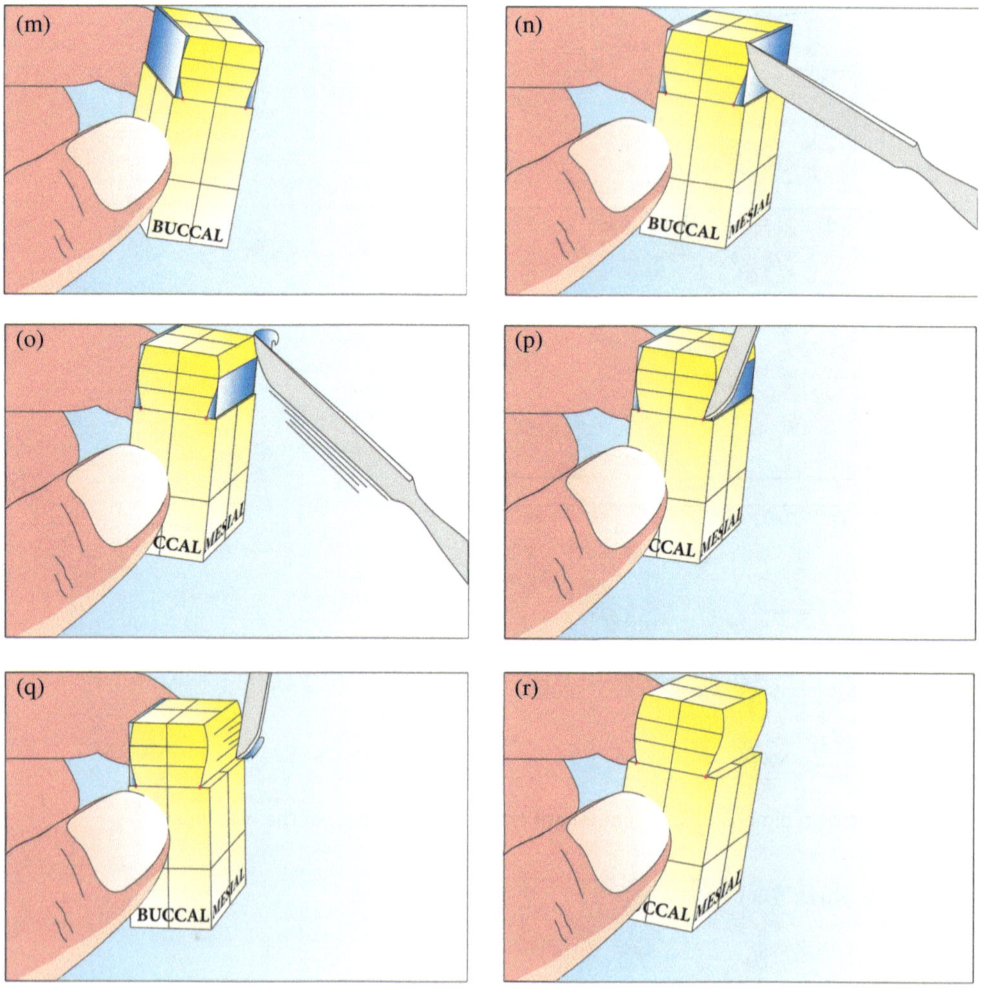

Figure 17.4 (m–r) Carving excess wax from mesial and distal side of the crown.

presence of deep developmental depression with the longitudinal groove [2, 4].

Distal Aspect

From this aspect, the outline of the tooth resembles that of the mesial aspect. But the crown appears narrower distally because of the convergence of buccal and lingual surfaces of the crown distally, the buccal being more convergent than the lingual (Figure 17.5f) [1, 3]. Most of the occlusal surface can be seen from this aspect due to the distal tilt or inclination of the crown on the root. The distal cusp seen from this aspect is placed slightly buccal to the centre of the crown. The distal marginal ridge is shorter. The cervical line shows little curvature compared to the mesial. The distobuccal developmental groove, the convex part of the buccal surface of the distobuccal and distal cusps, can be seen. The root also appears narrower than mesial. The lingual border of the mesial root may be seen from the distal aspect (Figure 17.5g) [1–3].

Carving from the Mesial Aspect

Exercise: Marking the Dimension and Outline of the Crown

On the mesial side of the wax, the buccolingual diameter of the crown of 10.5 mm (5.25 mm on either side of the midline) is marked near the occlusal end (Figure 17.6a and b). The buccolingual diameter of the crown at the cervix is marked near the cervical end about 9.0 mm (4.5 mm on either side of the midline; Figure 17.6c and d) [1]. The buccolingual outline (Figure 17.6e) is drawn with the features described in Figure 17.5b. Excess wax indicated in blue colour is carved out.

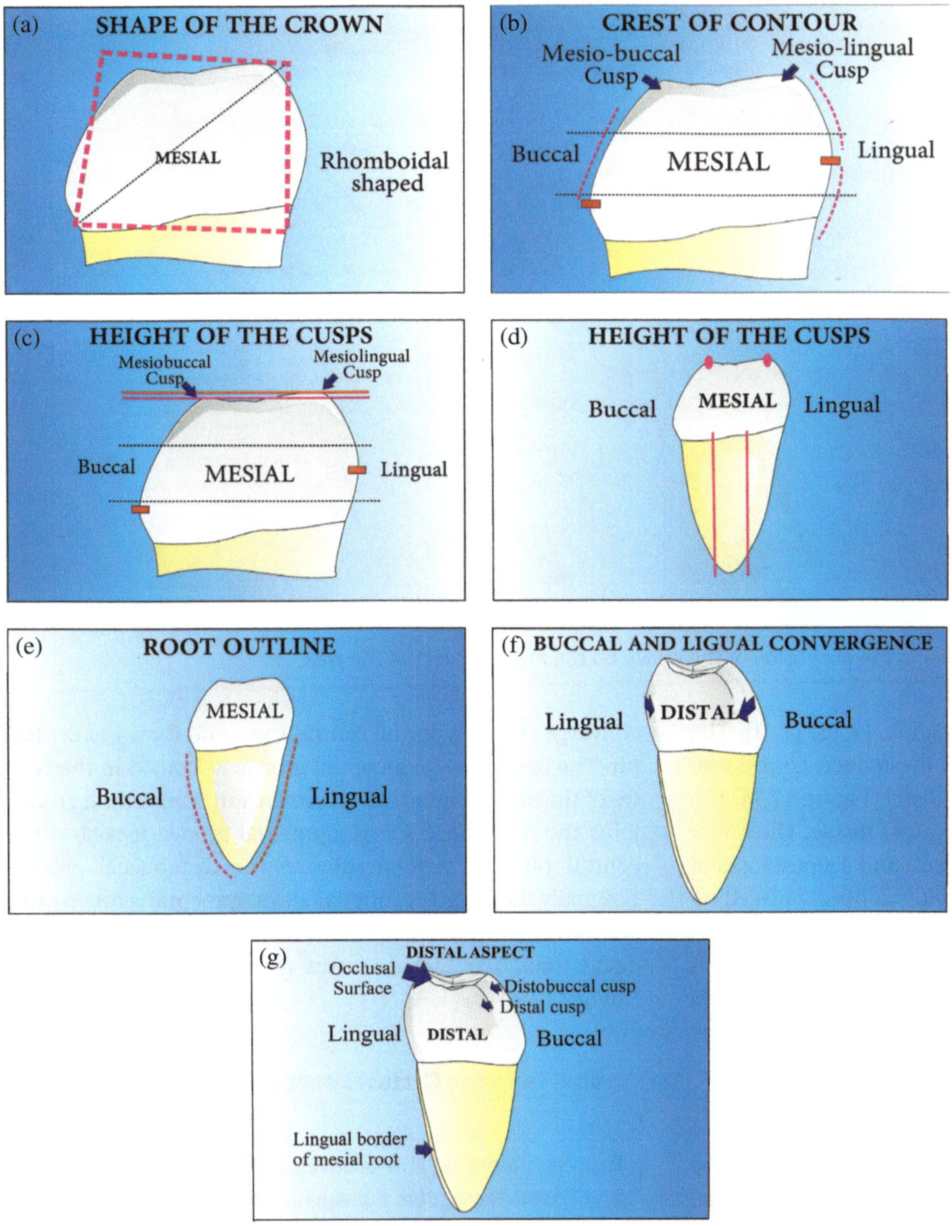

Figure 17.5 (a–g) Descriptive features of the permanent mandibular right first molar tooth from the mesial and distal aspects.

Exercise: Carving the Wax to Obtain the Lingual Outline

Because the crest of contour of the lingual outline is in the middle of the middle third, the curved part of the cutting edge of the carver is placed above it, facing the wax (Figure 17.6f). The carver is then moved in the mesiodistal direction until the lingual outline is reached (Figure 17.6g). The excess wax below the lingual crest of contour is carved by using the anterior part of the non-cutting side of the carver facing the wax (Figure 17.6h). The carver is then moved in the same direction as described previously (Figure 17.6i).

Exercise: Carving the Wax to Obtain the Buccal Outline

The excess wax on the buccal side, above (Figure 17.6j and k) and below (Figure 17.6l and m) the crest is carved in a similar manner as that done for the lingual surface (Figure 17.6n).

Occlusal Aspect

The tooth appears pentagonal in shape [2, 3]. The crown is greater mesiodistally than buccolingually [1–4]. The bucco-lingual measurement of the crown is greater on the mesial than on the distal side (Figure 17.7f). The crown converges

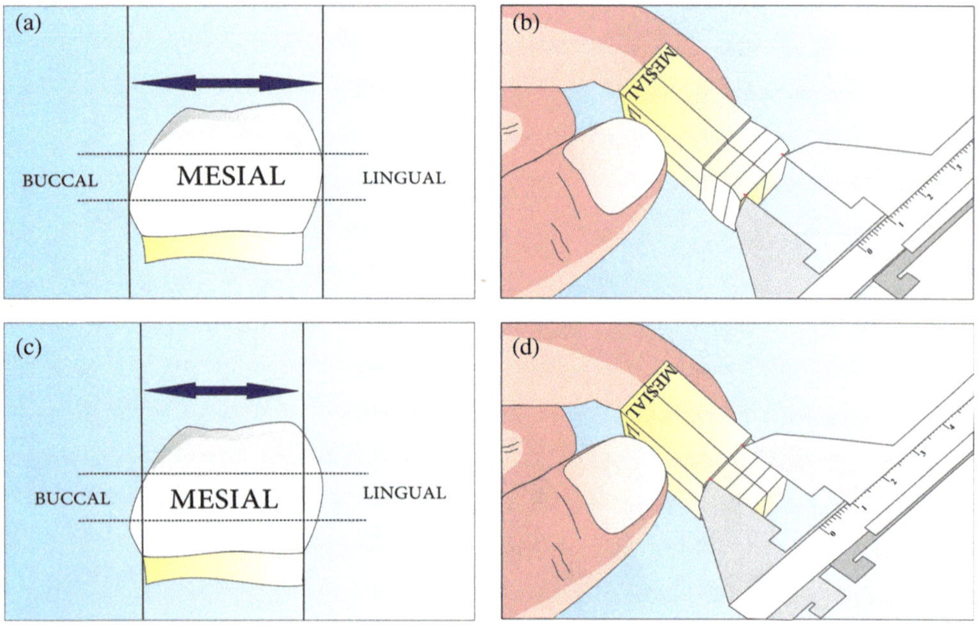

Figure 17.6 (a–d) Measuring and marking the dimension of the crown on the mesial aspect of the wax.

lingually from the contact areas (Figure 17.7g) [1, 2]. The cusps in decreasing order of size are mesiobuccal, mesiolingual, distolingual, distobuccal, and distal (Figure 17.7a) [3].

There is one major fossa and two minor fossae. The major fossa is the central fossa. It is the largest and deepest fossa of the three. It is roughly circular, and it is centrally placed on the occlusal surface between the buccal and lingual cuspal ridges. The central fossa is bounded buccally by the slopes of the distobuccal cusp, the mesial slope of the distal cusp, and the distal slope of the mesiobuccal cusp. Lingually the central fossa is bounded by the mesial slope of the distolingual cusp and the distal slope of the mesiolingual cusp. Mesiodistally the central fossa is bounded by the triangular ridges of all the major cusps [1, 3]. The two minor fossae are the *mesial triangular fossa*, immediately distal to the mesial marginal ridge, and the *distal triangular fossa*, immediately mesial to the distal marginal ridge (Figure 17.7b and c) [1].

The mesial triangular fossa is smaller than the central fossa and deeper than the distal triangular fossa. It bounded by the mesial marginal ridge, the mesial slope of the mesiobuccal cusp, and the mesiolingual cusp. The mesial part of the central groove unites with the buccal and lingual supplemental groove of the mesial fossa and forms the mesial pit [1–3].

The distal triangular fossa is the smallest fossa, bounded by the distal slope of the distal and distolingual cusps, the distal marginal ridge. The central groove terminates distally in this fossa [1–3].

The developmental grooves on the occlusal surface are the *central developmental groove*, the mesiobuccal developmental groove, the distobuccal developmental groove, and the lingual developmental groove. All developmental grooves converge centrally in the central fossa and form the central pit. The central developmental groove is located in the centre of the buccolingual crown dimension. The central groove joins the mesiobuccal developmental groove mesial to the central pit and distobuccally to the distobuccal groove. Lingually it joins the lingual developmental groove. The central developmental groove, before terminating in the distal triangular fossa, courses in a distolingual direction (Figure 17.7d–e) [1, 3].

Carving from the Occlusal Aspect

Exercise: Marking the Grooves and Carving the Mesial and Distal Triangular Fossae

After drawing the outline of grooves on the occlusal surface with the features mentioned, the carving step begins with the mesial and distal fossae. The fossa is carved by moving the tip of the carver along the buccal groove to the pit. The back of the carver (non-cutting edge) of the carver should be facing the wax. As the carver is moved towards the pit, force is applied by the carver on the wax to go deeper. Then the carver is moved towards the end of the lingual groove in the fossa (Figure 17.8a). During the latter movement, the carver is pulled outwards to surface from the deeper pit, so that the triangular depression is created (Figure 17.8b). While carving, the lower border or non-cutting end of the carver is angled from the occlusal surface of the wax. The fossa on the distal side is carved in a similar way as described for the mesial side.

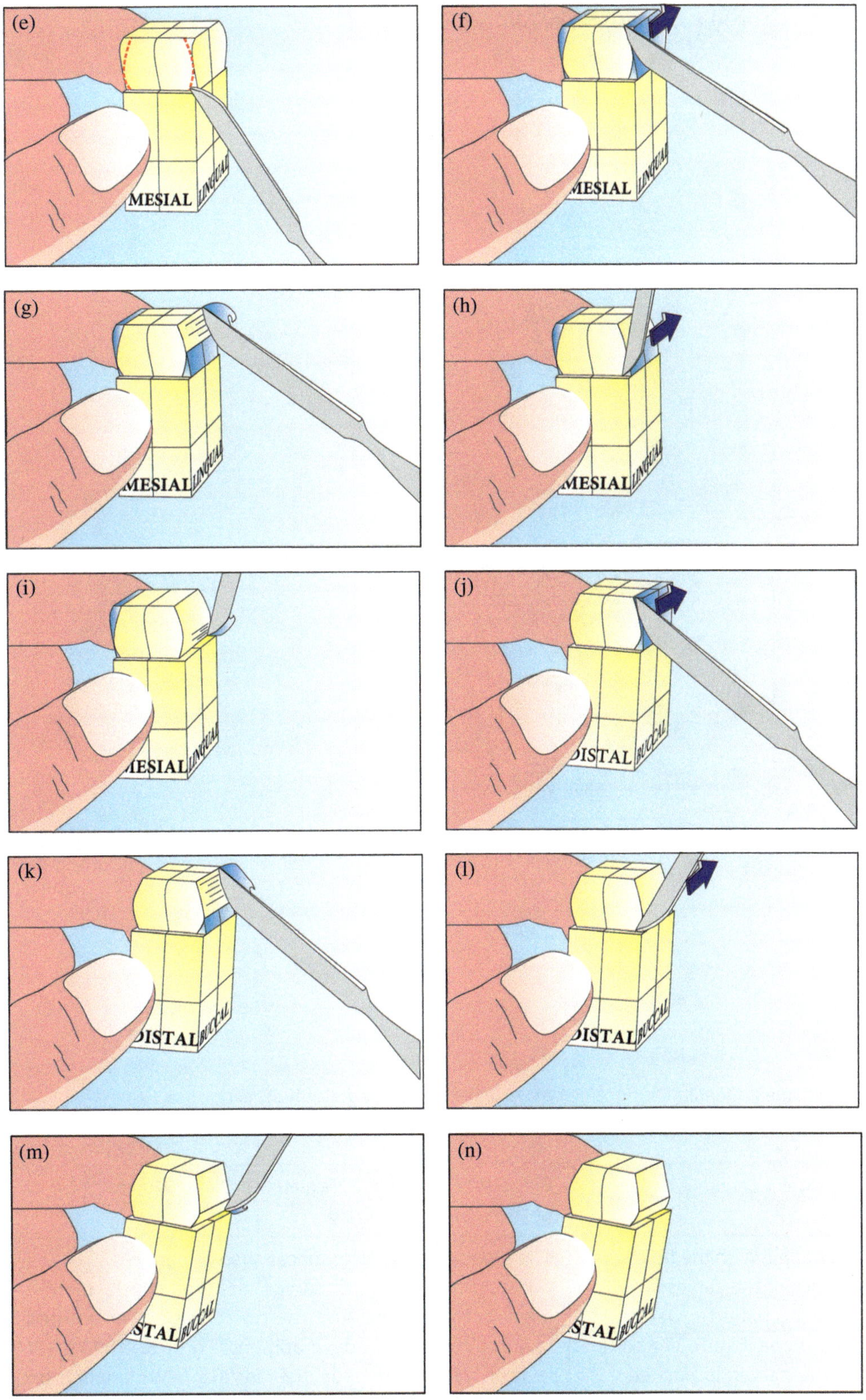

Figure 17.6 (e–n) Drawing the crown outline and carving excess wax from the buccal and lingual surfaces.

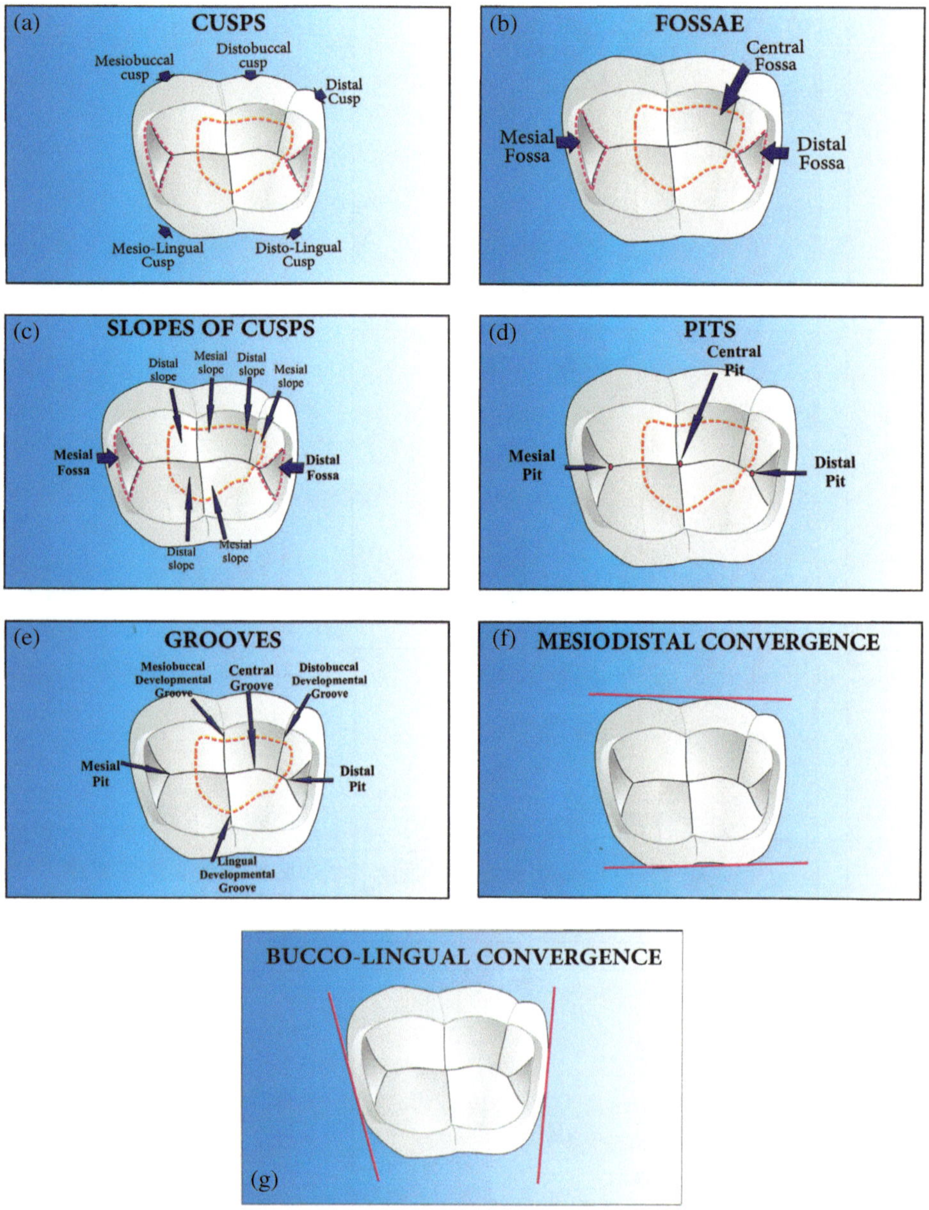

Figure 17.7 (a–g) Description of the permanent mandibular right first molar crown from the occlusal aspect.

Exercise: Carving the Mesial and Distal Slopes of the Mesiobuccal Cusp

The carving is initiated from the mesial pit. With the tip of the carver deep at the pit and the back of the carver facing the wax with at an angle, the carver is pulled upwards to the surface to complete the mesial slope (Figure 17.8c). Without altering the angulation, the carver is pushed deeper into the wax to create the distal slope that ends deep in area mesial to the central pit (Figure 17.8d).

With the formation of the mesial and distal slopes, the mesiobuccal triangular ridge is created. The triangular ridge is then smoothed so as to create the rounded cusp.

Exercise: Carving the Mesial and Distal Slopes of the Distobuccal Cusp

The slopes of the distobuccal cusp are carved with the non-cutting edge of carver at the depth of the mesiobuccal groove and the tip of the carver pointed towards the central developmental groove. The carver is then pulled towards the surface with angulation (Figure 17.8e). From here, the carver is pushed deep into the wax to the deepest point, where the distobuccal groove originates (Figure 17.8f).

Exercise: Carving the Distal Cusp

From the deep point on the distobuccal groove, the distal cusp is carved in a similar way as done for the mesiobuccal and distobuccal cusps (Figure 17.8g).

Exercise: Carving the Mesial and Distal Slopes of the Distolingual Cusp

The distolingual cusp is carved starting from the distal pit with the back of the carver facing the wax at the lingual groove of the distal fossa. The carver is moved towards the surface (Figure 17.8h) and then towards the central pit. The distolingual cusp is completed by moving the carver from the central pit along the lingual groove (Figure 17.8i).

Exercise: Carving the Mesial and Distal Slopes of the Mesiolingual Cusp

The mesiolingual cusp is carved starting from the central pit, moving towards the surface (Figure 17.8j) and then to the mesial pit (Figure 17.8k).

Exercise: Creating the Ridges on the Buccal and Lingual Surfaces

The ridges are created on the buccal and lingual surfaces (Figure 17.8m and n). The concavity of the marginal ridges is created on both the mesial (Figure 17.8o) and distal sides. Excess wax remaining on the distal side is carved out (Figure 17.8p and q) to complete the crown (Figure 17.8r).

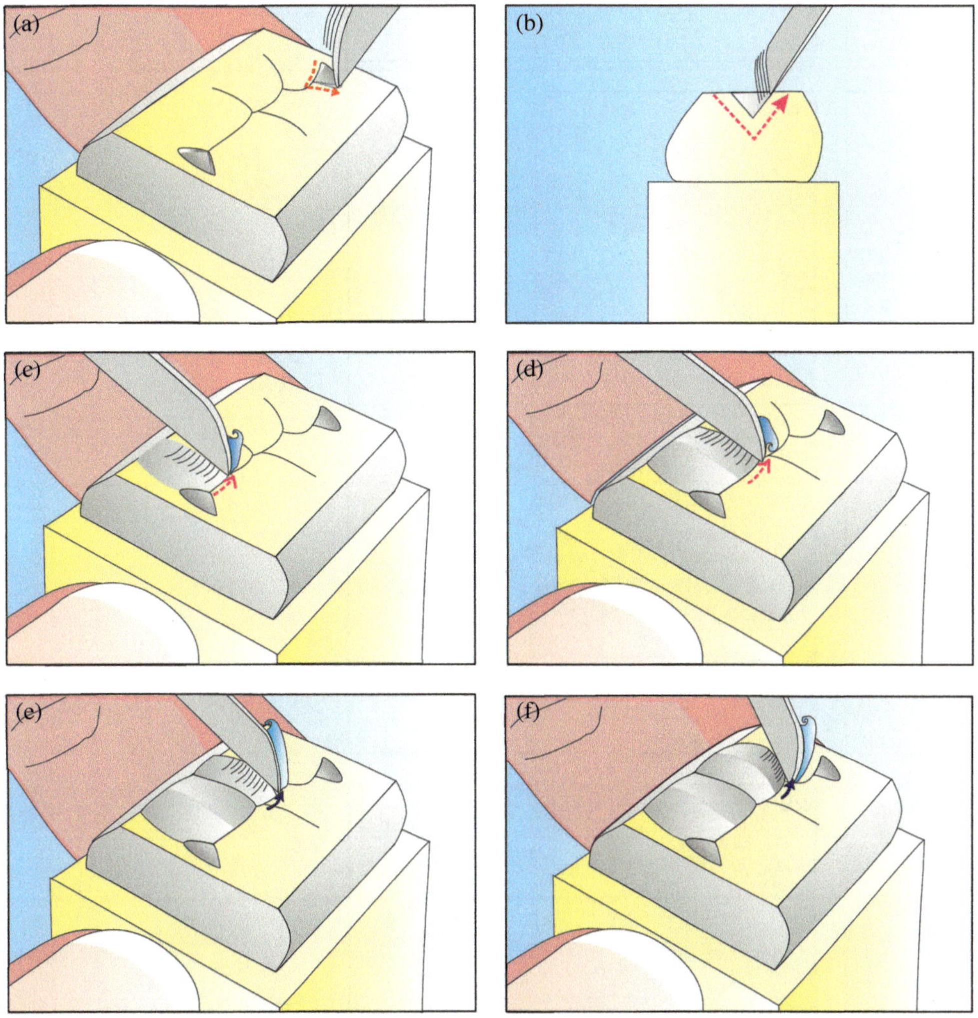

Figure 17.8 (a–r) Carving the occlusal features (cusps, their ridges, fossae, and grooves) and ridges on the buccal and lingual surfaces of the permanent mandibular right first molar.

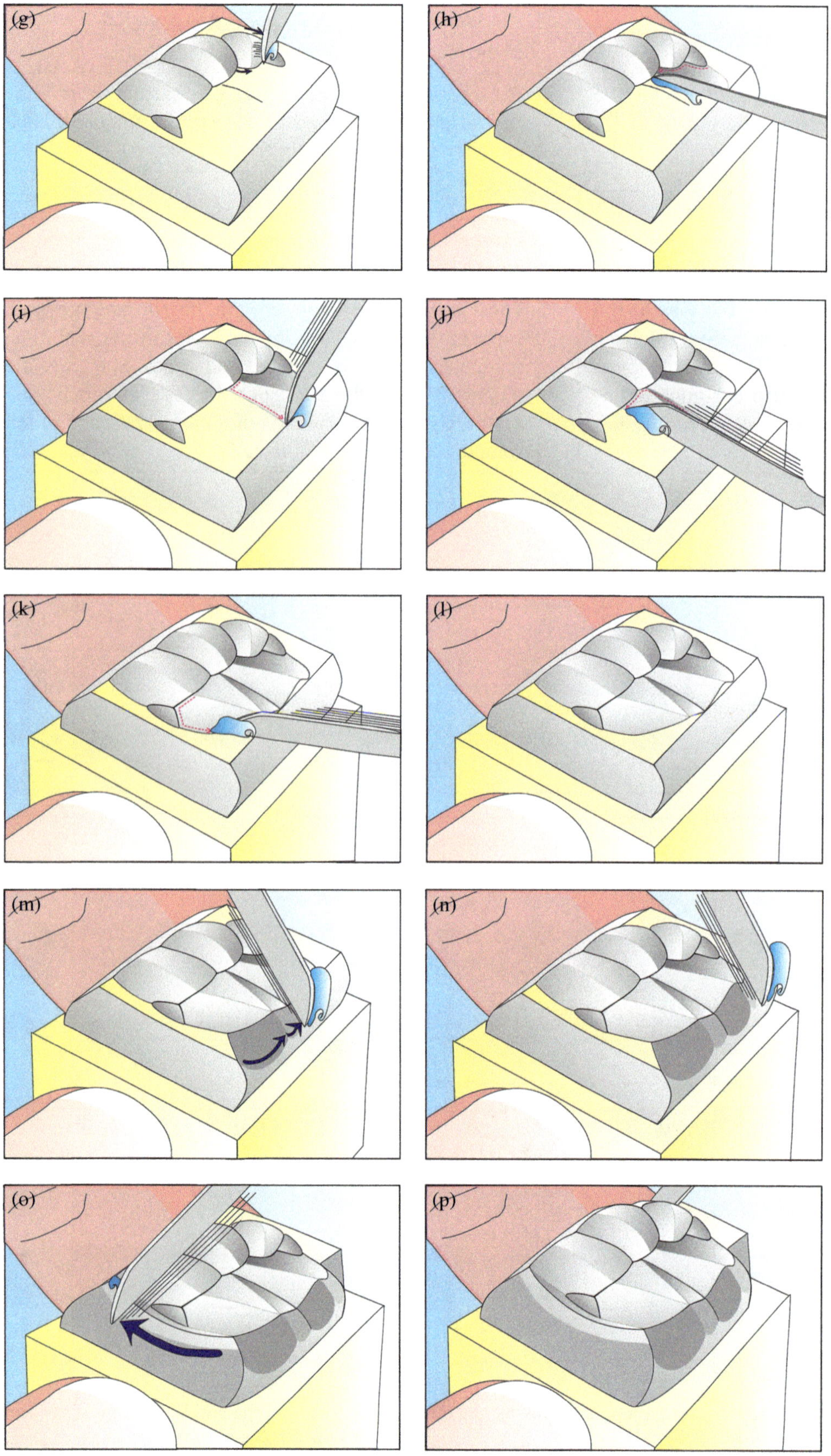

Figure 17.8 (Cont'd) (a–r)

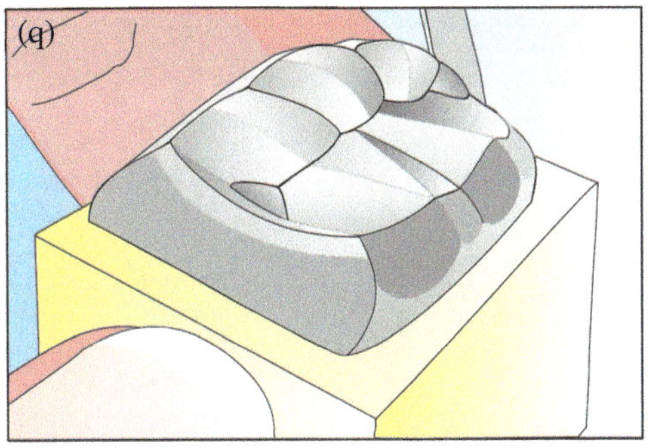

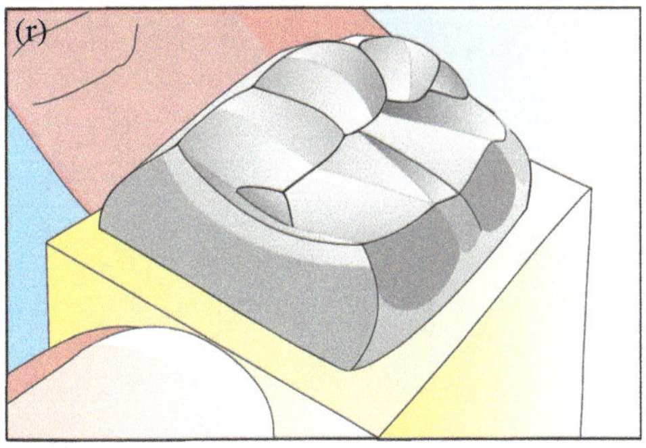

Figure 17.8 (Cont'd) (a–r)

Carving the Roots

Exercise: Carving the Roots from the Buccal Aspect

The outline of the mesial and distal roots (Figure 17.9a) is drawn with the features mentioned. The excess wax indicated in blue colour is carved from the sides and from the furcation (Figure 17.9b). The concavity on the mesial root surface is created by placing the curved or convex part of the carver facing the surface of excess wax (Figure 17.9c). The carver is then moved unidirectional from the buccal to the lingual, until the outline is reached (Figure 17.9d). The wax near the root apex is carved using the back of the carver facing the wax and the tip of the carver facing the apex (Figure 17.9e). The carver is then moved in the direction mentioned earlier (Figure 17.9f). The remaining wax is carved in a similar manner (Figure 17.9g and h). The excess wax on the distal side is also carved using techniques near the concavities and convexities already mentioned (Figure 17.9h).

Exercise: Carving at the Furcal Portion

The wax near the furcation area is carved by moving the anterior part of the carver along all the borders – distal outline of mesial root (Figure 17.9k and l), mesial outline of distal root (Figure 17.9i and j), and outline between the root apex, until the lingual surface is reached. Once the lingual surface on the other side is reached, the wax from the furcal area is carved (Figure 17.9m and n).

Exercise: Carving the Roots from the Proximal (Distal) Aspect

From the distal aspect, the outline of the root is drawn (Figure 17.9o). The excess wax on the buccal side is carved beginning at the cervical third, with the anterior part of the carver facing the wax and moved in a mesiodistal direction (Figure 17.9p). Then the wax on the middle and apical third on the distal root is carved using the anterior part of the carver, moving the carver cervico-apically (Figure 17.9q and r). The same step is repeated on the mesial root (Figure 17.9s and t). Once the root is completed, developmental depressions are created on the mesial and distal surface of the root. After the outline is drawn, the excavating end of the carver is moved cervico-apically (Figure 17.9u–w), deeper at the centre of the root and shallow near the periphery of the outline (Figure 17.9x).

Exercise: Carving the Cervical Line

At the end of the carving, the cervical line is drawn with the features mentioned. The curvature of the cervical line towards the occlusal surface on the mesial side is 1 mm and on distal side is 0 mm [1].

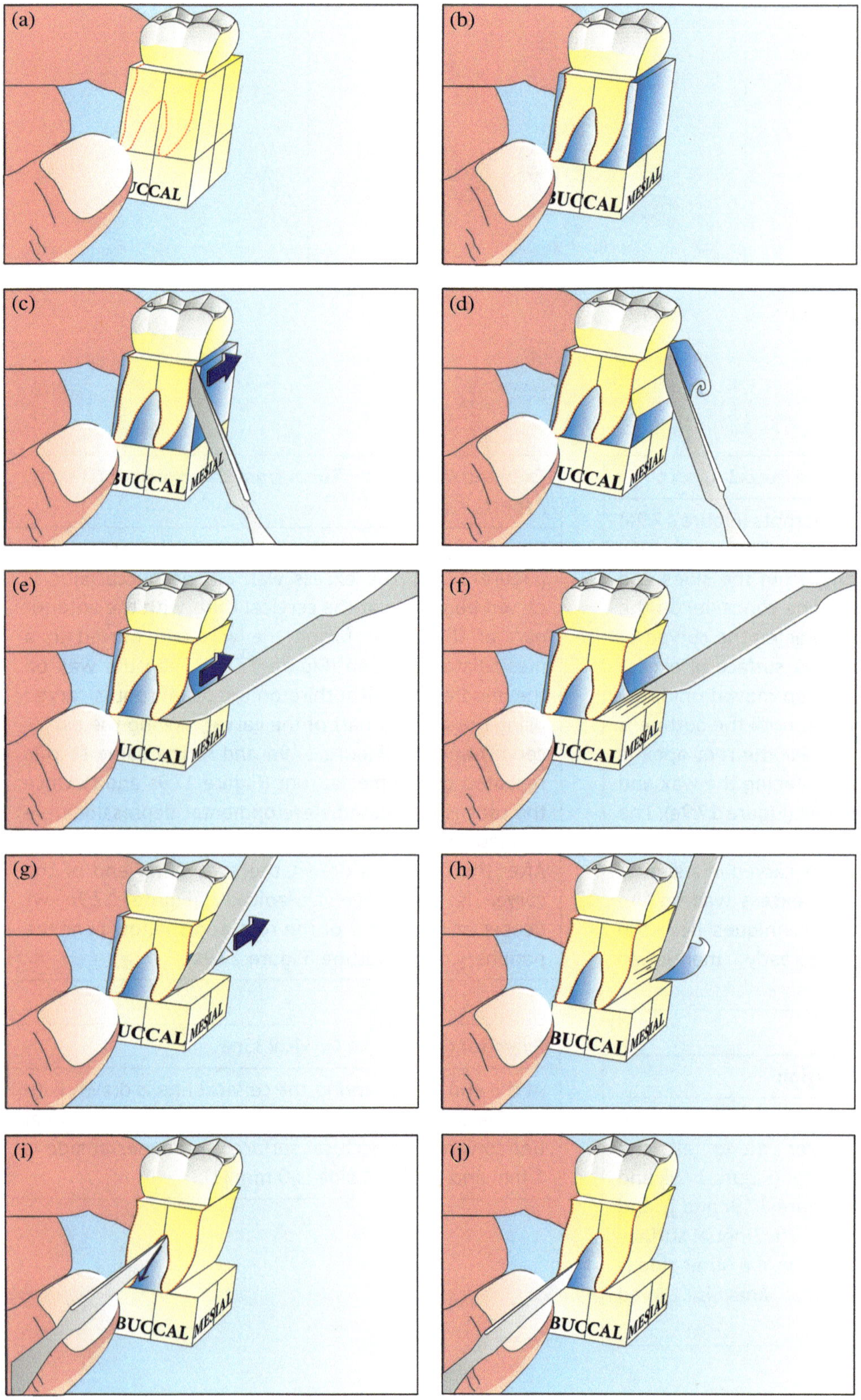

Figure 17.9 (a–x) Sequence of steps for carving the roots.

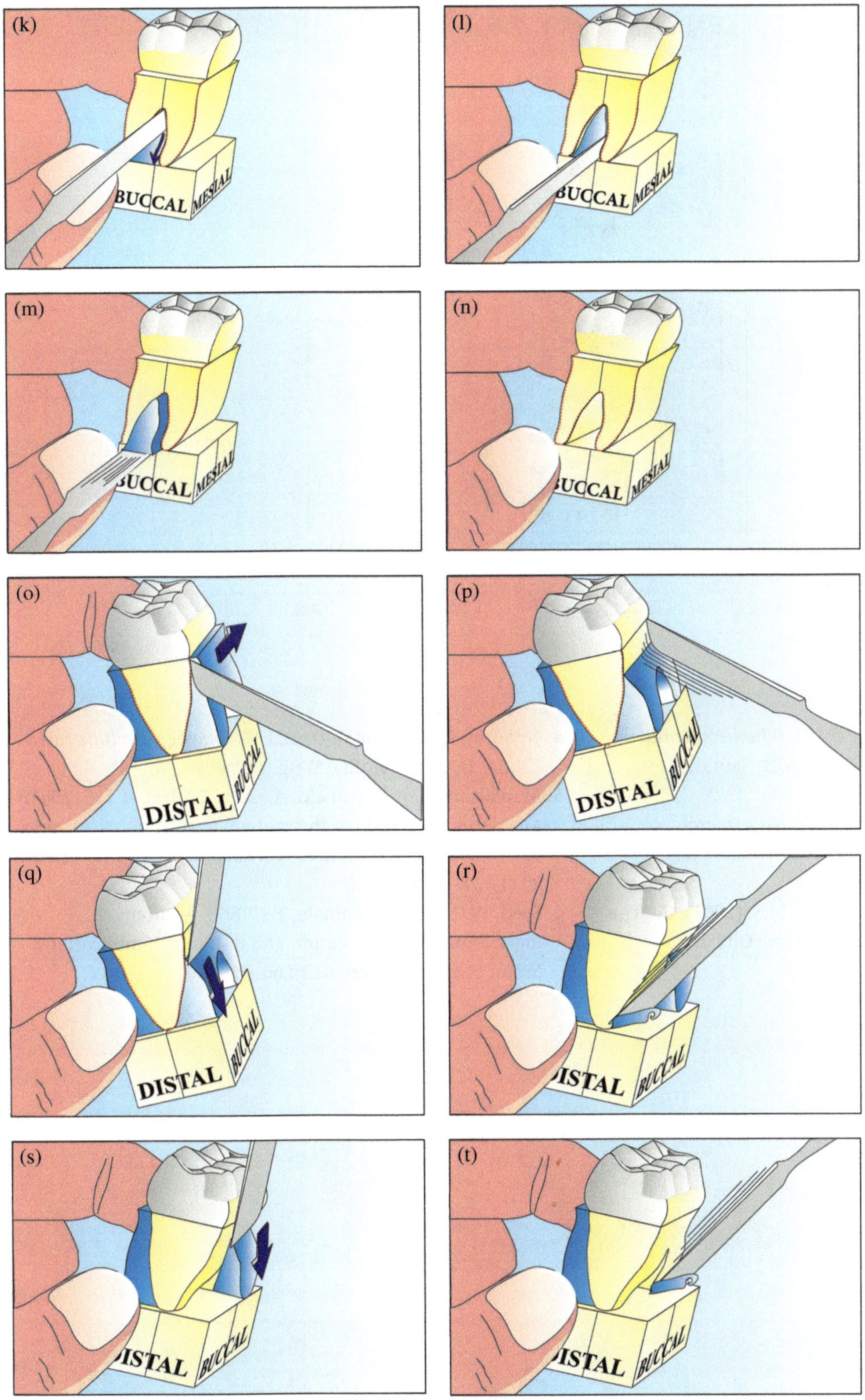

Figure 17.9 (Cont'd) (a–x)

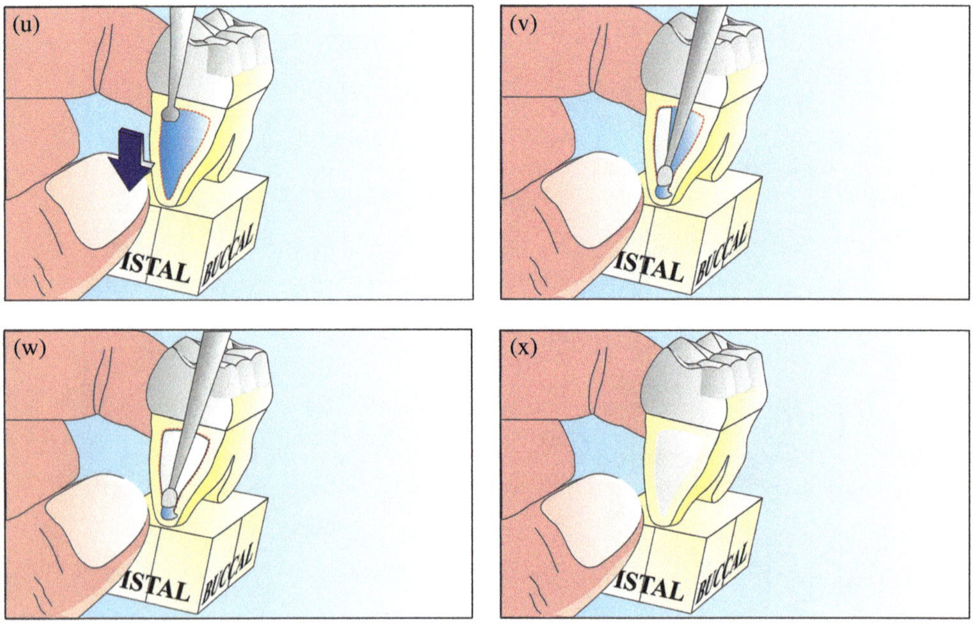

Figure 17.9 (Cont'd) (a–x)

References

1 Stanley, J.N. and Major, M.A.C. (2010). *Wheeler's Dental Anatomy and Occlusion*, 9e. St. Louis, MO: Saunders Elsevier.

2 Rickne, C.S. and Weiss, G. (2012). *Woelfel's Dental Anatomy*, 8e. Philadelphia: Lippincott Williams & Wilkins.

3 James, L.F., Gerald, E.D., and Thomas, M.S. (2001). *Concise Dental Anatomy and Morphology*, 4e. Iowa City, IA: University of Iowa College of Dentistry.

4 Geoffrey, C.V.B. (1983). *Dental Morphology. An Illustrated Guide*, 2e. Philadelphia: Wright Elsevier.

5 Marcaccini, A.A., Pavanelo, A., A. V. B, N. et al. (2012 Feb). Morphometric study of the root anatomy in furcation area of mandibular first molars. *Journal of Applied Oral Science* 20 (1): 76–81.

6 Syed, W.P. and Madhumala, T. (2007). Anatomy of mandibular molar furcation and its clinical implications. *Sebha Medical Journal* 6 (2): 66–69.

18

Permanent Mandibular Right Second Molar

LEARNING OBJECTIVE
At the end of the chapter, student should have knowledge of the permanent mandibular second molar and develop the psychomotor skills for carving and waxing the same.

Permanent Mandibular Right Second Molar

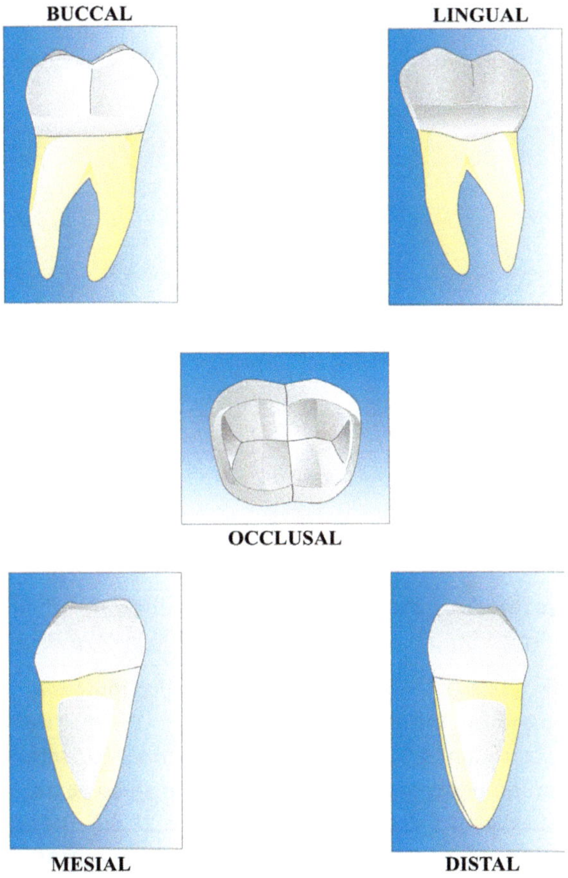

Buccal Aspect

The permanent mandibular second molar is the seventh tooth from the midline (Figure 18.1). The crown is narrower mesiodistally and shorter cervico-occlusally than the mandibular first molar (Figure 18.2a). From this aspect, the crown shows the presence of two buccal cusps: the mesiobuccal and distobuccal cusp. The buccal developmental groove forms a line of demarcation between the two cusps (Figure 18.2b) [1–3]. Prominence of the buccogingival ridge can be seen on the mesial side [2, 3]. There are two roots, mesial and distal. The cervical line points towards the furcation area of the root. The roots are shorter and closer, nearly parallel to each other [2–4]. The distal inclination of the root forms an acute angle to the occlusal plane (Figure 18.2c) [1].

An Illustrated Atlas of Tooth Carving and Wax-Up Techniques, First Edition. Anil Bangalore Shivappa.

Companion website: www.wiley.com/go/bangalore/toothcarving

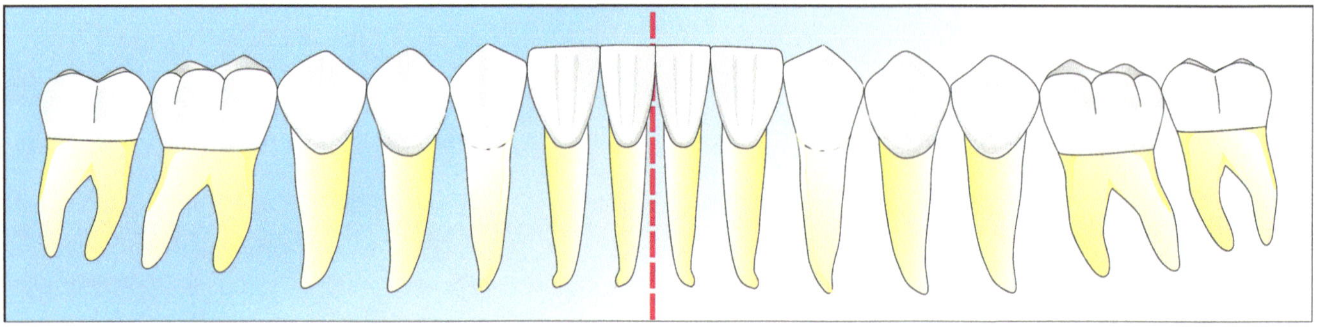

Figure 18.1 Position of the permanent mandibular second molar in relation to the midsagittal plane.

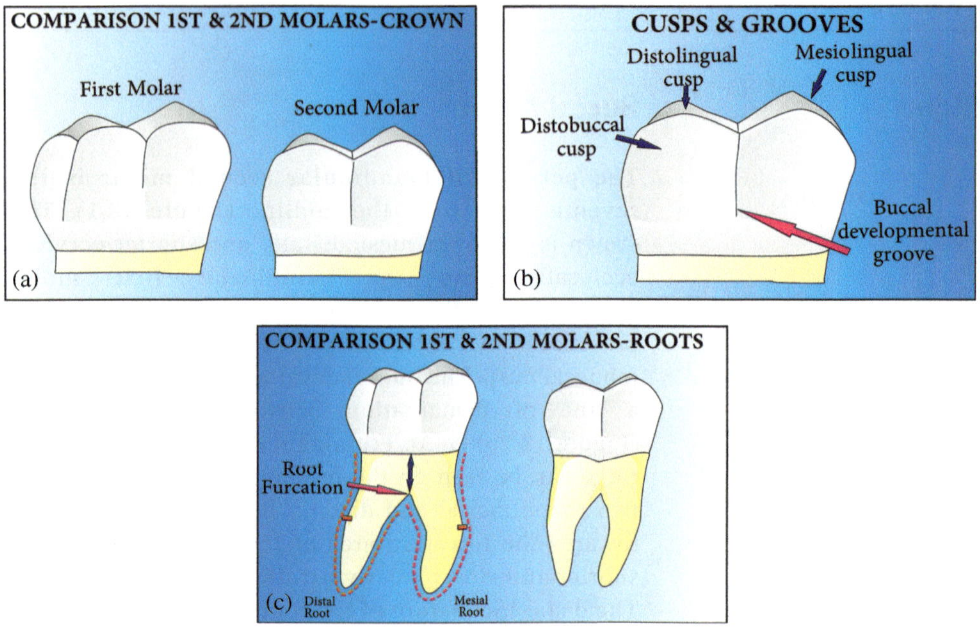

Figure 18.2 (a–c) Descriptive features of the permanent mandibular right second molar from the buccal aspect.

Carving from the Buccal Aspect

Exercise: Marking the Length of the Crown and Root on the Buccal Surface of the Wax Block

The length of the crown (7.0 mm) is marked from the occlusal edge of the prepared wax block (Figure 18.3a). The marking is extended to the remaining surfaces of the wax block (Figure 18.3b). Then the length of the root of 13.0 mm is marked from the cervical end of the crown measurement (Figure 18.3c) [1].

Exercise: Marking the Mesiodistal Dimension of the Crown on the Buccal Surface of the Wax Block

The crown part of the wax block is now divided into three equal parts on the buccal surface (Figure 18.3d). The mesiodistal diameter of the crown measuring 10.5 mm (5.25 mm on either side of the midline) is marked at the occlusal edge of the buccal surface (Figure 18.3e). Then the mesiodistal diameter of the crown at the cervix measuring 8.0 mm (4.0 mm on either side of the midline) is marked on the either side of the midline (Figure 18.3f) [1].

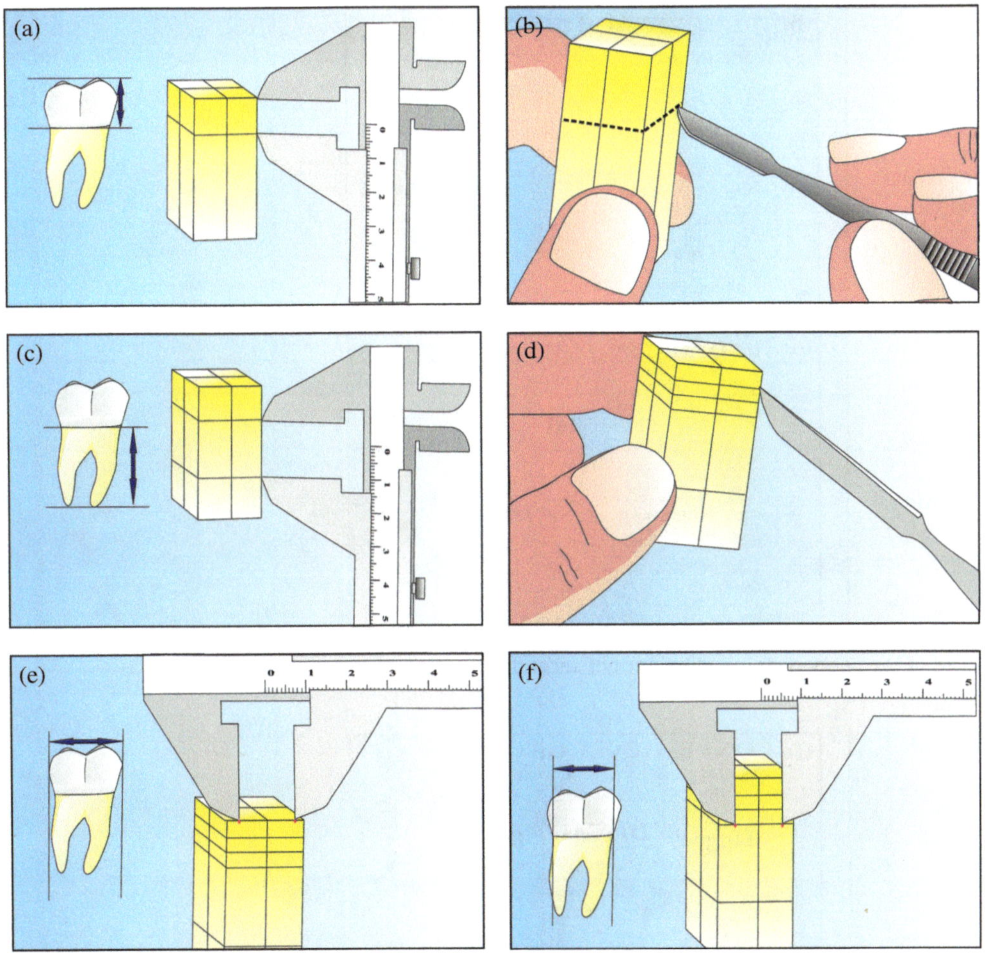

Figure 18.3 (a–f) Measuring and marking the dimension of the crown and length of the root.

Exercise: Marking the Outline and Carving on the Mesial and Distal Sides

NOTE: The marking and carving sequence is similar to that followed for the mandibular first molar. Students are directed to refer to Chapter 17 for this particular exercise.

Mesial Aspect

The cervico-occlusal and labiolingual dimension of the crown is reduced compared to that of the first molar. The buccal outline shows the reduced cervical ridge and narrower occlusal table. The cervical line is less pronounced. The mesial root is more pointed, and a part of the distal root can be seen buccally (Figure 18.4a–d).

Distal Aspect

From this aspect, the tooth has features to those of the first molar, except the absence of distal cusp and the distobuccal groove. The distal marginal ridge is placed more cervically than most of the occlusal surfaces (Figure 18.4e and f).

Carving from the Mesial Aspect

Exercise: Marking the Buccolingual Dimension on the Mesial Surface

The buccolingual diameter of the crown at the cervix measuring 9.0 mm (4.5 mm on either side of the midline) is marked at the cervical end of the crown measurement (Figure 18.5a and b). The buccolingual diameter of the crown of 10.0 mm (5.0 mm on either side of the midline) is marked at the occlusal edge of the buccal surface of the wax block (Figure 18.5c and d) [1].

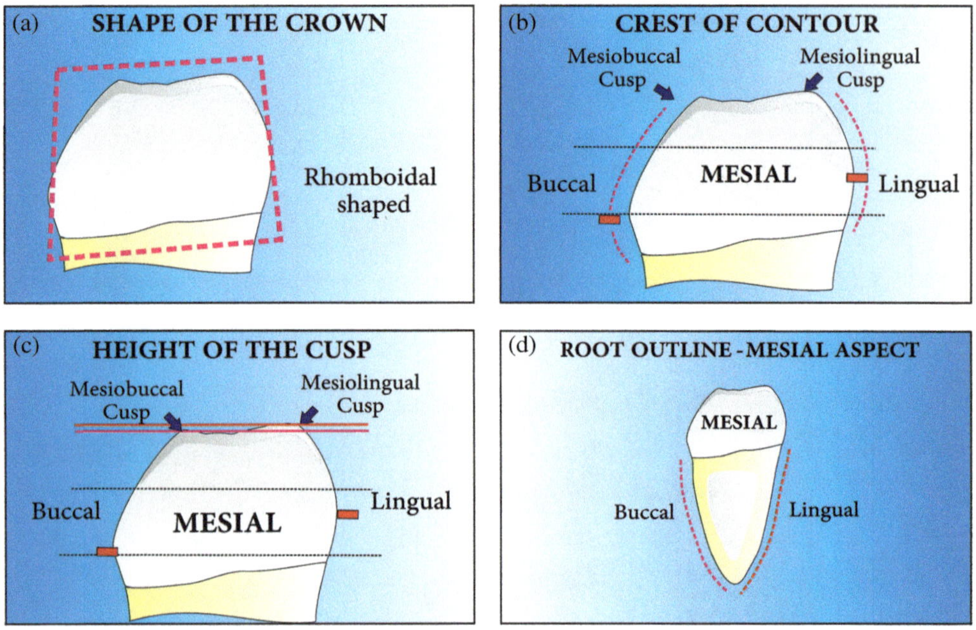

Figure 18.4 (a–d) Descriptive features of the permanent mandibular right second molar from the mesial aspect.

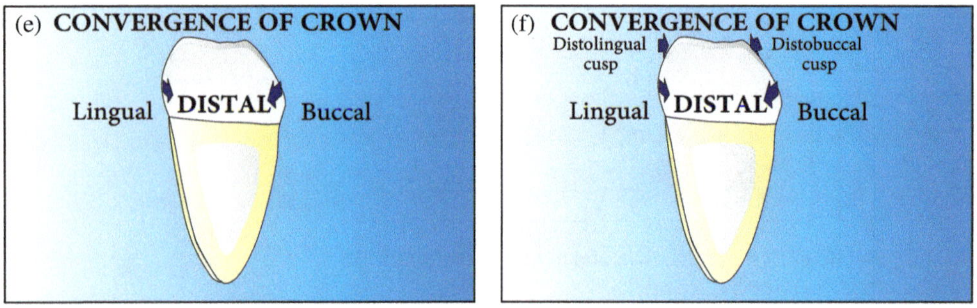

Figure 18.4 (e–f) Descriptive features of the permanent mandibular right second molar from the distal aspect.

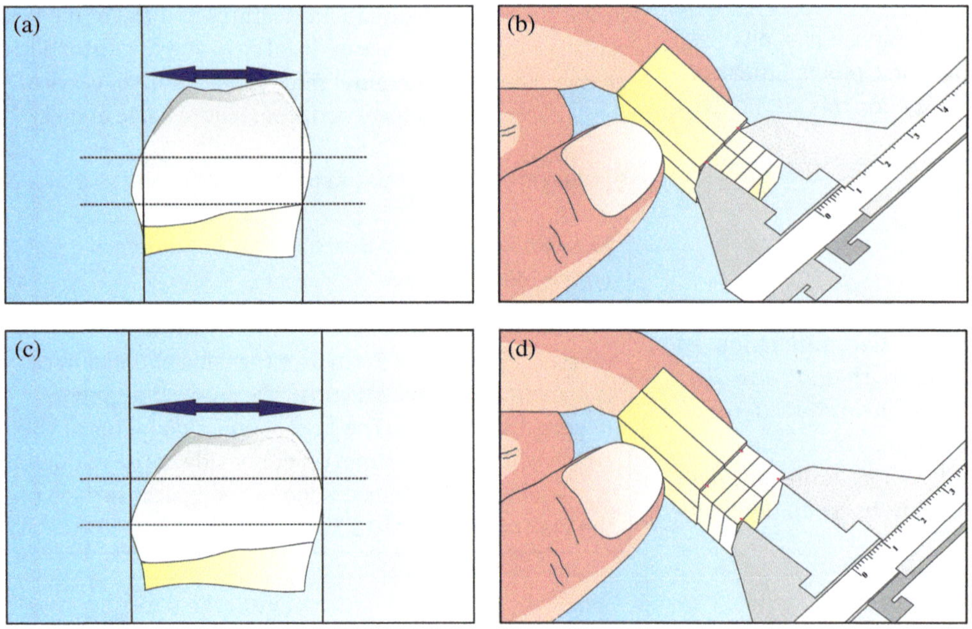

Figure 18.5 (a–d) Measuring and marking the dimension of crown on the mesial aspect of the wax.

Exercise: Marking the Outline and Carving on the Buccal and Lingual Sides

NOTE: The marking and carving sequence is similar to that followed for the maxillary first molar. Students are directed to refer to Chapter 17 for this exercise.

Lingual Aspect

From this aspect the crown is similar to that seen in the mandibular first molar. However, the crown and root exhibit less lingual convergence compared to that seen in the first molar, so less of the mesial and distal surfaces can be seen [1–3] (Figure 18.6a–e).

Occlusal Aspect

From this aspect, the tooth appears rectangular in shape (Figure 18.7a). The occlusal aspect differs from that of the first molar. The small distal cusp and the distobuccal groove are absent in the second molar. The central developmental groove unites with the buccal and lingual developmental groove at the central pit at a right angle (Figure 18.7b) [1, 2]. This union of grooves divides the occlusal surface into four equal parts that form the cusp (Figure 18.7c). Numerous supplementary grooves radiate from the central groove to the slopes of the cusp. The distal outline of the crown is rounded, and the mesial outline is roughly square. The mesiobuccal cervical ridge can be seen [1–4].

Carving from the Occlusal Aspect

Exercise: Creating the Groove Outline and Fossa

The grooves are created on the occlusal surface of the tooth such that the buccal and lingual grooves are perpendicular to the central developmental groove. The fossa is carved on the mesial and distal sides (Figure 18.8a and b).

NOTE: For detailed description of the steps, students are directed to refer to the occlusal carving exercise in Chapter 17.

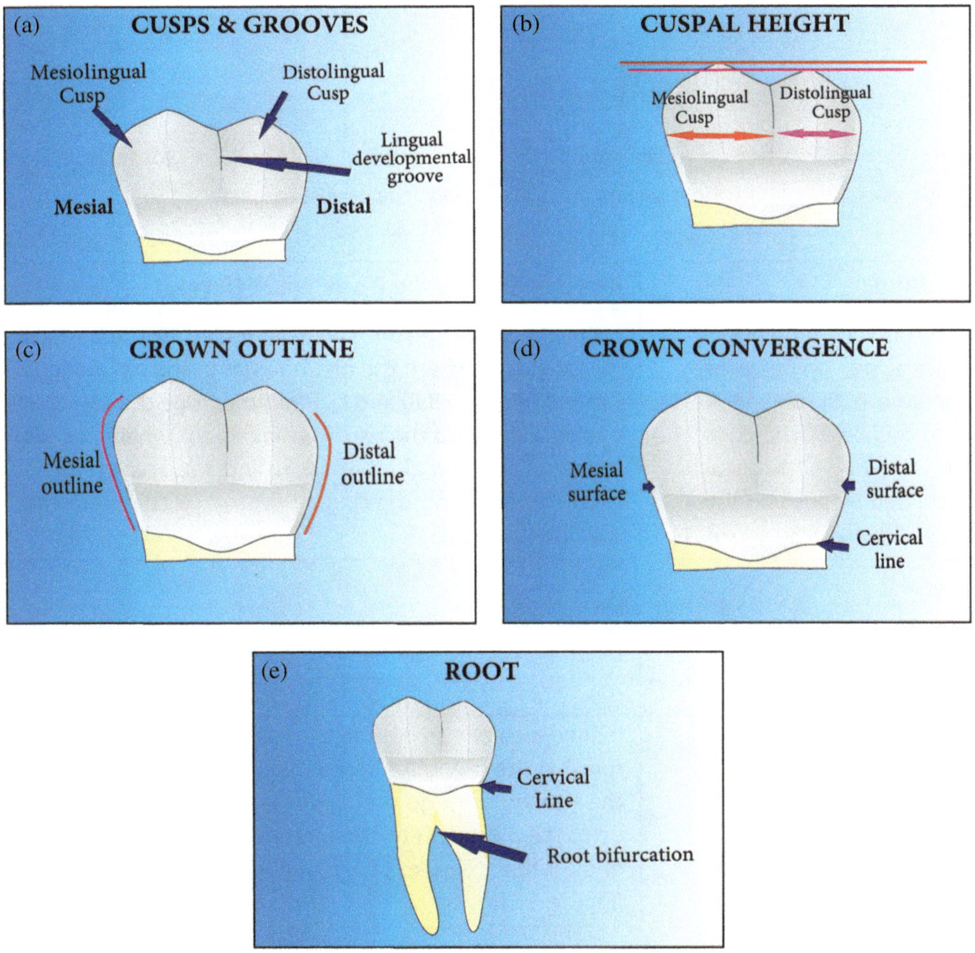

Figure 18.6 (a–e) Description of the permanent mandibular right second molar from the lingual aspect.

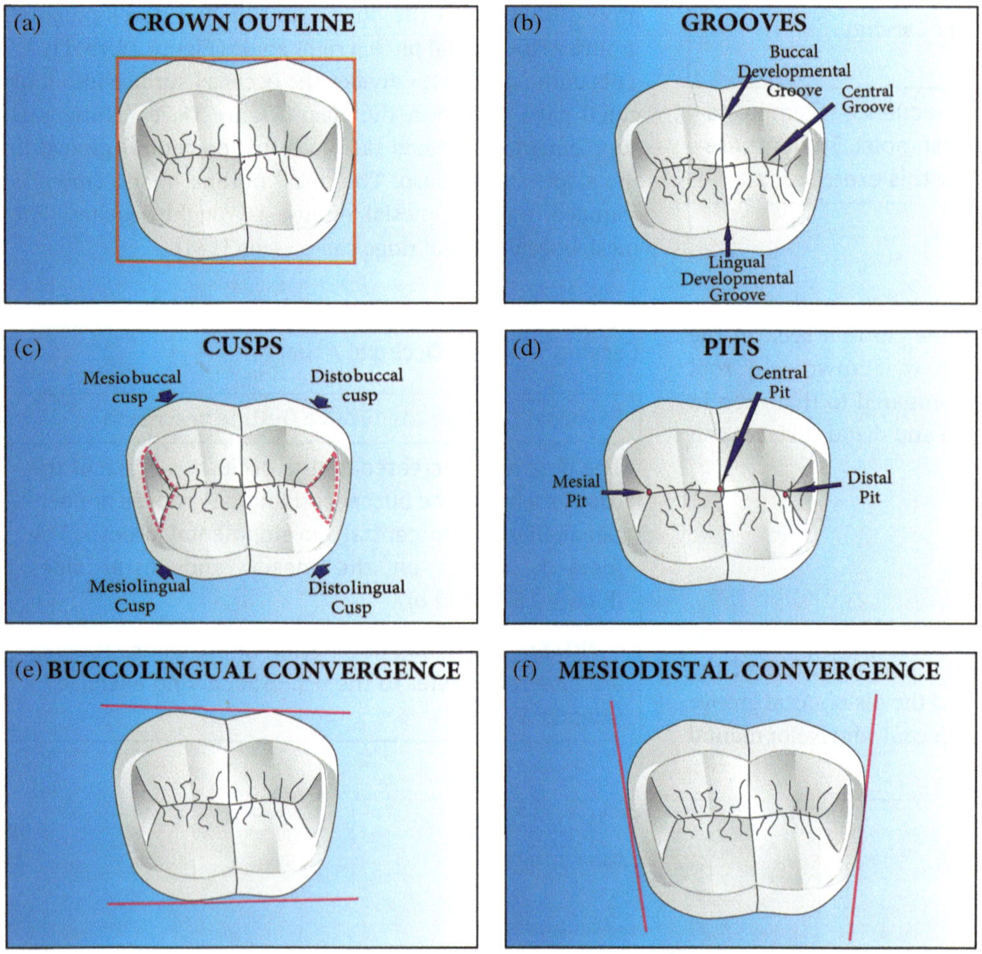

Figure 18.7 (a–f) Description of the permanent mandibular right second molar crown from the occlusal aspect.

Exercise: Carving the Mesiobuccal Cusp

With the back of the carver facing the buccal groove of the mesial fossa and the tip at the mesial pit, the carver is moved distally along the central groove by pulling it towards the surface of wax at the middle of the cusp (Figure 18.8c). This middle part forms the ridge. The distal surface of the triangular ridge is created by pushing the carver deep into the wax up to the pit (Figure 18.8d and e).

Exercise: Carving the Distobuccal Cusp

With the back of the carver facing the buccal developmental groove of the crown and the tip at the central pit, the carver is moved distally along the central groove and pulled out to the surface (mesial slope) where it forms the triangular ridge (Figure 18.8f and g). From this point the carver is moved deep into the wax, up to the distal pit in the distal fossa (Figure 18.8h and i).

Exercise: Carving the Distolingual Cusp

From the distal pit the carver is pulled to the surface (distal slope), where the distolingual triangular ridge is formed (Figure 18.8j and k). From the ridge the carver is pushed deep into the wax (mesial slope), where it ends in the central pit (Figure 18.8l and m). The carver is then moved along the lingual groove to complete the distolingual cusp.

Exercise: Carving the Mesiolingual Cusp

With the tip of the carver at the central pit, the carver is moved mesially by pulling the carver out to the surface, forming the triangular ridge (Figure 18.8n and o). From the triangular ridge the carver is pushed into the wax up to the mesial pit to complete the mesiolingual triangular ridge (Figure 18.8p and q) and all the cusps (Figure 18.8r).

Exercise: Creating the Buccal and Lingual Ridge on Surfaces

The midline is drawn on the buccal or lingual surface of the particular cusp from the cusp tip to the crest of contour. Slopes are created on either side of the midline of the particular cusp (Figure 18.8s).

Exercise: Carving Excess Wax from Other Surfaces

Excess wax is carved from the mesial, buccal, and distal surfaces (Figure 18.8t–w). Mesially and distally, marginal ridges are carved. Buccally the ridges on the surface are carved.

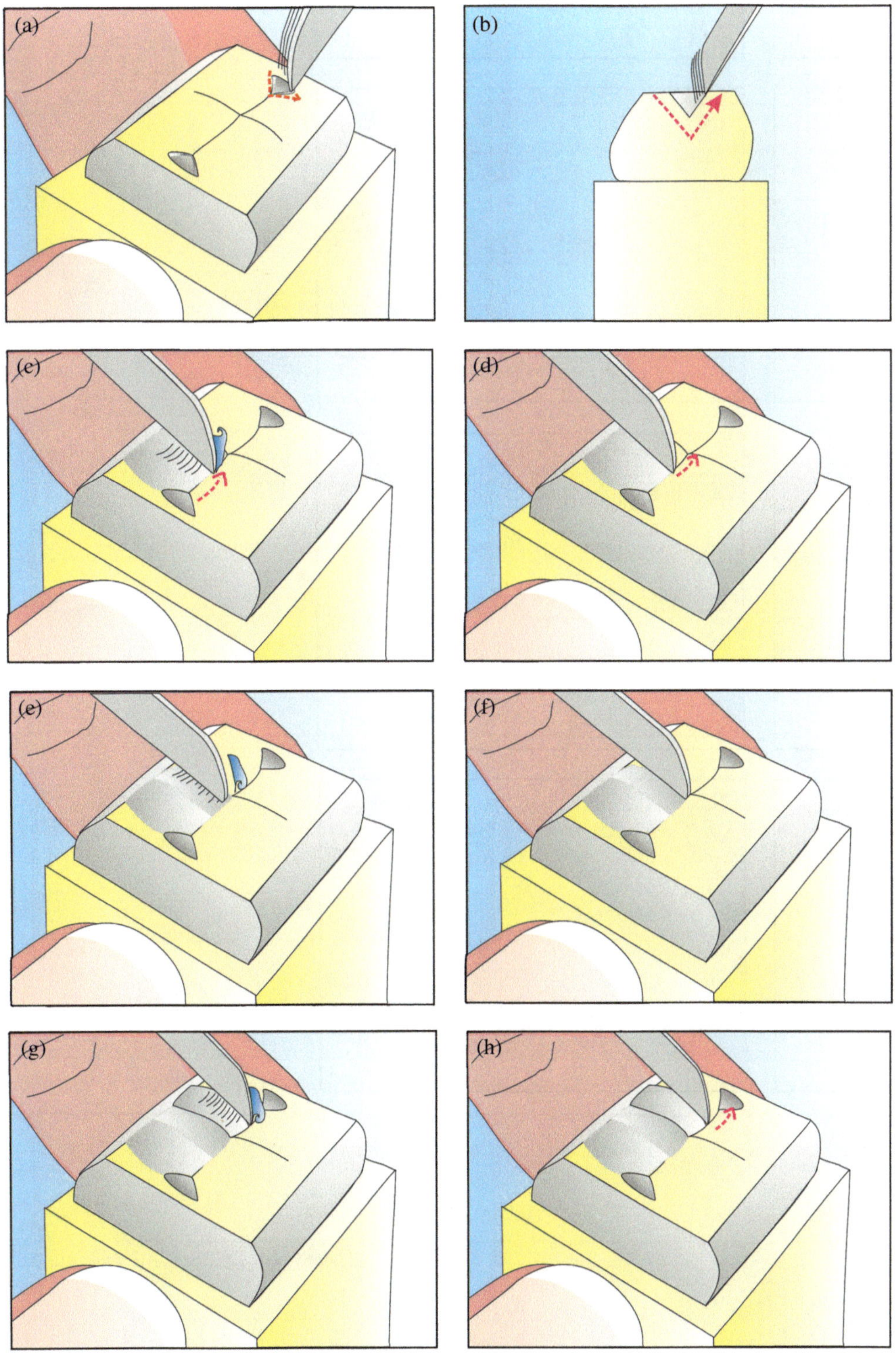

Figure 18.8 (a–w) Carving occlusal features of the permanent mandibular right second molar.

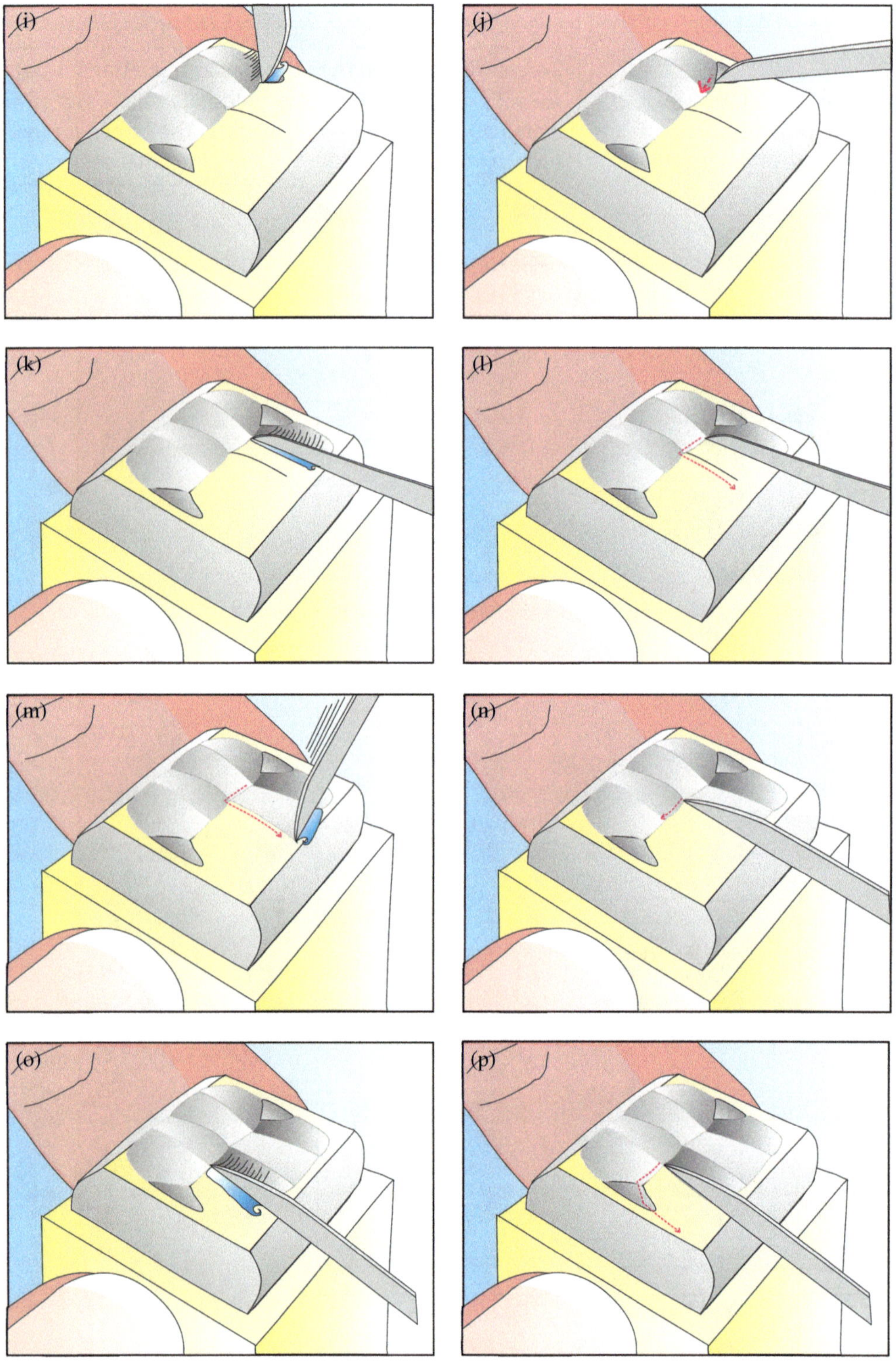

Figure 18.8 (Cont'd) (a–w)

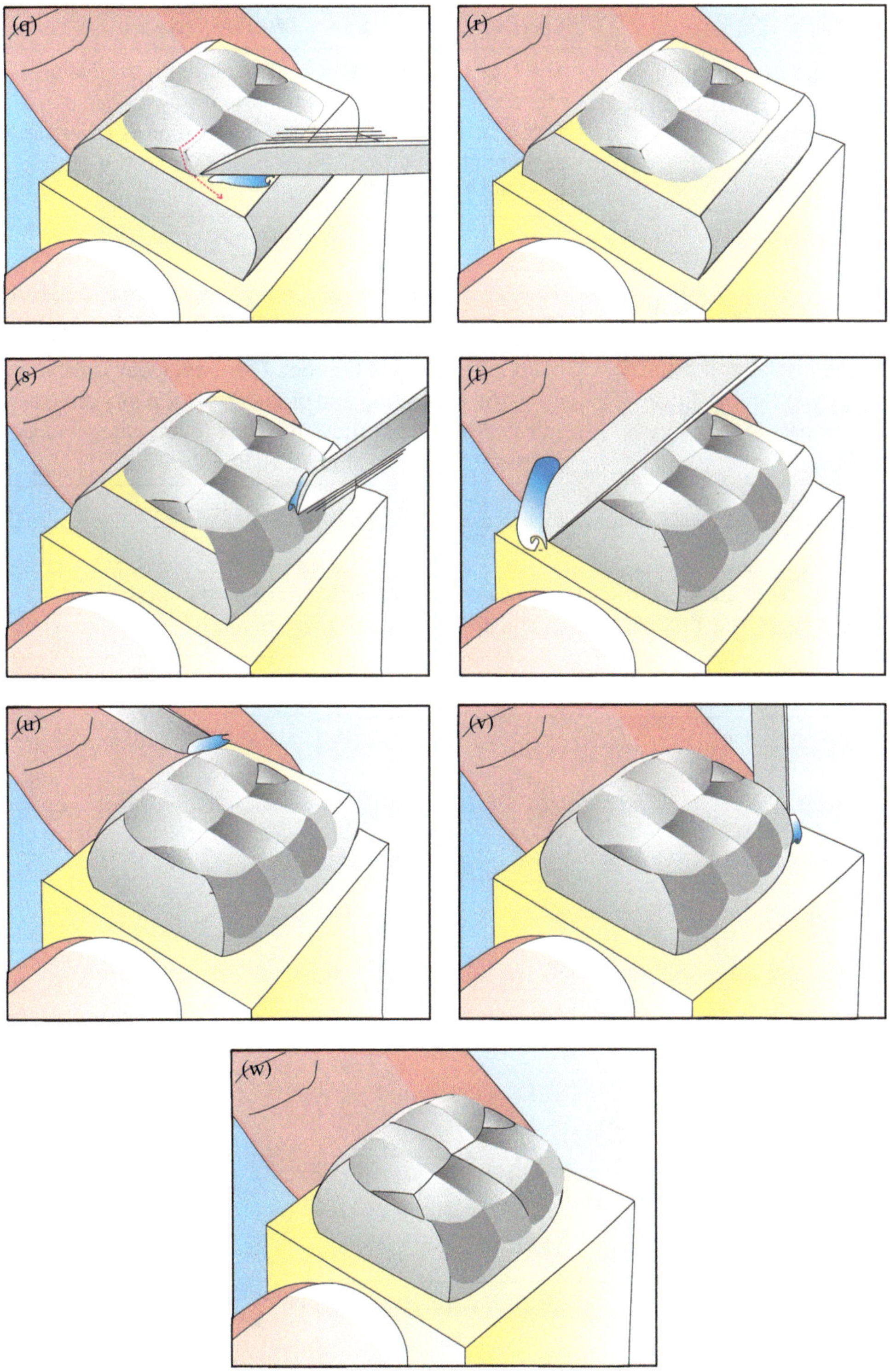

Figure 18.8 (Cont'd) (a–w)

Root Carving

The carving sequence for the root of the mandibular second molar is similar to that of the mandibular first molar, except for the change in outline.

Exercise: Carving from the Buccal Aspect

The outline of the root on the buccal surface of wax is drawn with the features mentioned earlier (Figure 18.9a). The excess wax outside the outline, indicated in blue, is carved on both the mesial and distal sides (Figure 18.9b–h). The excess wax at the furcal area is then carved using the anterior part of the carver along the root outline (Figure 18.9i–n).

Exercise: Carving from the Distal Aspect

The labiolingual outline of the root with the features mentioned earlier is drawn on the distal surface of the wax. The excess wax outside the outline is carved in sequential steps from the wax surface to the outline (Figure 18.9o–t).

Exercise: Creating the Depression on the Root Surfaces

The outline of the depression is marked at the centre of the outer surface of the root. The excess wax is carved using the excavating end of the carver run in a cervico-apical direction, shallow near the outer margin and deeper at the centre (Figure 18.9u–x).

Exercise: Carving the Cervical Line

At the end of the carving, the cervical line is drawn with the features mentioned. The curvature of the cervical line towards the occlusal surface on the mesial side is 1 mm and on the distal side is 0 mm [1].

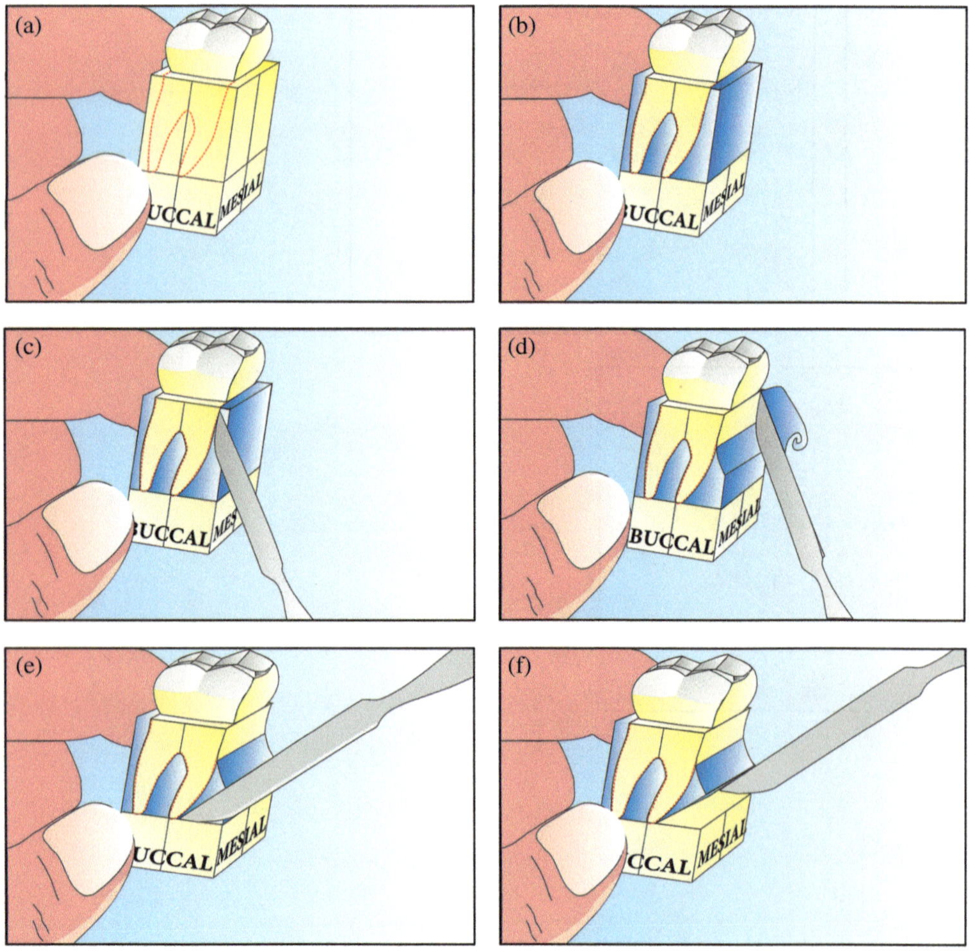

Figure 18.9 (a–x) Carving the roots from the buccal and distal aspects.

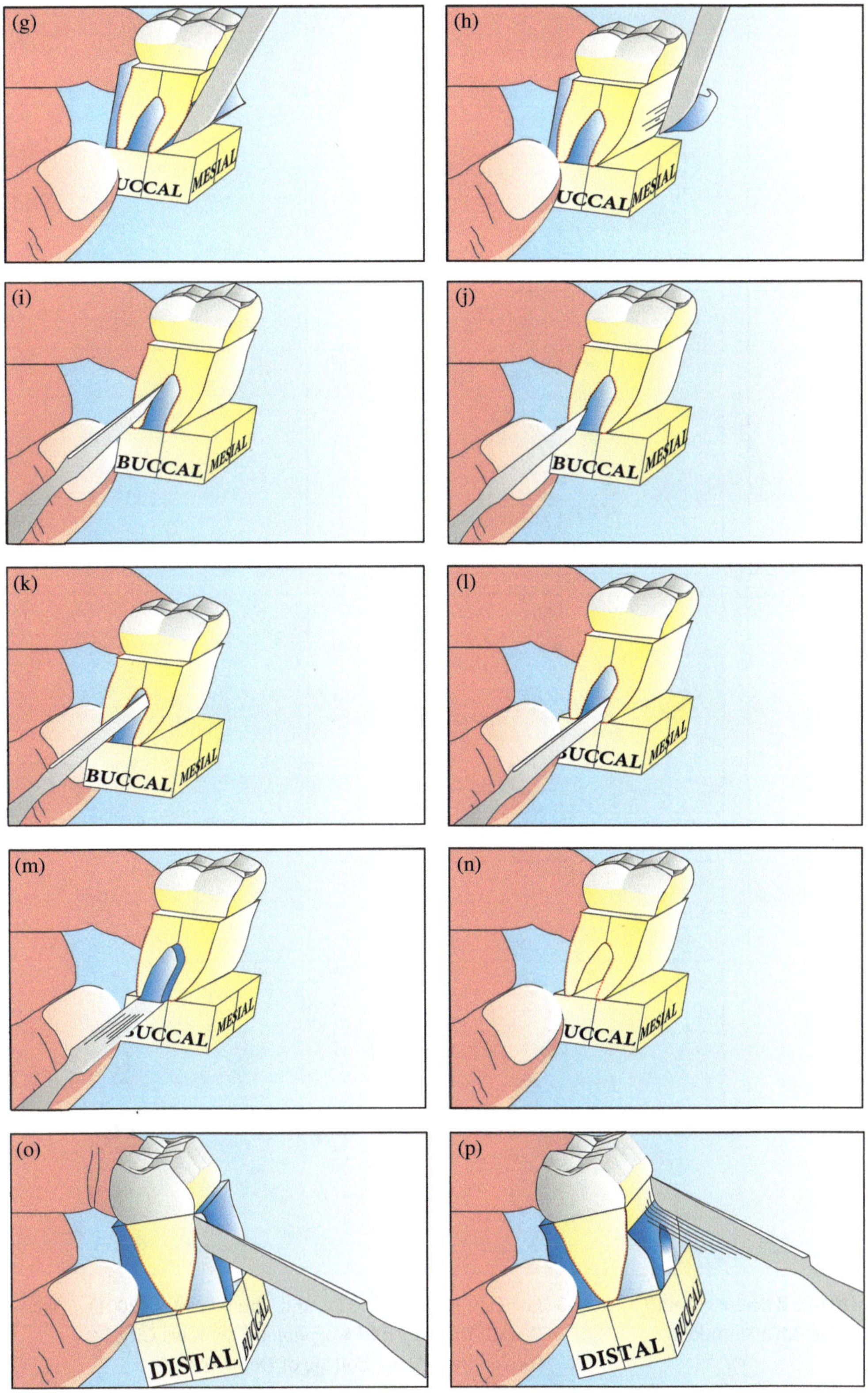

Figure 18.9 (Cont'd) (a–x)

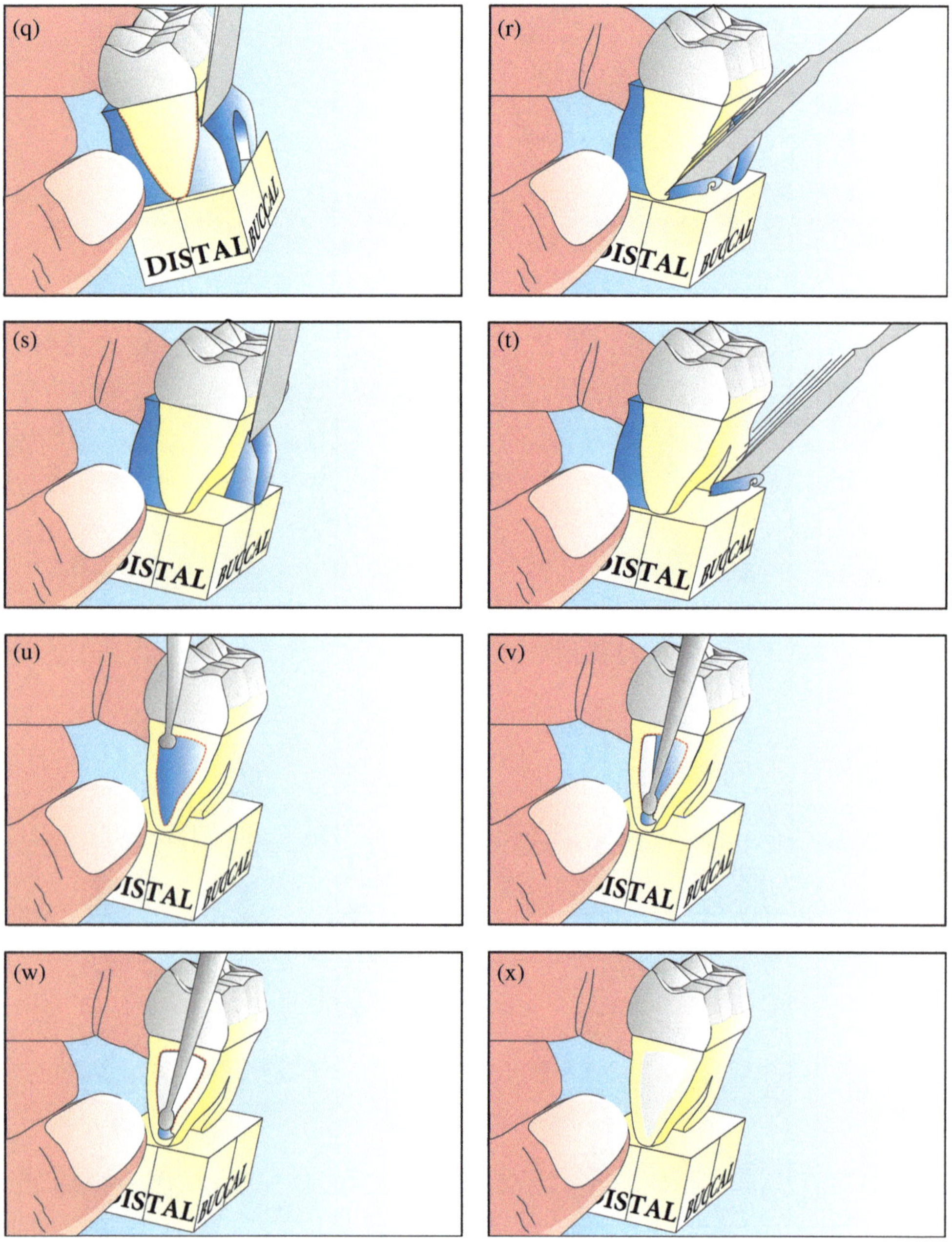

Figure 18.9 (Cont'd) (a–x)

References

1 Stanley, J.N. and Major, M.A.C. (2010). *Wheeler's Dental Anatomy and Occlusion*, 9e. St. Louis, MO: Saunders Elsevier.

2 Rickne, C.S. and Weiss, G. (2012). *Woelfel's Dental Anatomy*, 8e. Philadelphia: Lippincott Williams & Wilkins.

3 James, L.F., Gerald, E.D., and Thomas, M.S. (2001). *Concise Dental Anatomy and Morphology*, 4e. Iowa City, IA: University of Iowa College of Dentistry.

4 Geoffrey, C.V.B. (1983). *Dental Morphology. An Illustrated Guide*, 2e. Philadelphia: Wright Elsevier.

Part II

Wax-Up Technique

19

Waxing of the Maxillary Right Central Incisor

LEARNING OBJECTIVE
At the end of the chapter, the student should be able to wax up the permanent maxillary right central incisor.

Multiple coats of die lubricant are applied to the prepared tooth surface using a brush and allowed to dry. The sequence of waxing steps is then started [1].

Exercise: Initial Layer of Wax Application

The initial layer of wax is applied to cover the entire area of crown preparation. This is done using either large instruments like a wax spatula or using P.K. Thomas (PKT) no. 2 instrument. The wax should be in full molten state during wax application to prevent its solidification before application and also to prevent the distortion of the applied layer of wax or tag formation. The PKT instrument is moved from the rounded mesiolabial line angle to the distopalatal line angle along the labial surface (Figure 19.1a and b) and then from distopalatal line angle to the mesiolabial line angle along the palatal surface. Also, the wax is applied on the flat palatal surface [1].

Waxing the Labial Surface

Exercise: Waxing the Cervical Third of the Labial Surface

With the features of the crown of the maxillary central incisor in mind, the bulk waxing of the prepared tooth is started. The molten wax is added to the cervical part of the crown following the cervical line mesiodistally to create the height of contour (Figure 19.1c–e).

Exercise: Placing the Cones and Contour Bars on the Labial Surface

Incisal cones are placed at the mesial and distal sides of the incisal ridges (Figure 19.1f and g) forming the reference points for application of contour bars. The contour bars are the wax bars created to represent the developmental lobes of natural teeth. The contour bars are placed at the mesiobuccal line angle, distobuccal line angle (that are reduced during crown preparation), and at the position of the buccal lobe. The mesiobuccal contour bar is created at its line angle by placing the molten wax at the cervical part of the preparation and extending in a cervico-incisal direction to join the respective cone (Figure 19.1h and i). The same steps are followed for the buccal and the mesiobuccal contour bars (Figure 19.1j–o).

Exercise: Filling the Gaps between the Contour Bars and Placement of the Incisal Ridge Bar

After the contour bars are placed, the surface between the contour bars is filled with wax in increments to get smooth labial surface (Figure 19.1p and q).

The incisal ridge bar is created by joining the mesiobuccal cuspal cone with the distobuccal cuspal cone using PKT no. 1 or 2 instrument (Figure 19.1r and s) [2].

An Illustrated Atlas of Tooth Carving and Wax-Up Techniques, First Edition. Anil Bangalore Shivappa.

Companion website: www.wiley.com/go/bangalore/toothcarving

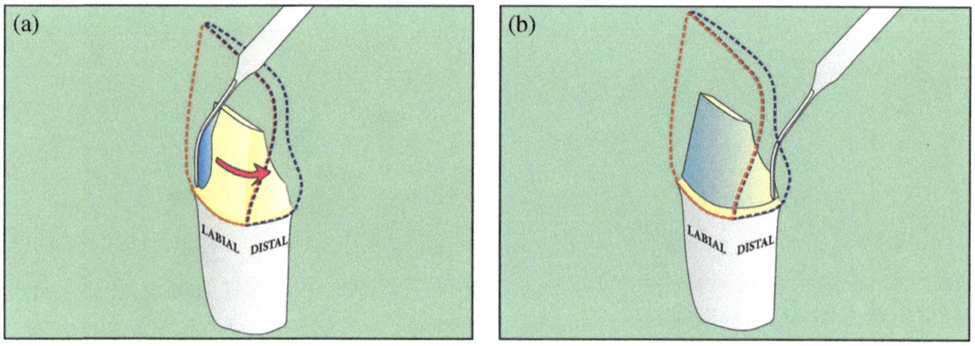

Figure 19.1 (a–b) Application of the initial layer of wax on all prepared surfaces of tooth.

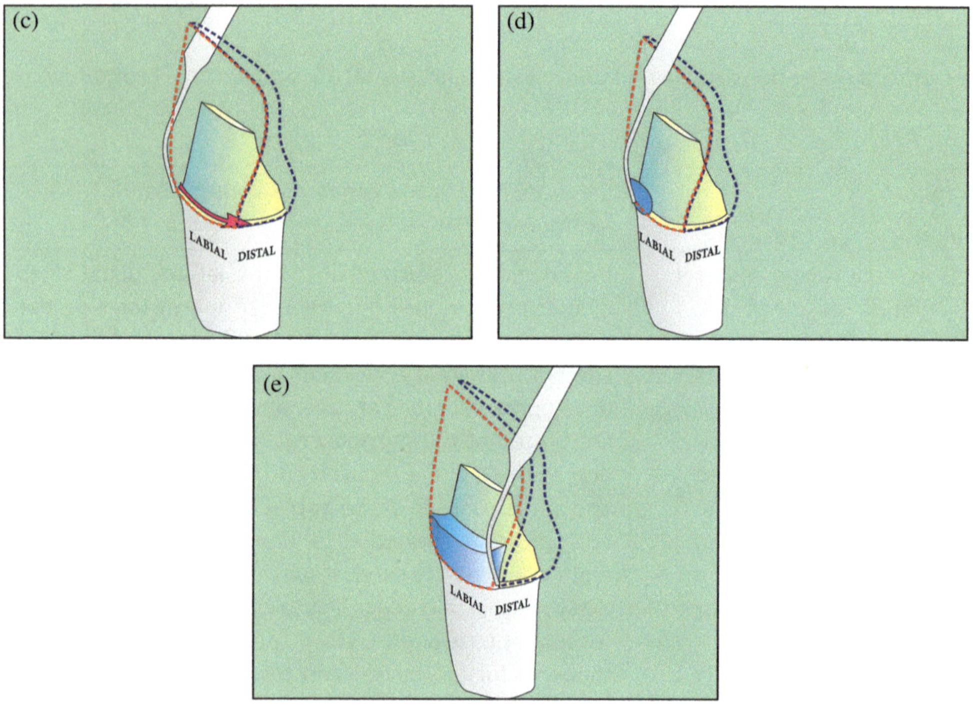

Figure 19.1 (c–e) Waxing the cervical part of the labial surface.

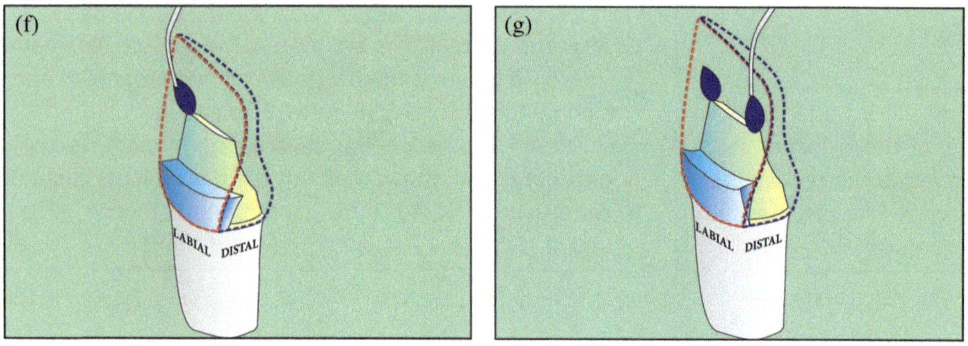

Figure 19.1 (f–g) Placing the molten wax cones at the mesio-incisal and disto-incisal angles.

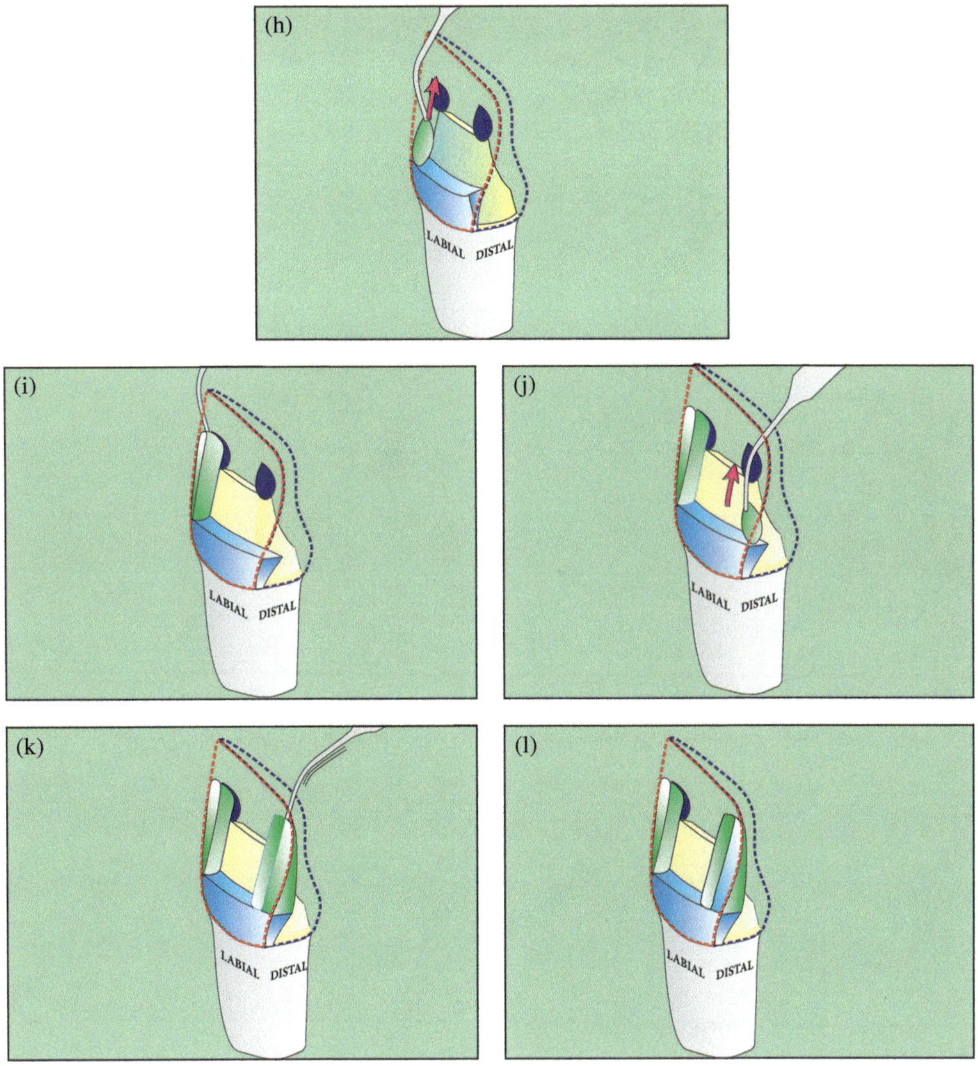

Figure 19.1 (h–l) Placing the molten wax contour bars at the mesio-incisal and disto-incisal angles.

Waxing the Palatal Surface

Exercise: Waxing the Cervical Third of the Palatal Surface
Palatally, the wax is added at the cervical third to create a part of the bulk contour of the cingulum. The wax is added incrementally by passing the PKT no. 1 instrument from the distopalatal to the mesiopalatal line angle (Figure 19.2a–f).

Exercise: Waxing to Create the Mesial and Distal Marginal Ridges and Bulk of the Cingulum
The contour bars are placed at the distal (Figure 19.2g and h) and mesial marginal ridge areas (Figure 19.2i and j). The bulk of the wax is added at the cingulum area (Figure 19.2k and l).

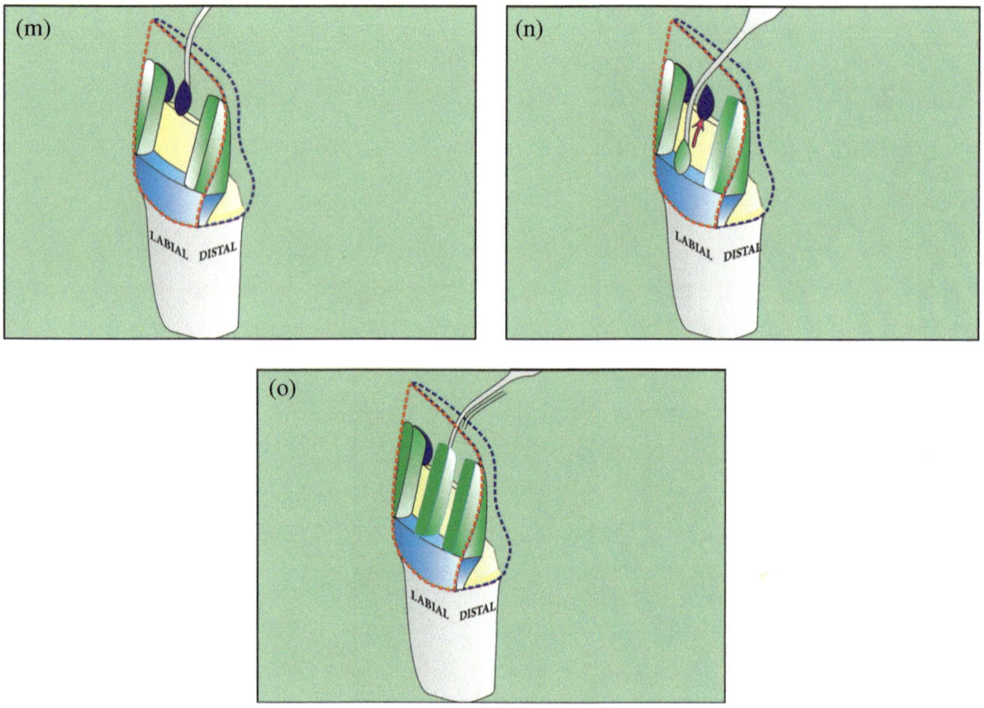

Figure 19.1 (m–o) Placing the molten wax beads and contour bars at the midbuccal lobe position of the prepared tooth.

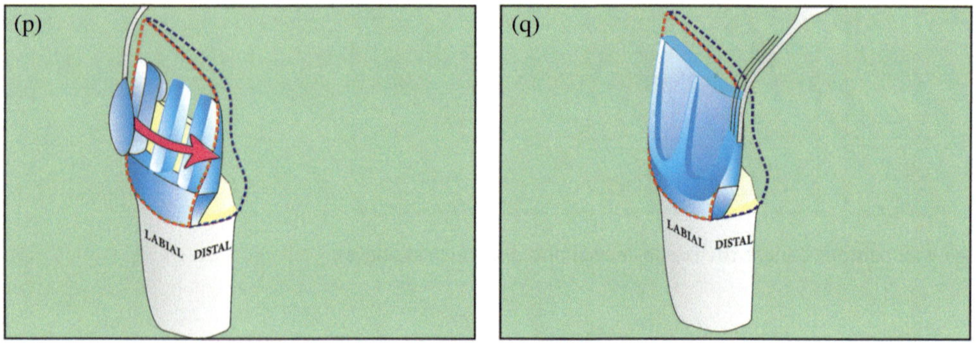

Figure 19.1 (p–q) Filling the space between the contour bars with molten wax.

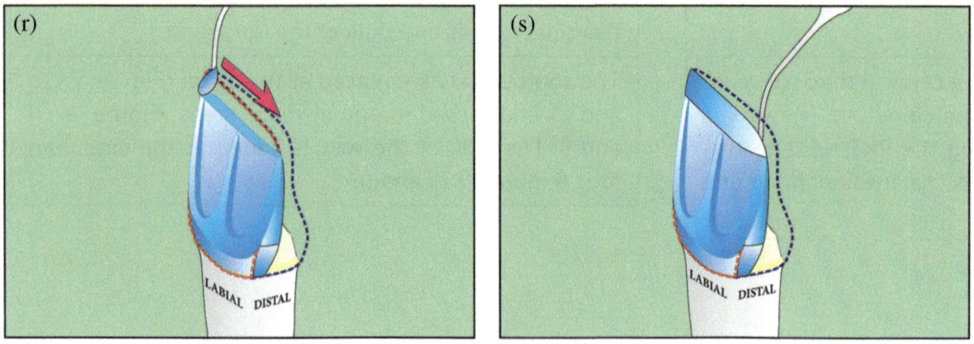

Figure 19.1 (r–s) Contouring and filling the incisal edge.

Exercise: Waxing the Middle Part (Fossa Area) of the Palatal Surface and Creating the Incisal Ridge

The molten wax is added to the middle part (fossa area) of the palatal surface incrementally, to get a smooth flow of marginal ridges, fossa, and cingulum. Care should be taken to seal the marginal areas properly and carve the excess (Figure 19.2m and n). A thin layer of wax is added at the incisal edge to create the incisal ridge (Figure 19.2o and p).

Exercise: Application of the Final Layer of Molten Wax on the Labial and Palatal Surfaces

Finally, a layer of wax is applied on the labial surface to get a smooth surface (Figure 19.2q and r). Excess wax is carved and polished to achieve a smooth and shiny surface (Figure 19.2s) [2].

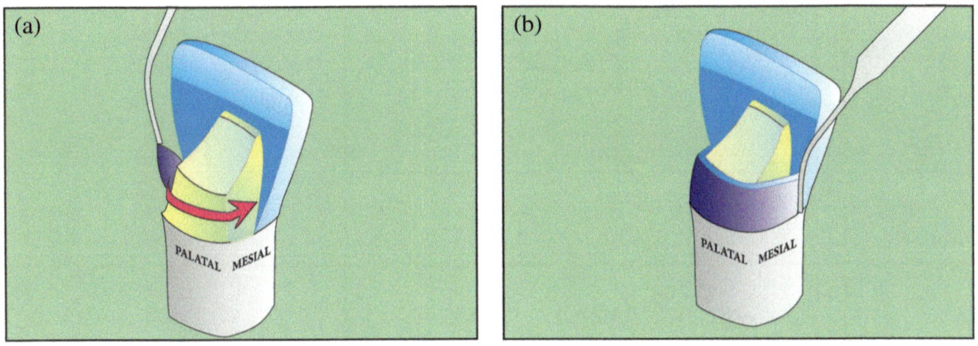

Figure 19.2 (a–b) Waxing the initial layer on the cervical third of the palatal surface.

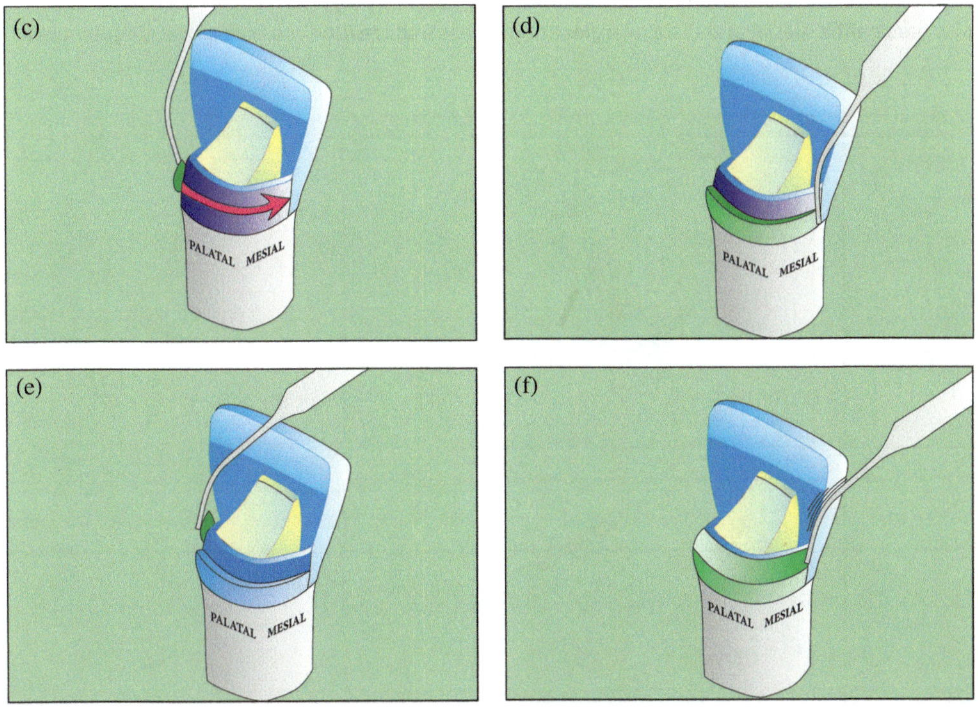

Figure 19.2 (c–f) Waxing to create the bulk contour (of the cingulum) on the cervical third of the palatal surface.

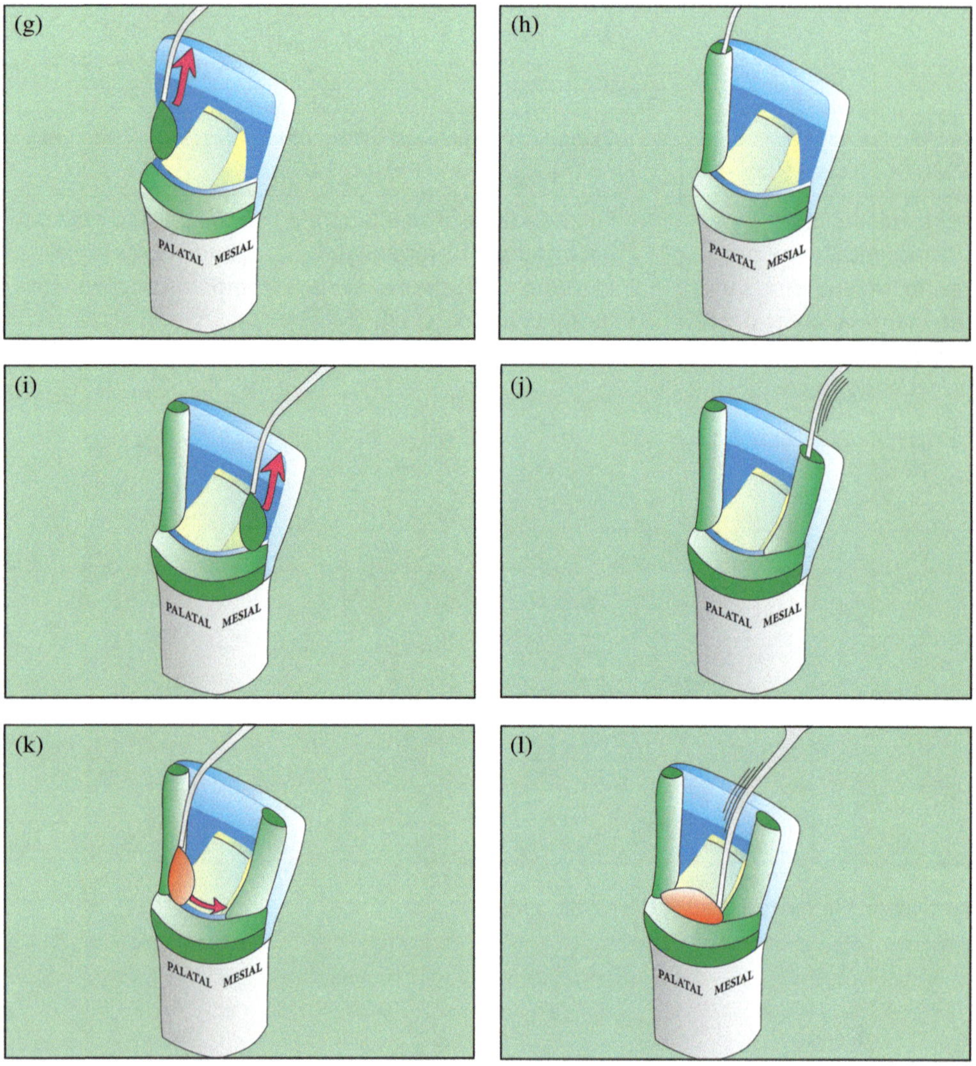

Figure 19.2 (g–l) Placing the contour bars on the mesial and distal marginal ridge areas and creating the bulk of the cingulum near the palatal fossa.

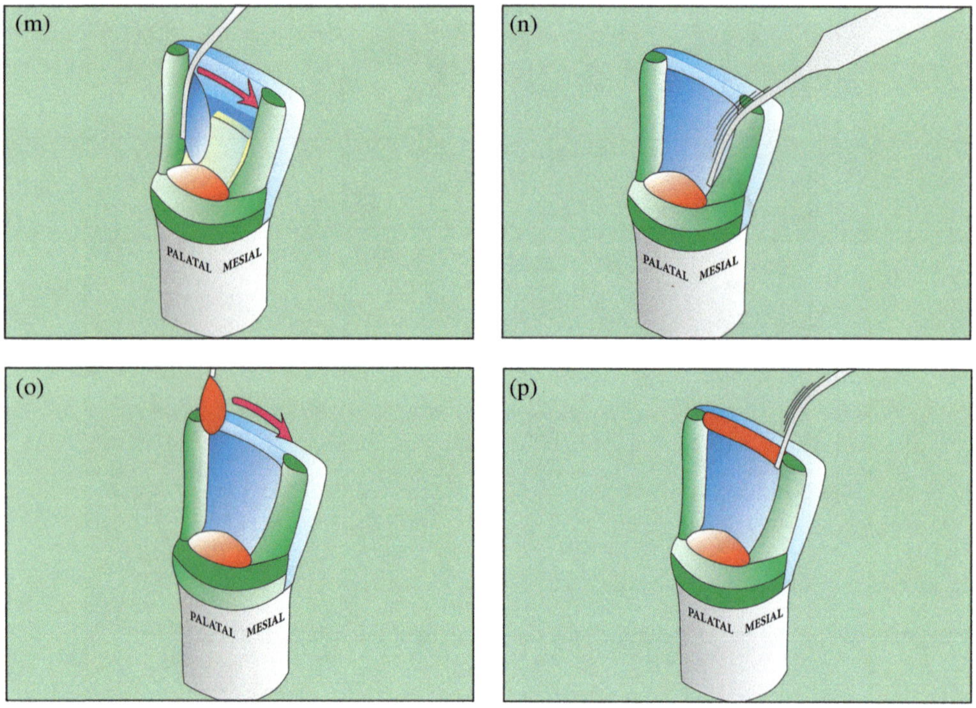

Figure 19.2 (m–p) Placing the molten wax in the fossa area and placing the incisal ridge bar to create the incisal ridge.

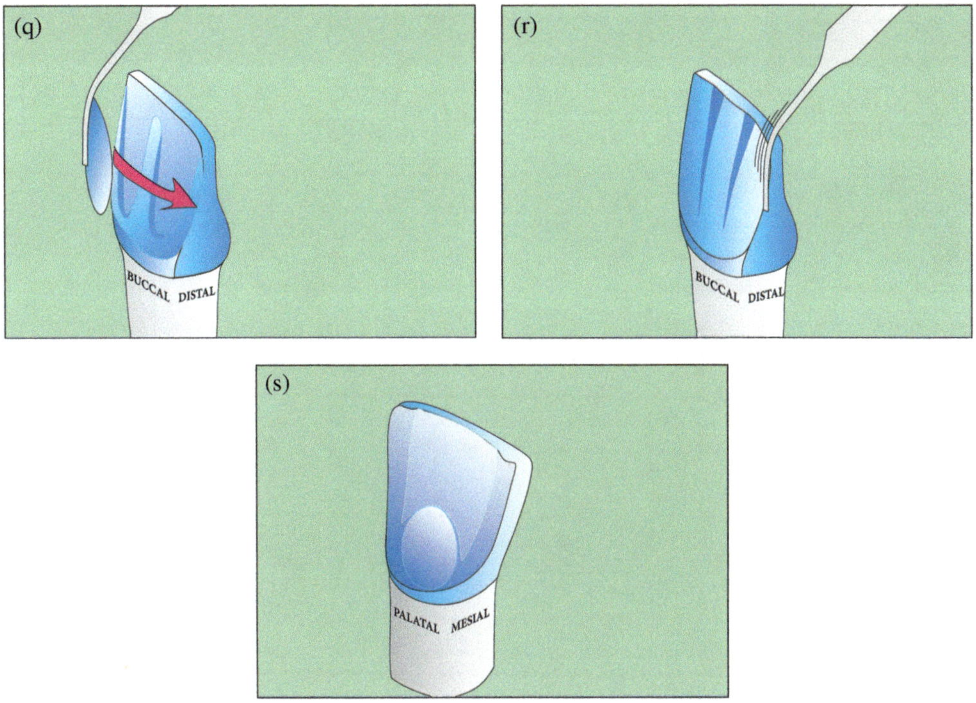

Figure 19.2 (q–s) Direction for application of the final layer of molten wax on the labial and palatal surfaces.

References

1 Stephen, F.R., Martin, F.L., and Junhei, F. (2016). *Contemporary Fixed Prosthodontics*, 5e. St. Louis, MO: Elsevier.

2 Rowida, A. (2019). *The Art of Occlusal and Esthetic Waxing*. Kindle Edition: Quintessence Publishing Co IncBatavia, IL. Co Inc.

20

Waxing of the Permanent Mandibular Right Central Incisor

LEARNING OBJECTIVE

At the end of the chapter, the student should be able to wax up the permanent mandibular right central incisor.

Exercise: Application of Die Lubricant

The die lubricant is applied to the prepared tooth surface using a brush and allowed to dry. The second coat is applied to ensure no voids form. Once the lubricant is dried, the waxing procedure is initiated.

Waxing the Labial Surface

Exercise: Initial Layer of Wax Application

The initial layer of wax is applied to cover the entire area of crown preparation. This is done using either large instruments like a wax spatula or using P. K. Thomas (PKT) no. 2 instrument. The wax should be in full molten state during wax application to prevent its solidification before its application and to prevent the distortion of the applied layer of wax or tag formation. The PKT instrument is moved from the rounded distobuccal line angle to the mesiolingual line angle along the labial surface (Figure 20.1a and b) and then from the mesiolingual line angle to the distobuccal line angle along the lingual surface. Also, the wax is applied on the prepared lingual surface of the preparation [1].

Exercise: Waxing the Cervical Portion of the Labial Surface

The molten wax is added to the cervical part of the crown using a PKT instrument, following the cervical line mesiodistally to create the height of contour (Figure 20.1c and d) [2].

Exercise: Placing the Cones and Contour Bars on the Labial Surface and Incisal Edge

Incisal cones are placed at the mesio-incisal and disto-incisal angles of the incisal preparation (Figure 20.1e and f). These form the reference points for application of the contour bars. The contour bars are the wax bars created to represent the developmental lobes of natural teeth. The contour bars are placed at the mesiobuccal line angle, the distobuccal line angle (that are reduced during crown preparation), and the position of buccal lobe. The distobuccal contour bar is created at its line angle by placing the molten wax at the cervical part of the preparation and extending in a cervico-incisal direction to join the respective cone (Figure 20.1g and h). The same steps are followed for the buccal and the mesiobuccal contour bars (Figure 20.1i). The incisal ridge bar is created by joining the distobuccal cuspal cone with the mesiobuccal cuspal cone using PKT no. 1 or 2 instrument (Figure 20.1j) [1, 2].

Exercise: Waxing the Space Between the Contour Bars

After the formation of boundaries, the area of the prepared crown between the contour bars is filled with wax in increments up to the surface of bars to get a smooth labial surface (Figure 20.1k–n) [2].

An Illustrated Atlas of Tooth Carving and Wax-Up Techniques, First Edition. Anil Bangalore Shivappa.

Companion website: www.wiley.com/go/bangalore/toothcarving

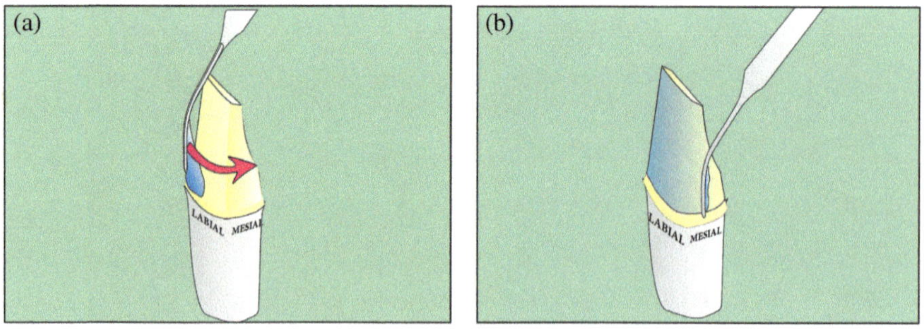

Figure 20.1 (a–b) Application of the initial layer of wax on the prepared tooth surface.

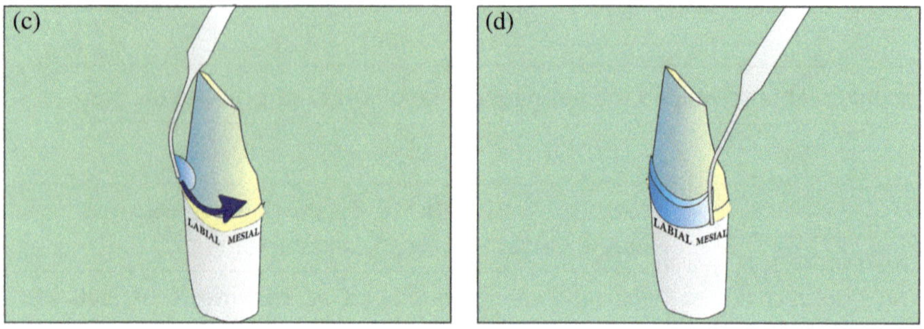

Figure 20.1 (c–d) Direction of movement of the instrument with molten wax to wax up the cervical portion of the labial surface of prepared tooth.

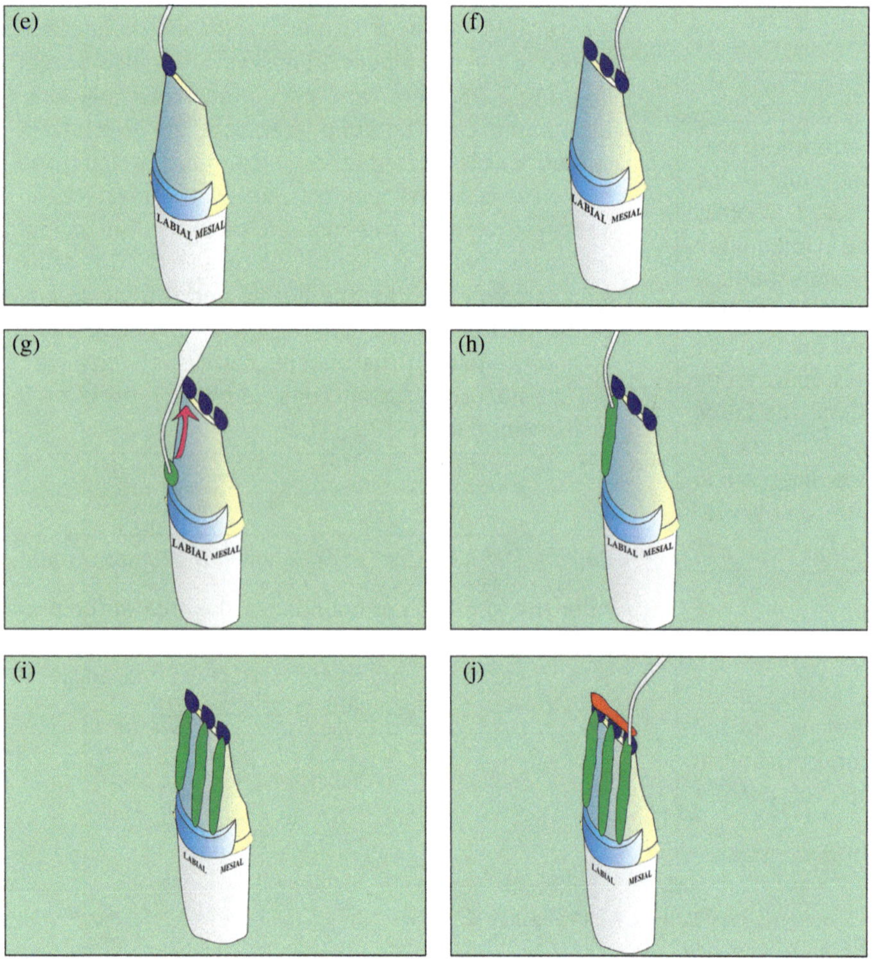

Figure 20.1 (e–j) Step sequence in adding bulk to the tooth structure on the labial surface by placing cones and contour bars.

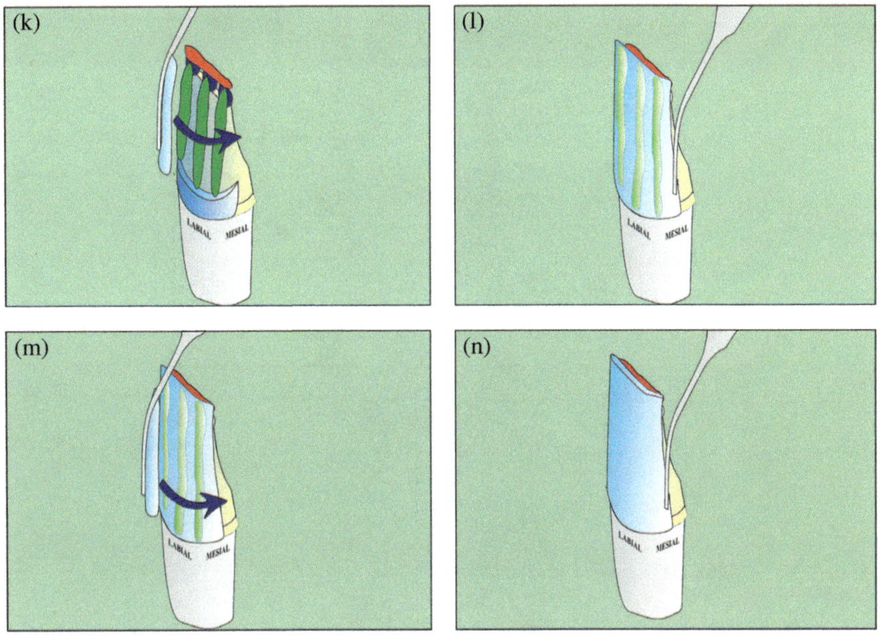

Figure 20.1 (k–n) Flushing the surface of the prepared tooth between the contour bars with molten wax.

Waxing the Lingual Surface

Exercise: Waxing the Cervical Portion of the Lingual Surface

Lingually, the wax is added at the cervical third to create a part of the cingulum bulk. The wax is added incrementally by passing the PKT no. 1 instrument from the mesiolingual to the distobuccal line angle (Figure 20.1p and q) [2].

Exercise: Creating Ridges on the Lingual Surface of the Prepared Crown

The contour bars are placed at the mesial and distal marginal ridge areas (Figure 20.1r–t). Also contour bars are placed on the incisal edge (Figure 20.1u). The molten wax is added to the area of the prepared tooth between the ridges incrementally, to get smooth marginal ridges, fossa, and cingulum (Figure 20.1v). Care should be taken to seal the marginal areas properly and remove the excess. The surfaces of the tooth are then polished to get smooth surface [2].

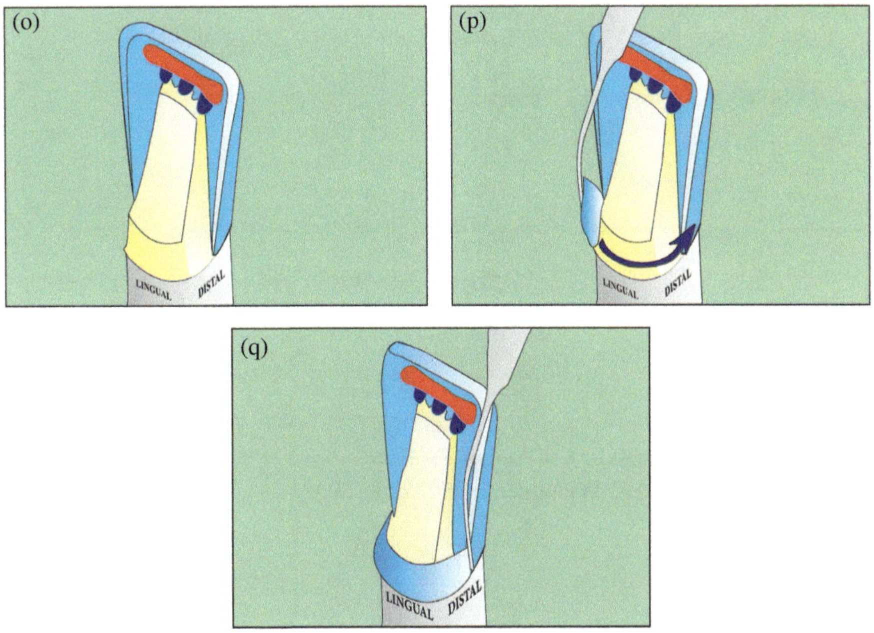

Figure 20.1 (o–q) Direction of movement of the instrument with molten wax to wax up the cervical portion of the lingual surface of the prepared tooth.

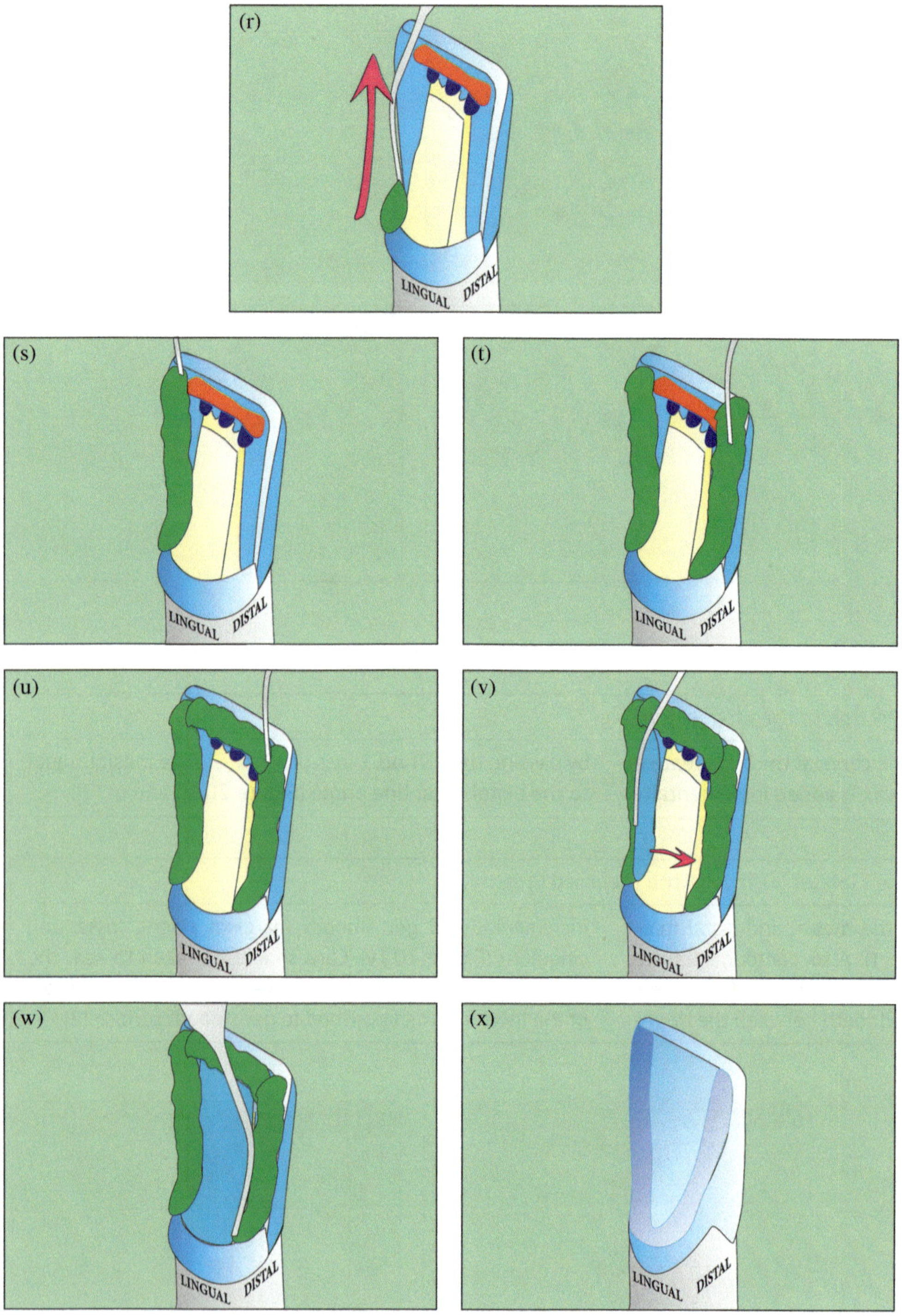

Figure 20.1 (r–x) Waxing on the lingual surface to create ridges, fossa, and cingulum.

References

1 Stephen, F.R., Martin, F.L., and Junhei, F. (2016). *Contemporary Fixed Prosthodontics*, 5e. St. Louis, MO: Elsevier.

2 Rowida, A. (2019). *The Art of Occlusal and Esthetic Waxing*, Kindle Edition. Kindle Edition: Quintessence Publishing Co IncBatavia, IL.

21

Waxing of the Permanent Maxillary Left Canine

LEARNING OBJECTIVE
At the end of the chapter, the student should be able to wax up the permanent maxillary left canine.

Exercise: Application of Die Lubricant

The die lubricant is applied to the prepared tooth surface using a brush and allowed to dry. The second coat is applied to ensure no voids form. Once the lubricant is dried, the waxing procedure is started [1].

Waxing the Labial Surface

Exercise: Initial Layer of Wax Application

The initial wax application is done to cover the entire area of crown preparation. This can be done using large instruments like either a wax spatula or using P. K. Thomas (PKT) no. 2 instrument. The wax should be in full molten state during wax application to prevent its solidification before its application and also to prevent the distortion of the applied layer of wax or tag formation. The PKT instrument is moved from the rounded distolabial line angle to the mesiopalatal line angle along the labial surface (Figure 21.1a and b) and then from the mesiopalatal line angle to the distolabial line angle along the lingual surface (Figure 21.1c and d). In addition, the wax is applied on the flat palatal surface [1].

Exercise: Waxing the Cervical Portion of the Labial Surface

The molten wax is applied to the cervical part of the crown that follows the cervical line mesiodistally to create the height of contour (Figure 21.1e and f).

Exercise: Placing the Cones and Contour Bars on the Labial Surface and Creating the Mesial and Distal Cuspal Ridges

The cuspal or the incisal cones are placed at the end of the mesial and the distal cuspal ridges and at the cusp tip areas (Figure 21.1g and h) that form the reference points for application of the contour bars. The contour bars are the wax bars created, representing the developmental lobes of natural teeth. The contour bars are placed at the mesiobuccal line angle, distobuccal line angle (that are reduced during crown preparation), and the buccal ridge. Depressions are found between the contour bars. The distobuccal contour bar is created at its line angle by placing the molten wax at the cervical part of the preparation and extending in a cervicoincisal direction to join the cone (Figure 21.1i). The same steps are followed for the buccal and the mesiobuccal contour bars (Figure 21.1j).

The distal cuspal ridge bar is created by joining the distobuccal cuspal cone with the buccal cuspal cone using PKT no. 1 or 2 instrument. In a similar way, the mesial cuspal ridge bar is created (Figure 21.1k).

Exercise: Waxing the Space Between the Contour Bars

After the formation of boundaries with ridge bars and contour bars, the gaps between them are filled with wax in increments to the level of the surface of the bars, to get a smooth labial surface and buccal ridge (Figure 21.1l–n) [2].

An Illustrated Atlas of Tooth Carving and Wax-Up Techniques, First Edition. Anil Bangalore Shivappa.

Companion website: www.wiley.com/go/bangalore/toothcarving

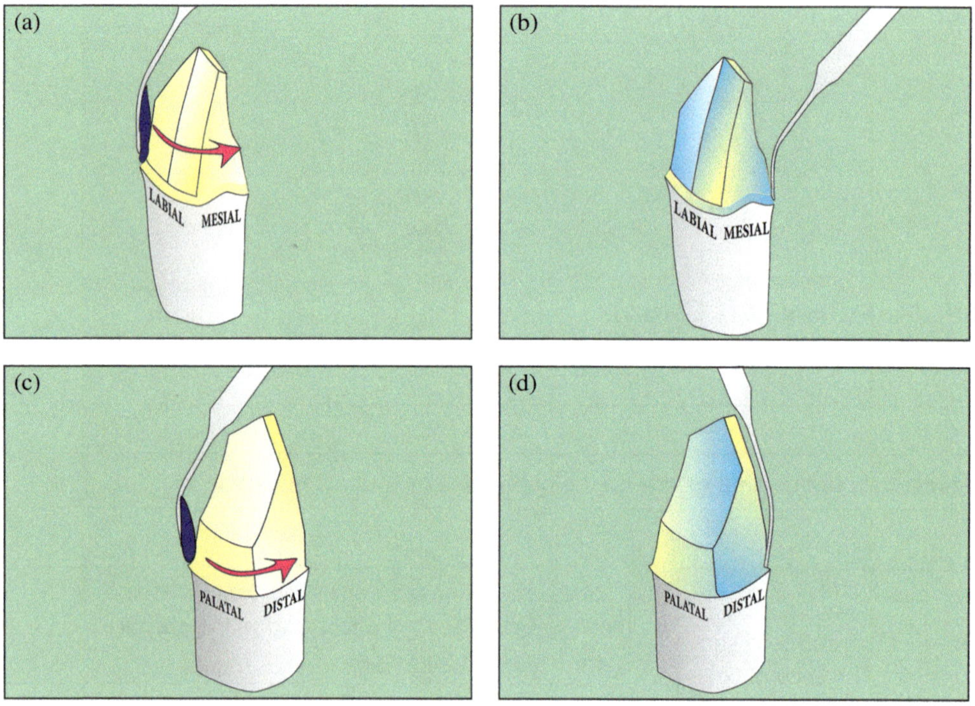

Figure 21.1 (a–d) Direction for application of the initial layer of wax on the labial and palatal surfaces of the prepared tooth.

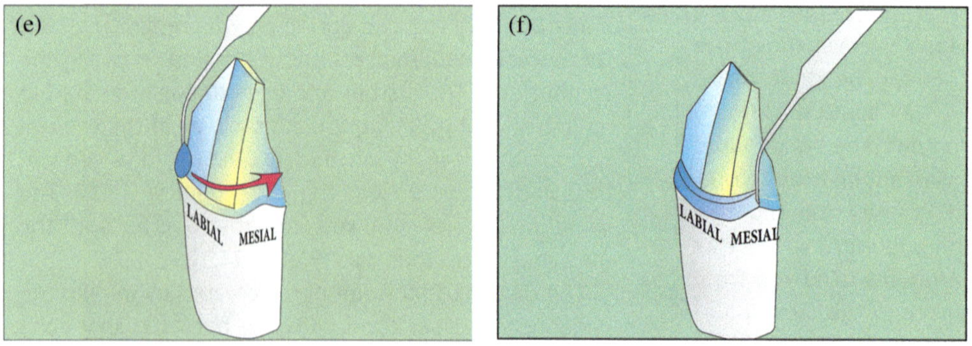

Figure 21.1 (e–f) Direction of movement of the PKT instrument with molten wax to wax up the cervical portion of the labial surface of the prepared tooth.

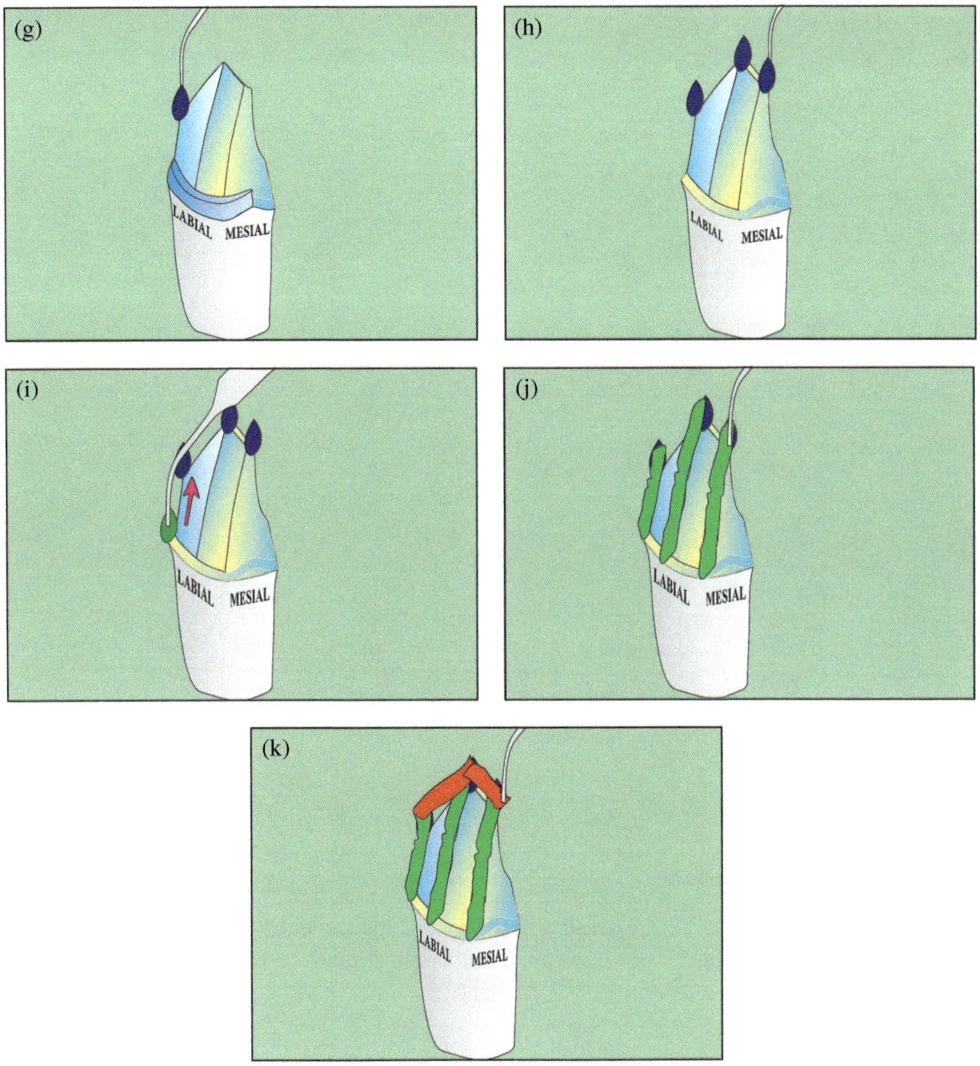

Figure 21.1 (g–k) Placing the molten wax cones and the contour bars of the marginal ridges and cuspal ridges.

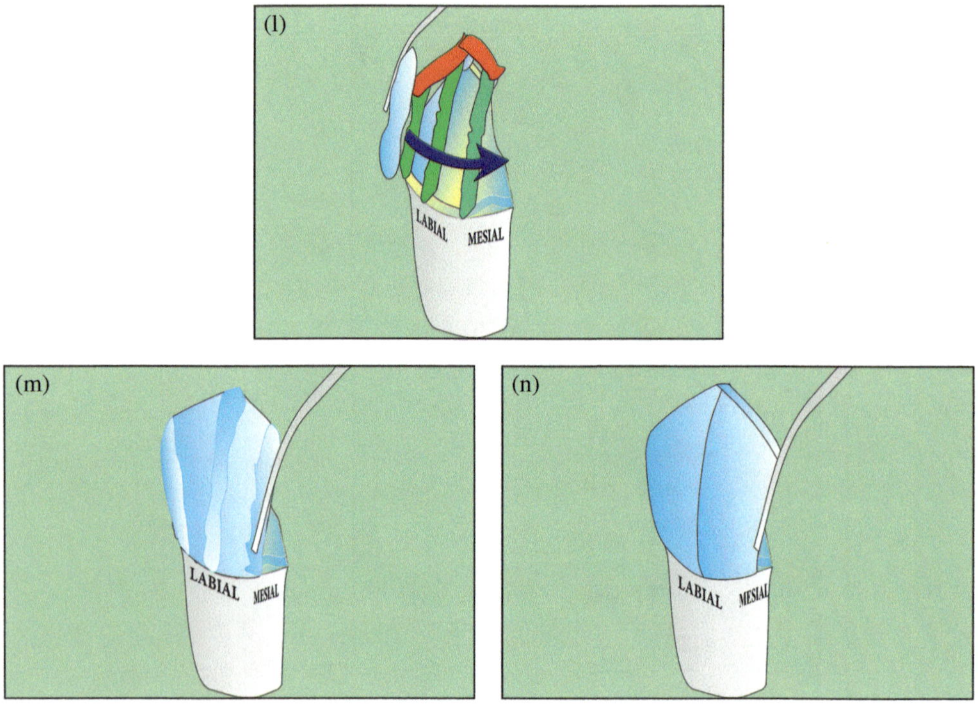

Figure 21.1 (l–n) Filling the space between the contour bars with molten wax.

Waxing the Palatal Surface

Exercise: Waxing the Cervical Portion of the Palatal Surface
Palatally, the wax is added at the cervical third to create part of the bulk of the cingulum. The wax is added incrementally by passing the PKT no. 1 instrument from the mesiolabial to the distolabial line angle (Figure 21.1p and q).

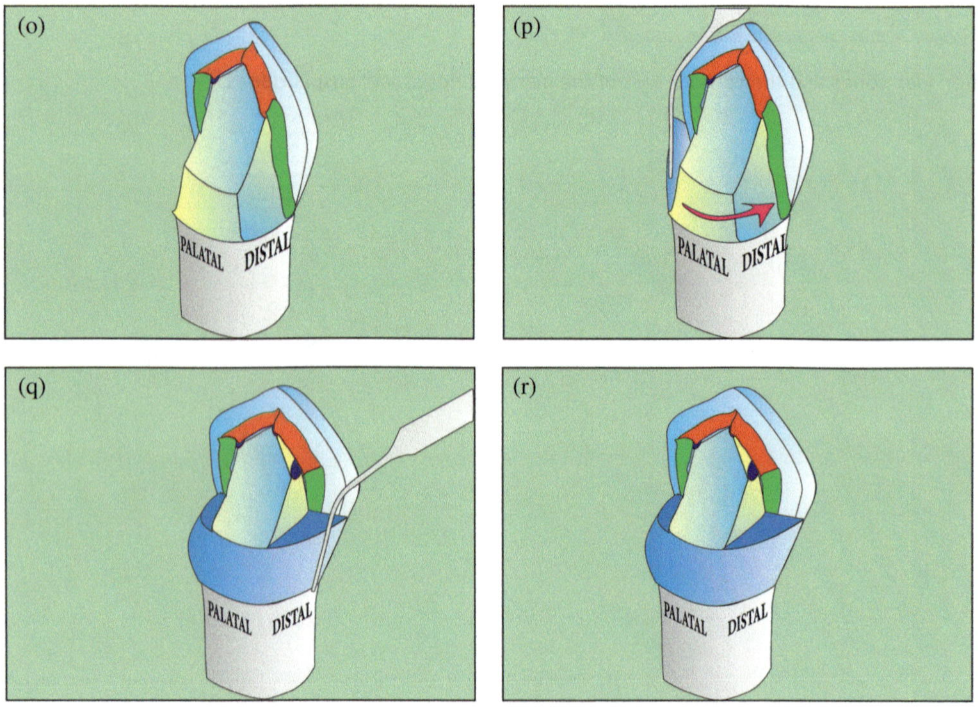

Figure 21.1 (o–r) Waxing the cervical third of the palatal surface.

Exercise: Waxing to Create the Mesial and Distal Marginal Ridges, Palatal Ridge, and Bulk of the Cingulum

The contour bars are placed at the mesial and distal marginal ridge areas and at the lingual or palatal ridge areas of the prepared tooth (Figure 21.1s–u). The bulk of the cingulum is contoured by adding wax at its incisal portion (Figure 21.1v). The molten wax is added to the middle and the incisal third of the palatal surface incrementally to fill the gap between bars and to get smooth marginal ridges and fossa. Care should be taken to seal the marginal areas properly and remove the excess (Figure 21.1w) [2].

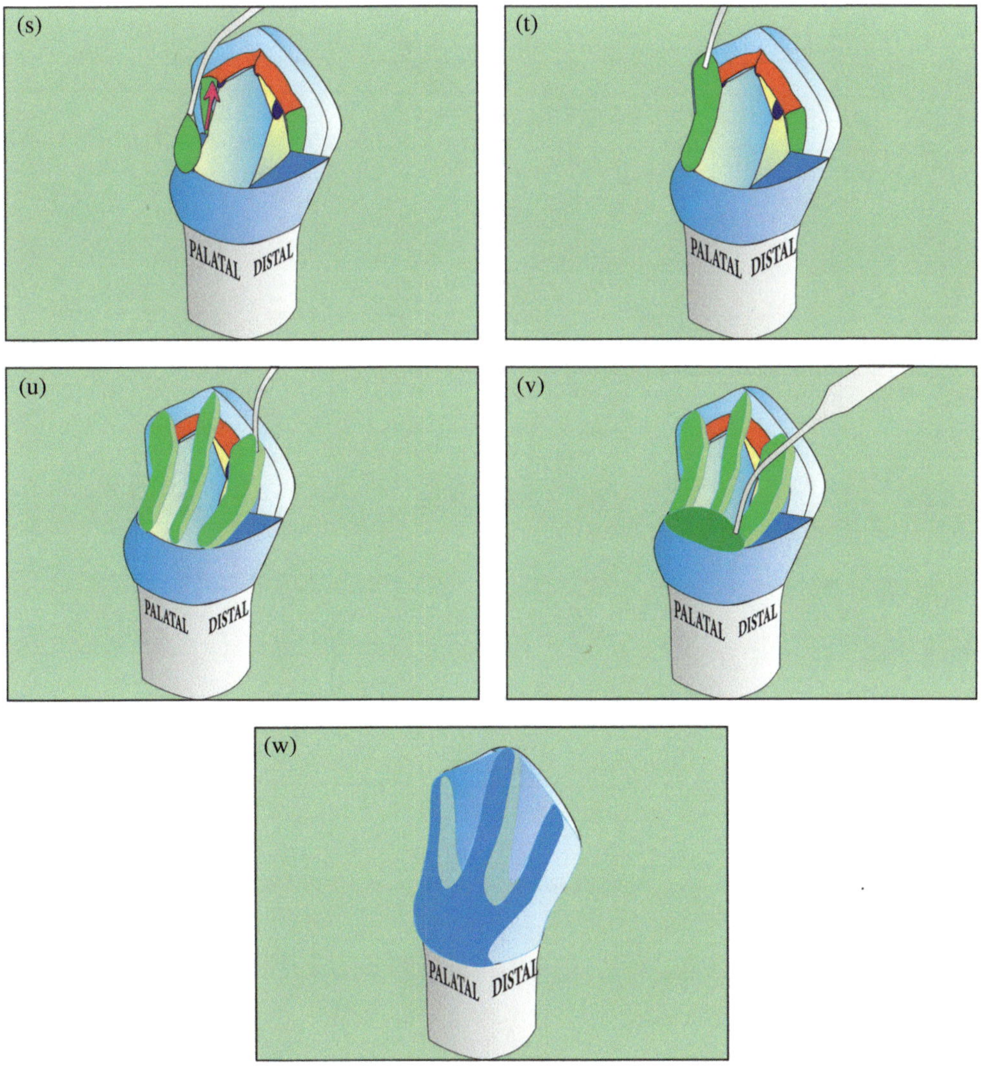

Figure 21.1 (s–w) Placing the contour bars on the mesial and distal marginal ridge areas along with the palatal ridge and creating the bulk of cingulum near the palatal fossa.

References

1 Stephen, F.R., Martin, F.L., and Junhei, F. (2016). *Contemporary Fixed Prosthodontics*, 5e. St. Louis, MO: Elsevier.

2 Rowida, A. (2019). *The Art of Occlusal and Esthetic Waxing*. Kindle Edition. Batavia: IL: Quintessence Publishing Co Inc.

22

Waxing of the Permanent Maxillary Left First Premolar

LEARNING OBJECTIVE
At the end of the chapter, the student should be able to wax up the permanent maxillary left first premolar.

Exercise: Initial Layer of Wax Application

After the tooth preparation, multiple coats of the die lubricant are applied to get a smooth surface. Using the P. K. Thomas (PKT) no. 2 waxing instrument, the initial layer of wax is applied on the prepared surfaces. The PKT instrument is moved from the distobuccal line angle of the prepared tooth along the buccal and mesial surfaces, up to the mesiopalatal line angle (Figure 22.1a and b). In a similar way, the initial layer of wax is applied starting from the mesiopalatal line angle along the palatal and distal surfaces to the distobuccal line angle (Figure 22.1c and d). An initial layer of wax is also applied on the slopes of the buccal and palatal triangular ridges (Figure 22.1e and f) [1].

Exercise: Placing the Cones and Contour Bars

The wax cones are placed at the buccal cusp tip and at the ends of the mesial cuspal ridge and distal cuspal ridge (Figure 22.1g and h) which represent the buccal developmental lobes. The contour bars are placed at the distobuccal line angle by placing the molten wax from the cervical preparation connected to the cone of the particular buccal cusps (Figure 22.1i and j). Remaining contour bars are placed at the buccal ridge and mesiobuccal line angle of the prepared tooth (Figure 22.1k) [1, 2].

An Illustrated Atlas of Tooth Carving and Wax-Up Techniques, First Edition. Anil Bangalore Shivappa.

Companion website: www.wiley.com/go/bangalore/toothcarving

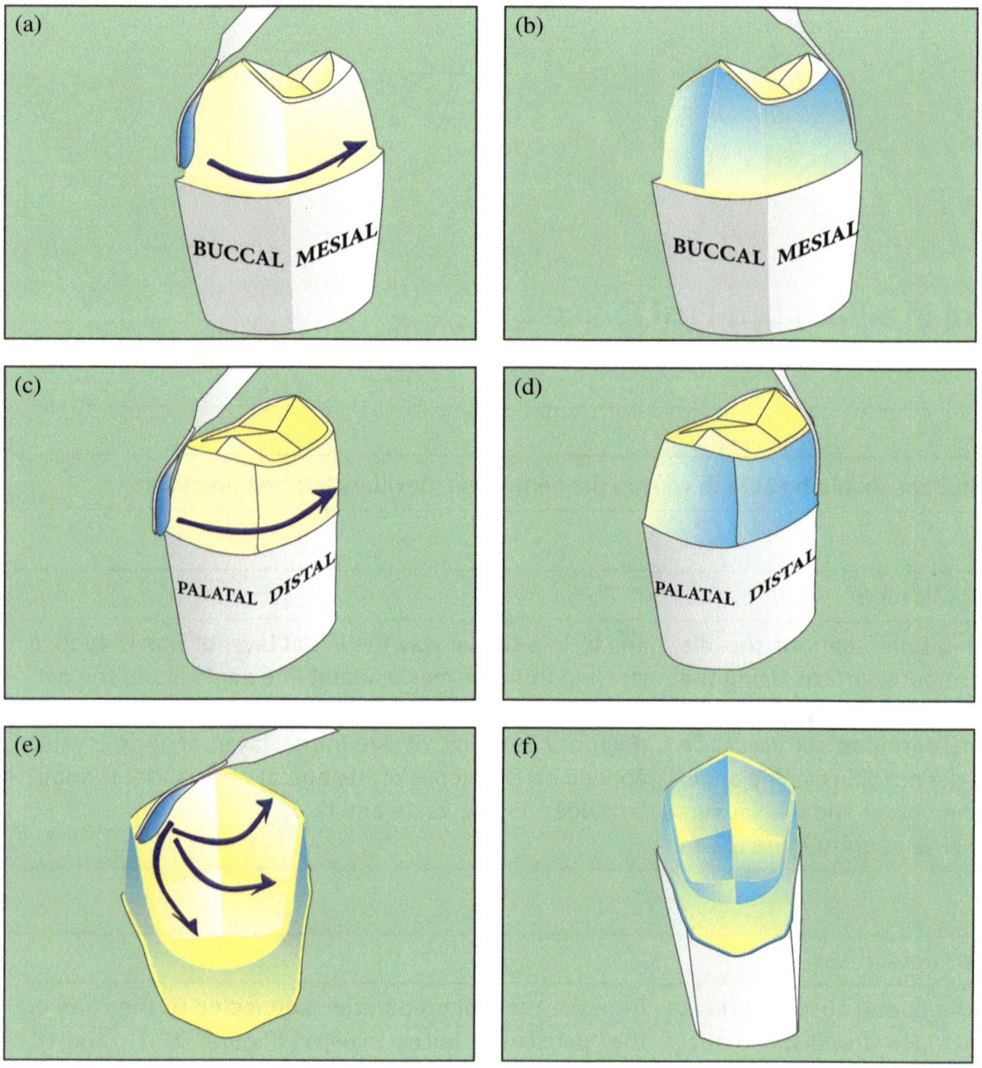

Figure 22.1 (a–f) Application of the initial layer of wax on all prepared tooth surfaces.

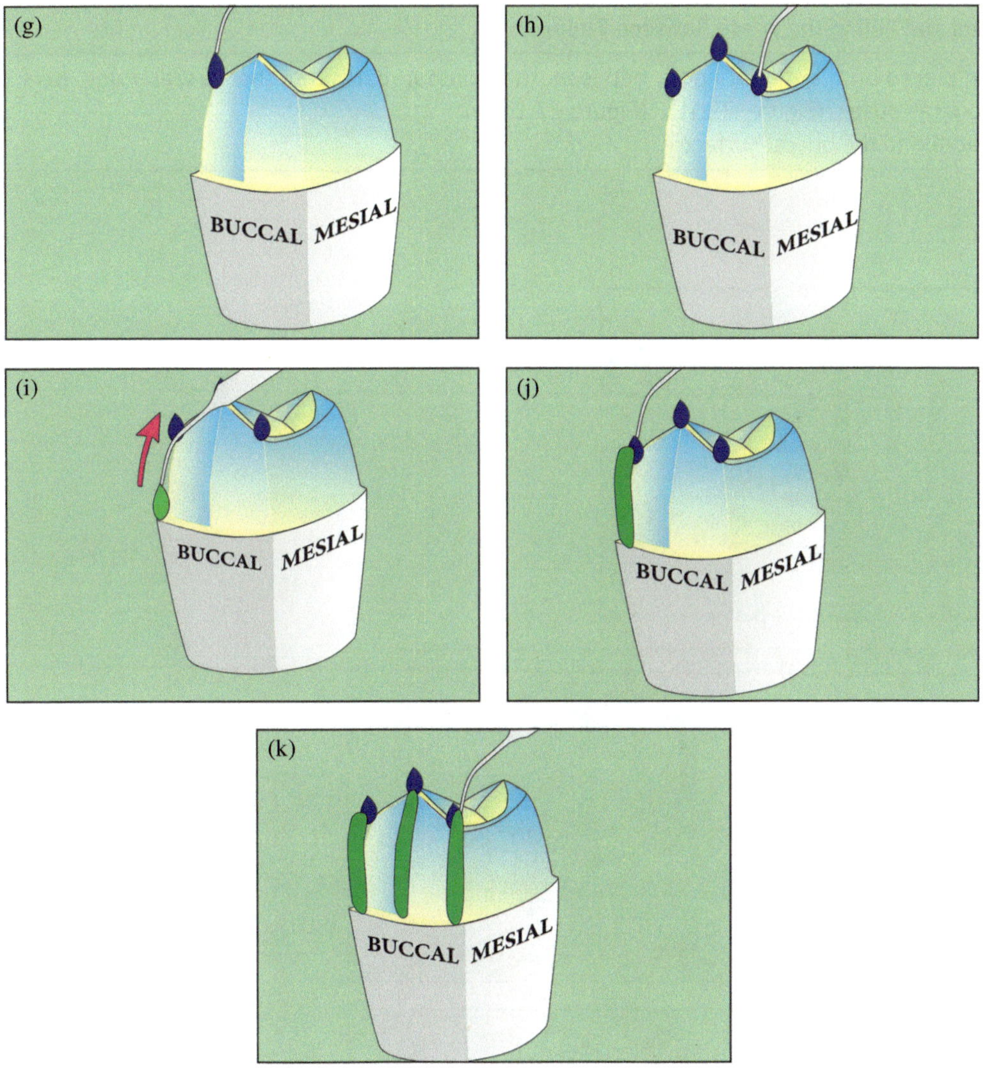

Figure 22.1 (g–k) Placing the molten wax cones at the mesio-incisal and disto-incisal angles and the cusp tip portion along with the contour bars.

Exercise: Placing the Ridge Bars and Filling the Space Between Them

The cuspal ridge (red) bars are placed on the mesial and distal cuspal ridges of the buccal cusps (Figure 22.1l and n). The bulk of the wax is added to the buccal surface between the contour bars and the cuspal ridge bars (Figure 22.1o–p).

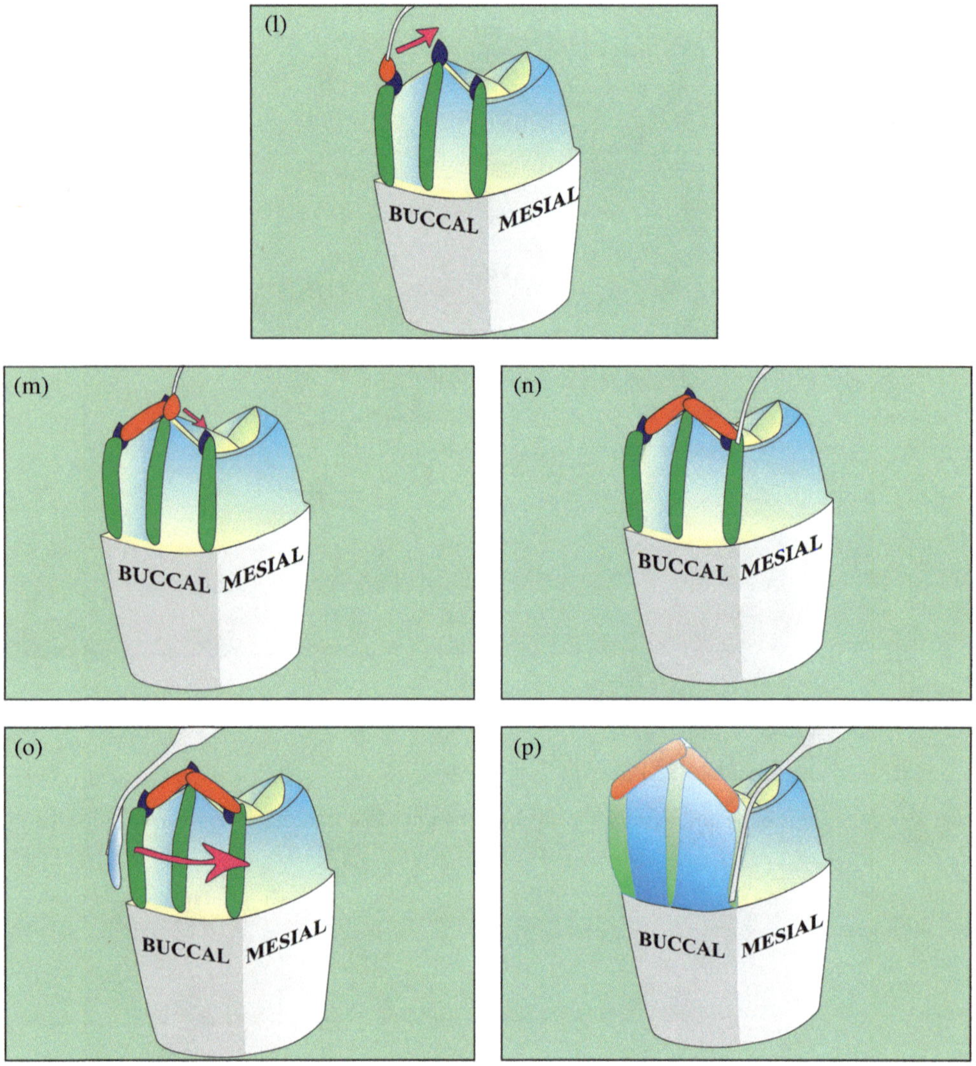

Figure 22.1 (l–p) Movement of the instrument with molten wax for placing the mesial and distal cuspal ridge bars and filling the space between the contour bars with molten wax.

Exercise: Adding the Bulk of the Wax on the Proximal (Mesial and Distal) and Palatal Surfaces

The bulk of the wax is added using the PKT no. 2 instrument from the mesiobuccal line angle to the palatal ridge and then from the palatal ridge to the distobuccal line angle (Figure 22.1q–u) [1, 2].

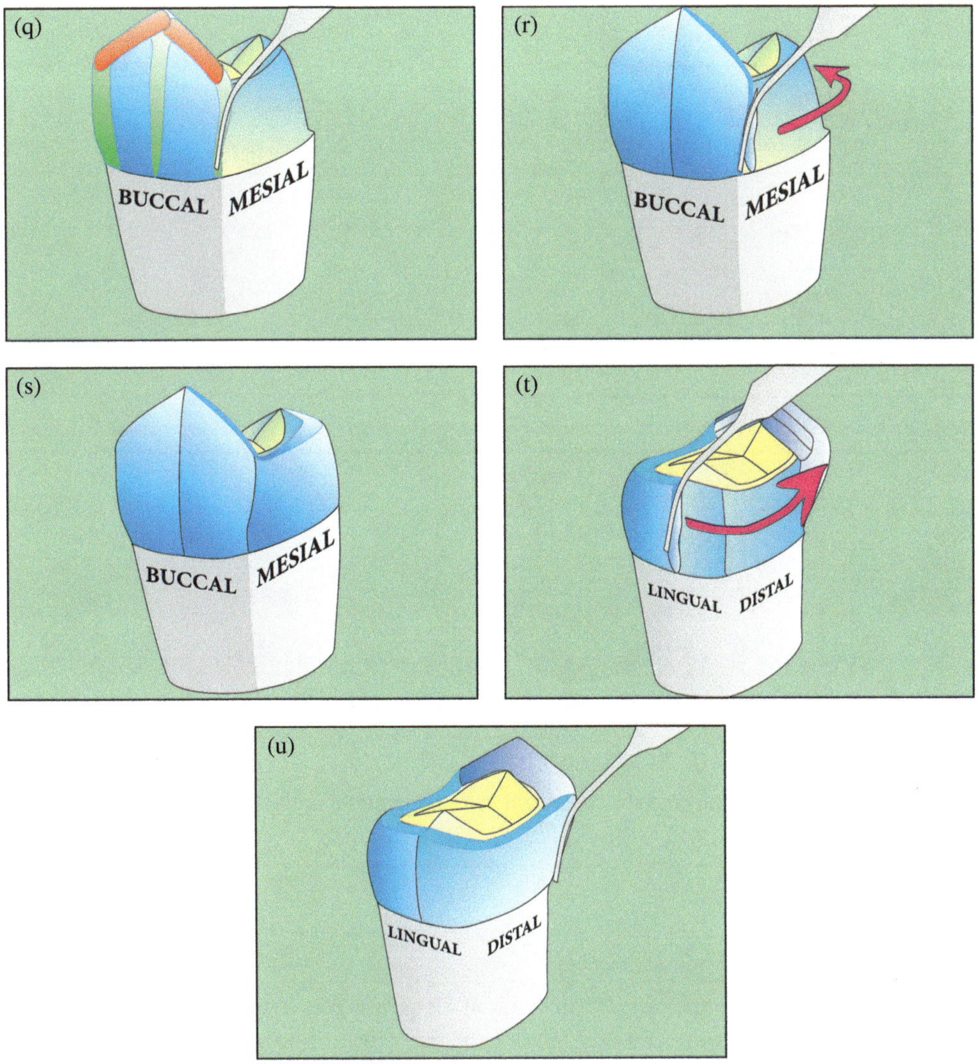

Figure 22.1 (q–u) Direction of movement of the instrument with molten wax on the proximal and palatal surfaces.

Exercise: Placing the Palatal Ridge Bars on the Occlusal Surface

The palatal cuspal ridge (red) wax is added near the bevel (Figure 22.1v). The triangular ridge bars (green) are placed on the buccal and palatal triangular ridge region of the prepared tooth (Figure 22.1w). Marginal ridge bars (blue) are placed on the particular ridge area of the prepared tooth (Figure 22.1x) [1, 2].

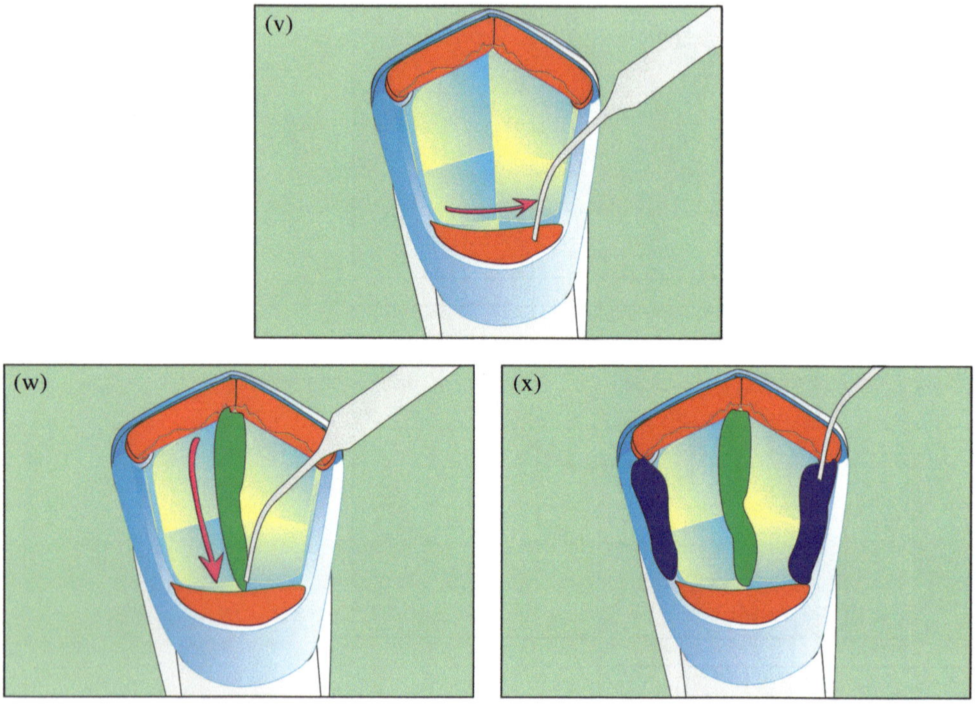

Figure 22.1 (v–x) Placing the molten wax to create the palatal cuspal ridges, transverse ridge, and marginal ridges.

Exercise: Waxing the Slopes of the Triangular Ridges on the Occlusal Surface

Wax bars are also placed at the central groove region (Figure 22.2a). The bulk of the wax is now added to obtain the mesial and distal slopes of the buccal triangular ridge (Figure 22.2b and c). In the same way, the slopes of the palatal triangular ridge are created (Figure 22.2d and e). Finally, waxing of the mesial and distal marginal ridge along with the fossae is done (Figure 22.2f and g) [1, 2].

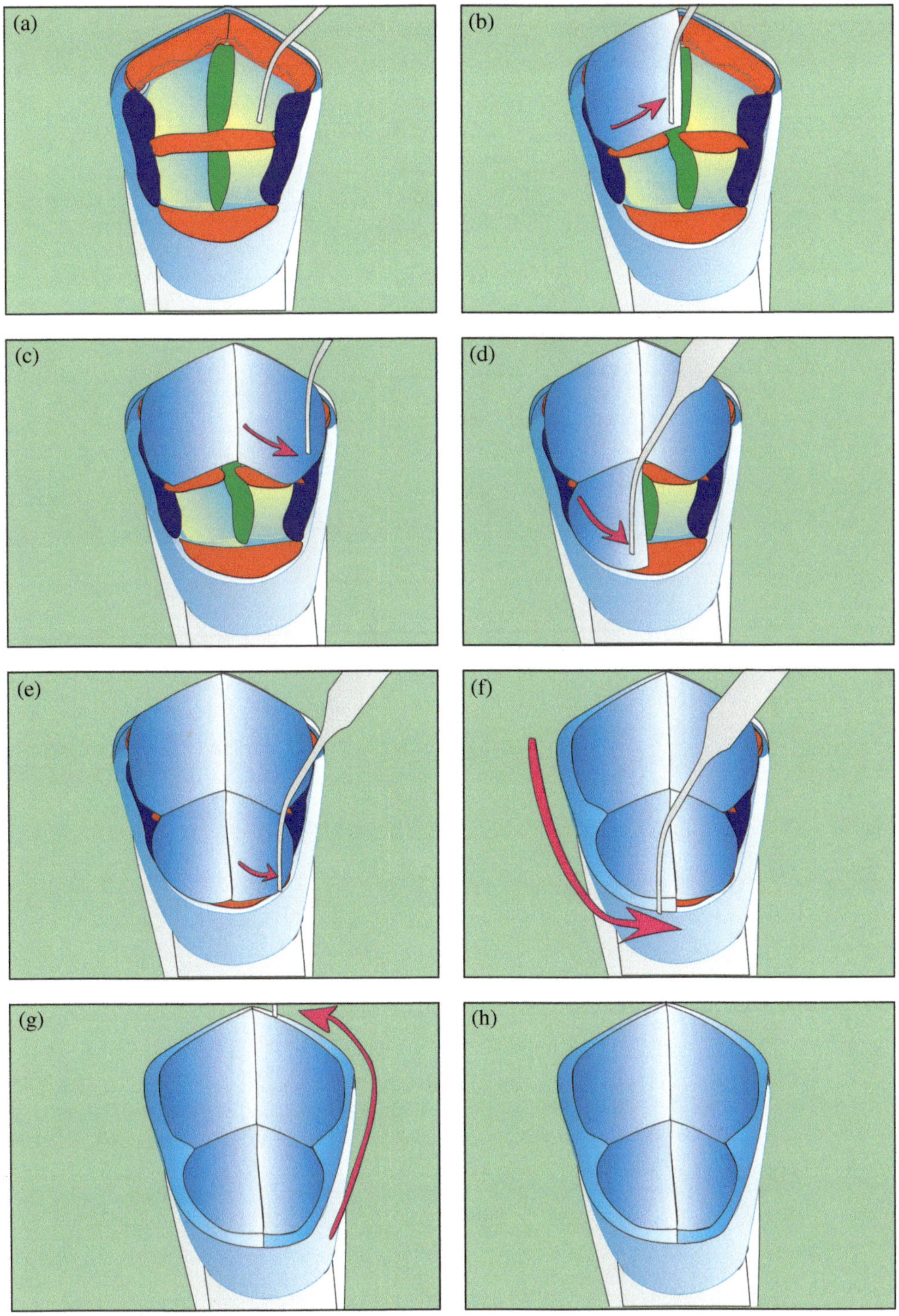

Figure 22.2 (a–h) Creating the slopes of the buccal and palatal triangular ridges and waxing the marginal ridges.

References

1 Stephen, F.R., Martin, F.L., and Junhei, F. (2016). *Contemporary Fixed Prosthodontics*, 5e. St. Louis, MO: Elsevier.

2 Rowida, A. (2019). *The Art of Occlusal and Esthetic Waxing*. Kindle Edition. Batavia, IL: Quintessence Publishing Co Inc.

23

Waxing of the Permanent Maxillary Right First Molar

LEARNING OBJECTIVE
At the end of the chapter, the student should be able to wax up the permanent maxillary right first molar.

Exercise: Application of the Initial Layer of Wax

After the application of multiple coats of die lubricant, a thin layer of wax is applied to all prepared surfaces. With molten wax taken in P.K. Thomas (PKT) instrument no. 2, the instrument is passed from the distopalatal line angle along the palatal surface to the mesiobuccal line angle (Figure 23.1a and b). Then in a similar way, the instrument carrying the molten wax is passed from the distopalatal line angle along the buccal surface to the mesiobuccal line angle (Figure 23.1c and d). Using the wax spatula, the molten wax is applied to the occlusal surface of the prepared tooth surface (Figure 23.1e) [1].

Exercise: Placing the Cones and Contour Bars

The wax cones are placed at the cusp tips of all the four major cusps (Figure 23.1f–h). The contour bars are placed at the distopalatal surface ridge by applying molten wax from the cervical preparation connected to the cone of the particular cusp (Figure 23.1i–j). Contour bars for the remaining cusps are placed in a similar way (Figure 23.1k–o).

An Illustrated Atlas of Tooth Carving and Wax-Up Techniques, First Edition. Anil Bangalore Shivappa.

Companion website: www.wiley.com/go/bangalore/toothcarving

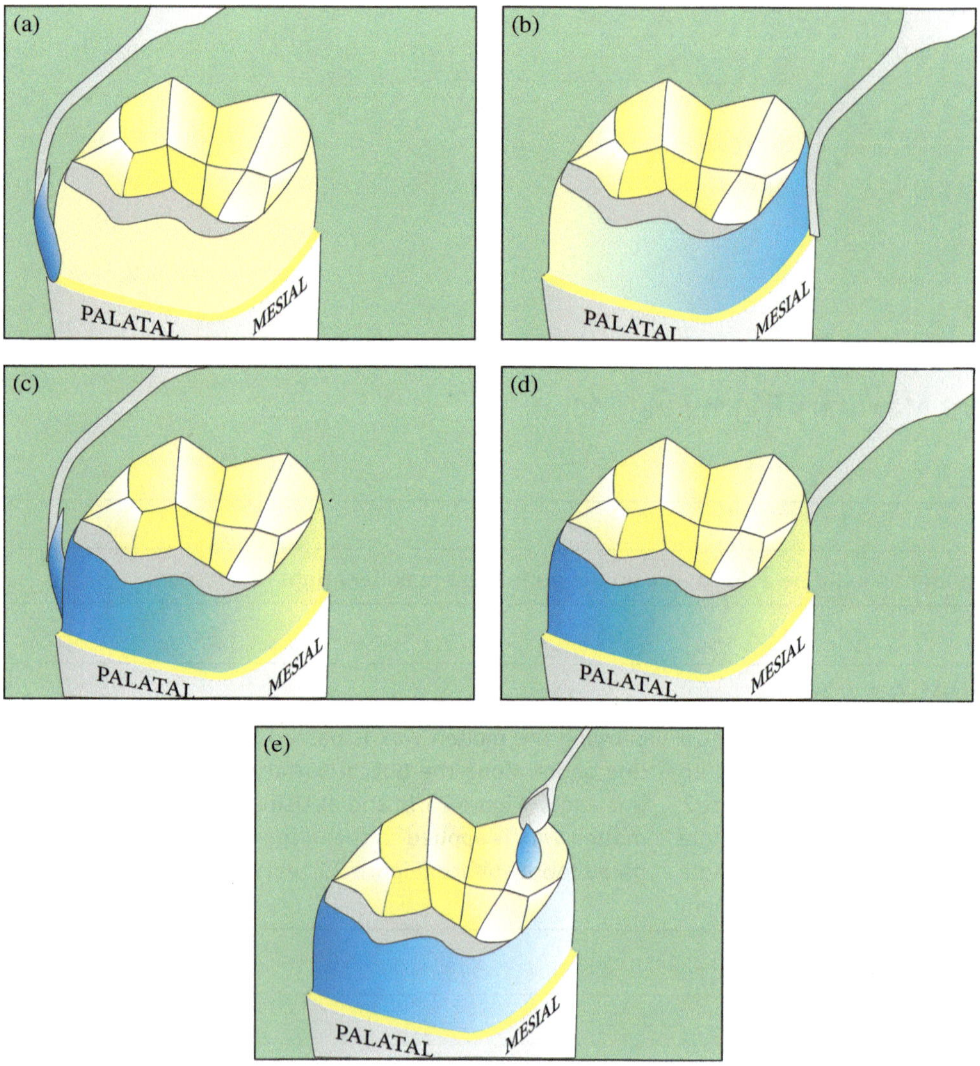

Figure 23.1 (a–e) Application of the initial layer of wax on all prepared tooth surfaces.

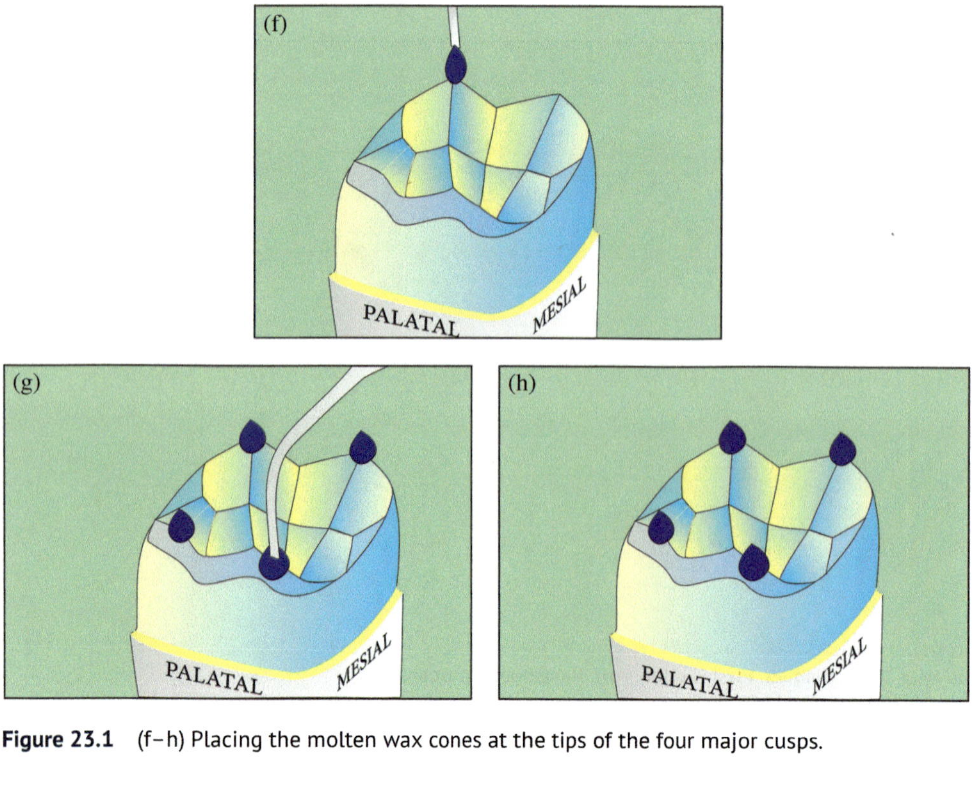

Figure 23.1 (f–h) Placing the molten wax cones at the tips of the four major cusps.

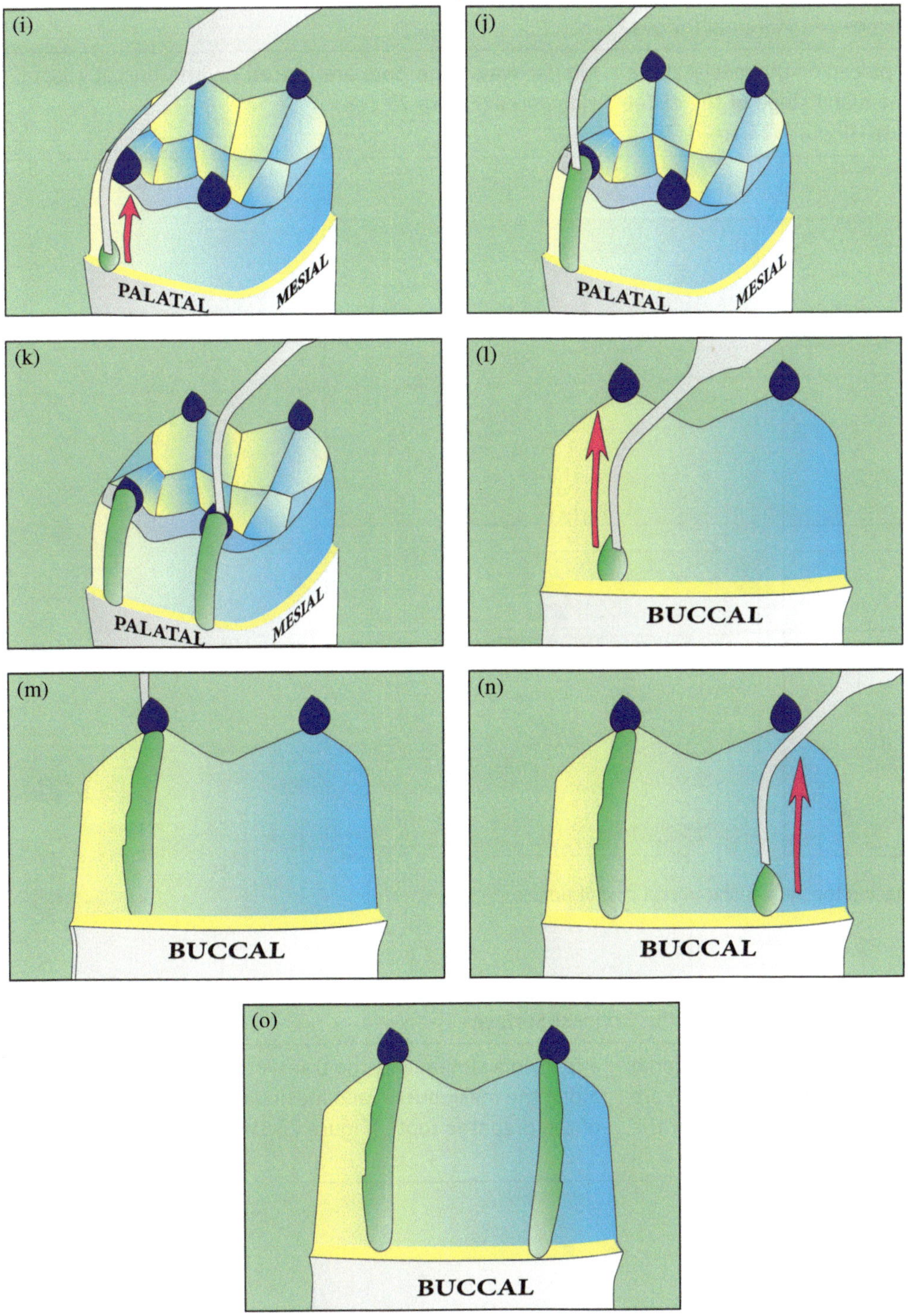

Figure 23.1 (i–o) Placing the contour bars on the buccal and palatal prepared surfaces, using the cones as a guide.

Exercise: Placing the Cuspal Ridges and Marginal Ridges

The cuspal ridge (red) bars are placed on the mesial slope of the distopalatal cusp and the distal slope of the distal ridge of the mesiopalatal cusp (Figure 23.1p–r). In a similar way ridge bars are placed on the buccal cuspal ridge area (Figure 23.1s).

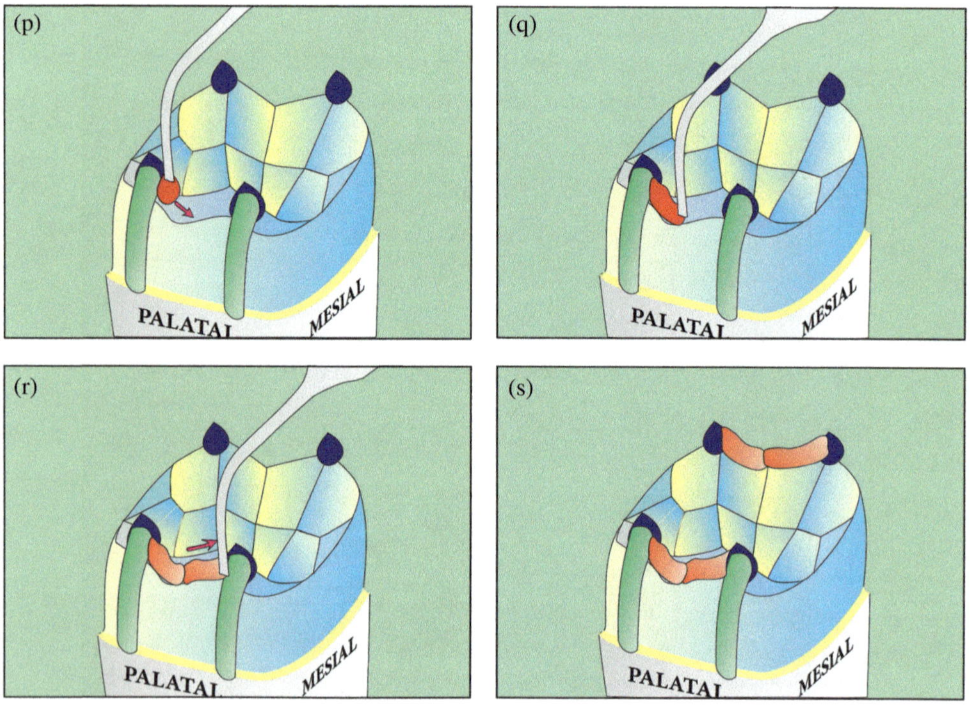

Figure 23.1 (p–s) Directions for placing the palatal and buccal cuspal ridges.

Exercise: Placing the Marginal Ridges and Ridges of the Occlusal Surface

The bars are created on the distal and mesial marginal ridges (Figure 23.1t). The triangular ridge bars (green) are placed on the mesiopalatal and distobuccal ridges of the prepared tooth to form the oblique ridge bar (Figure 23.1u and v). In a similar way the transverse ridge bar is created along the mesiobuccal and mesiopalatal triangular ridges of the prepared tooth (Figure 23.1w–x) [1, 2].

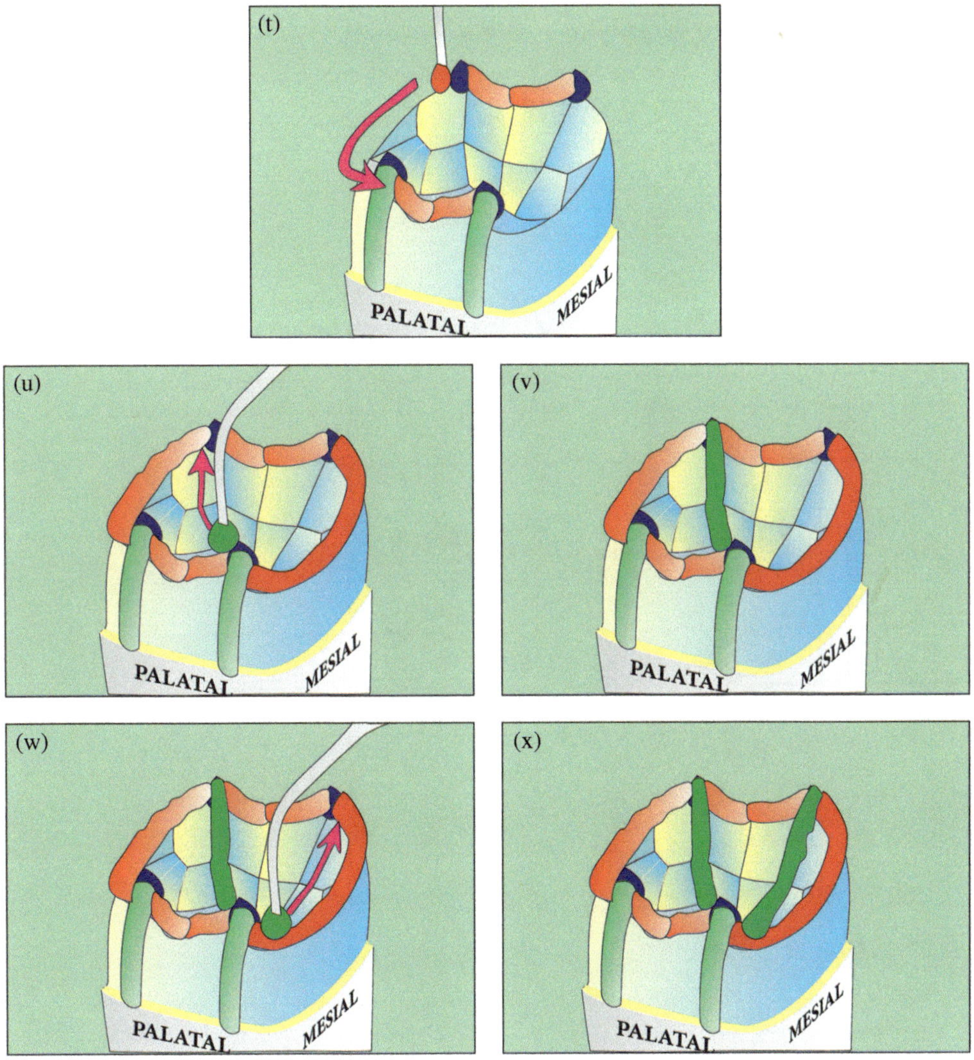

Figure 23.1 (t–x) Direction for placing the marginal ridges, oblique ridge, and transverse ridge.

Exercise: Bulk Waxing of the Buccal, Palatal, and Proximal Surfaces

Molten wax is then applied on surfaces using the PKT no. 2 instrument to create the bulk of the surfaces. The instrument with molten wax is passed from the distopalatal line angle along the palatal surface to the mesiobuccal line angle, while adding the bulk of the wax in increments (Figure 23.2a–c). Bulk is added to the distal and buccal surfaces in a similar way (Figure 23.2d–f) [1, 2].

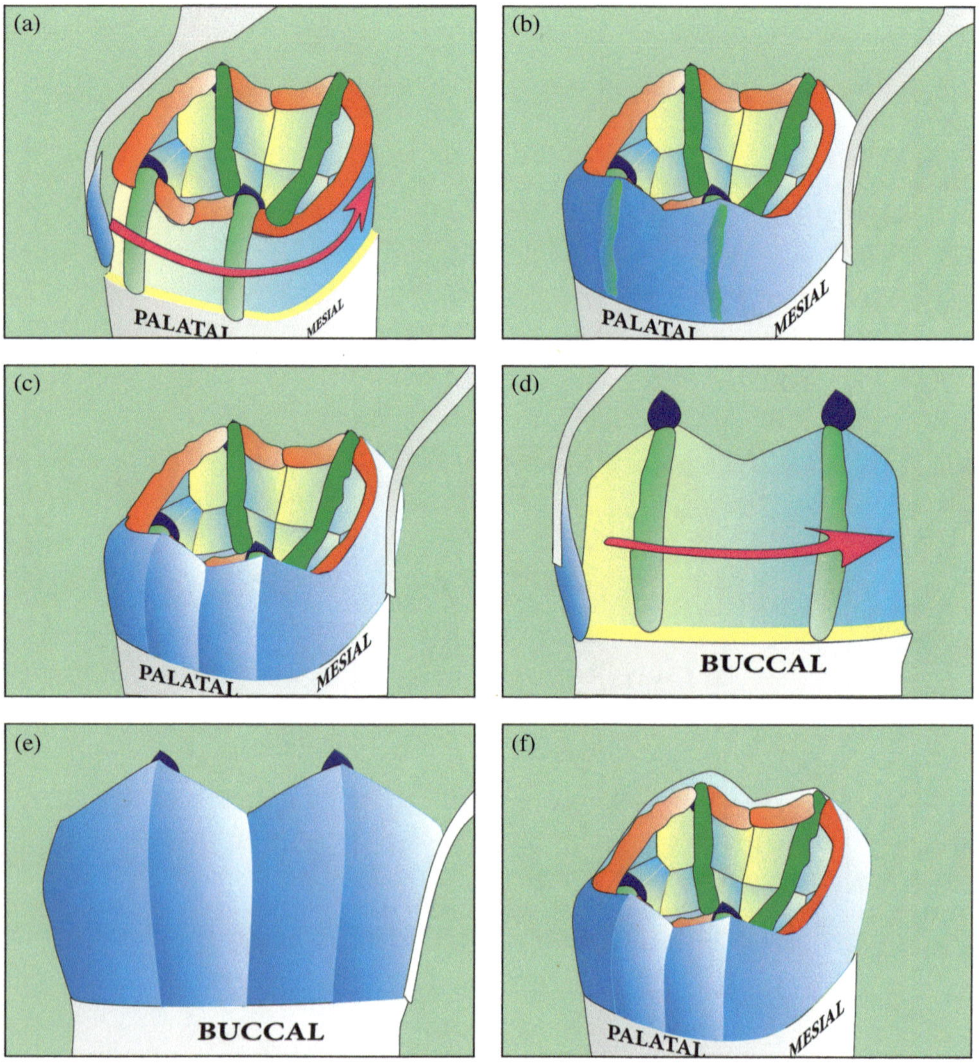

Figure 23.2 (a–f) Directions for placing the molten wax on the mesiopalatal and distobuccal surfaces.

Exercise: Waxing the Slopes of the Triangular Ridges, Oblique Ridge, and Transverse Ridge on the Occlusal Surface

The bulk of the wax is added to create the slopes of the triangular ridges on the occlusal surface. The PKT no. 2 instrument carrying molten wax is passed from distal slope of the distobuccal cusp to the distal slope of the distal ridge of the mesiopalatal cusp. This creates the distal slope of the oblique ridge (Figure 23.2g and h).

The instrument with molten wax is then passed from the mesial slope of the distobuccal cusp to the mesial slope of the distal cuspal ridge of the mesiopalatal cusp and then to the distal slope of the mesial triangular ridge of mesiopalatal cusp (Figure 23.2i and j).

The bulk of the wax is applied to obtain the mesial and distal slopes of the mesiobuccal triangular ridge (Figure 23.2k–m) and on the mesial slope of the mesial triangular ridge of the mesiopalatal cusp to complete the triangular ridge (Figure 23.2n).

The distopalatal triangular ridge is created with its slopes (Figure 23.2o and p). Finally the wax is applied to create the mesial and distal fossae and the cusp of Carabelli (Figure 23.2q–v). The rough surfaces are carved and polished to get smooth and shiny surfaces [1, 2].

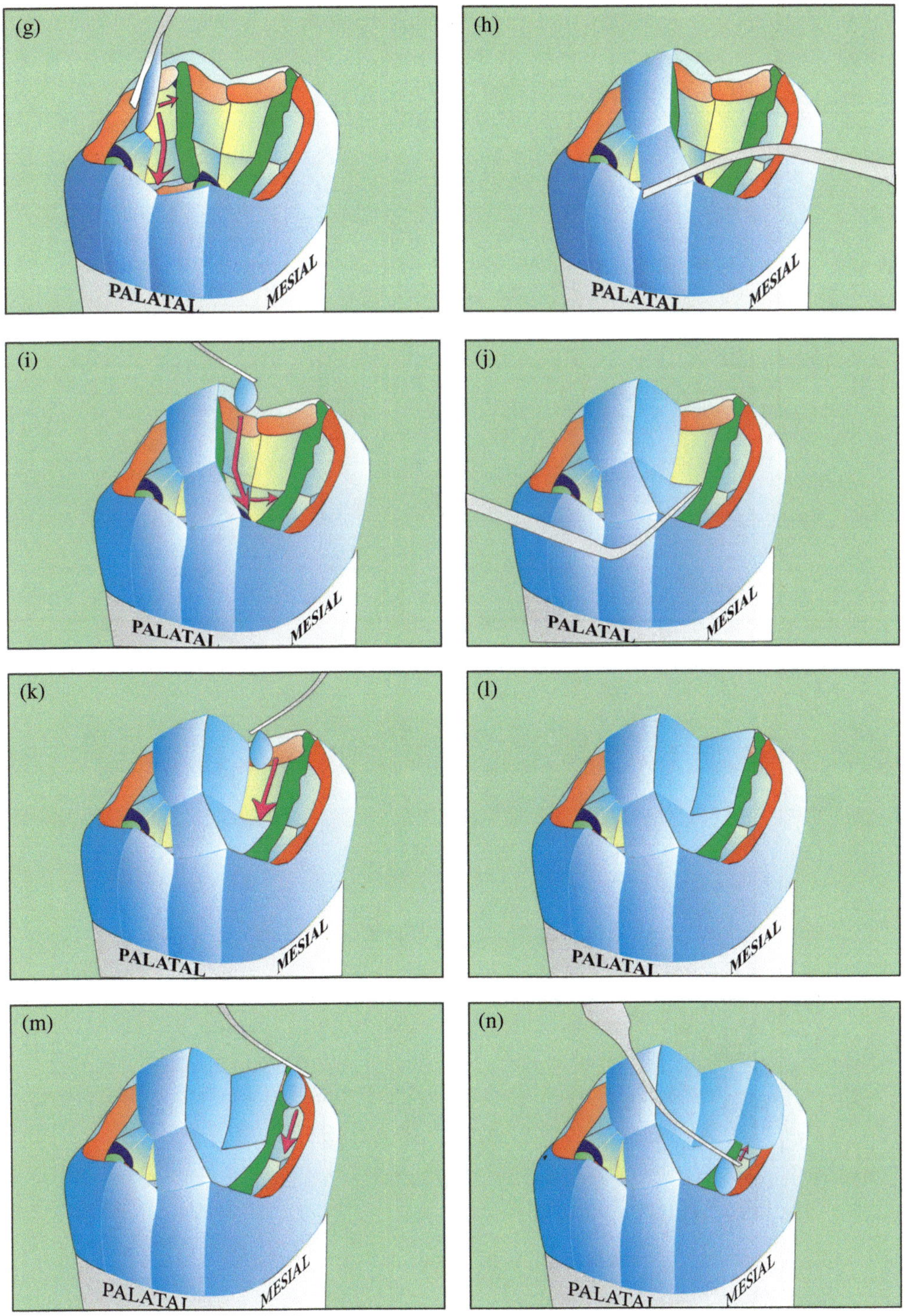

Figure 23.2 (g–v) Directions for placing the bulk of molten wax to create the slopes of the ridges of the occlusal surface.

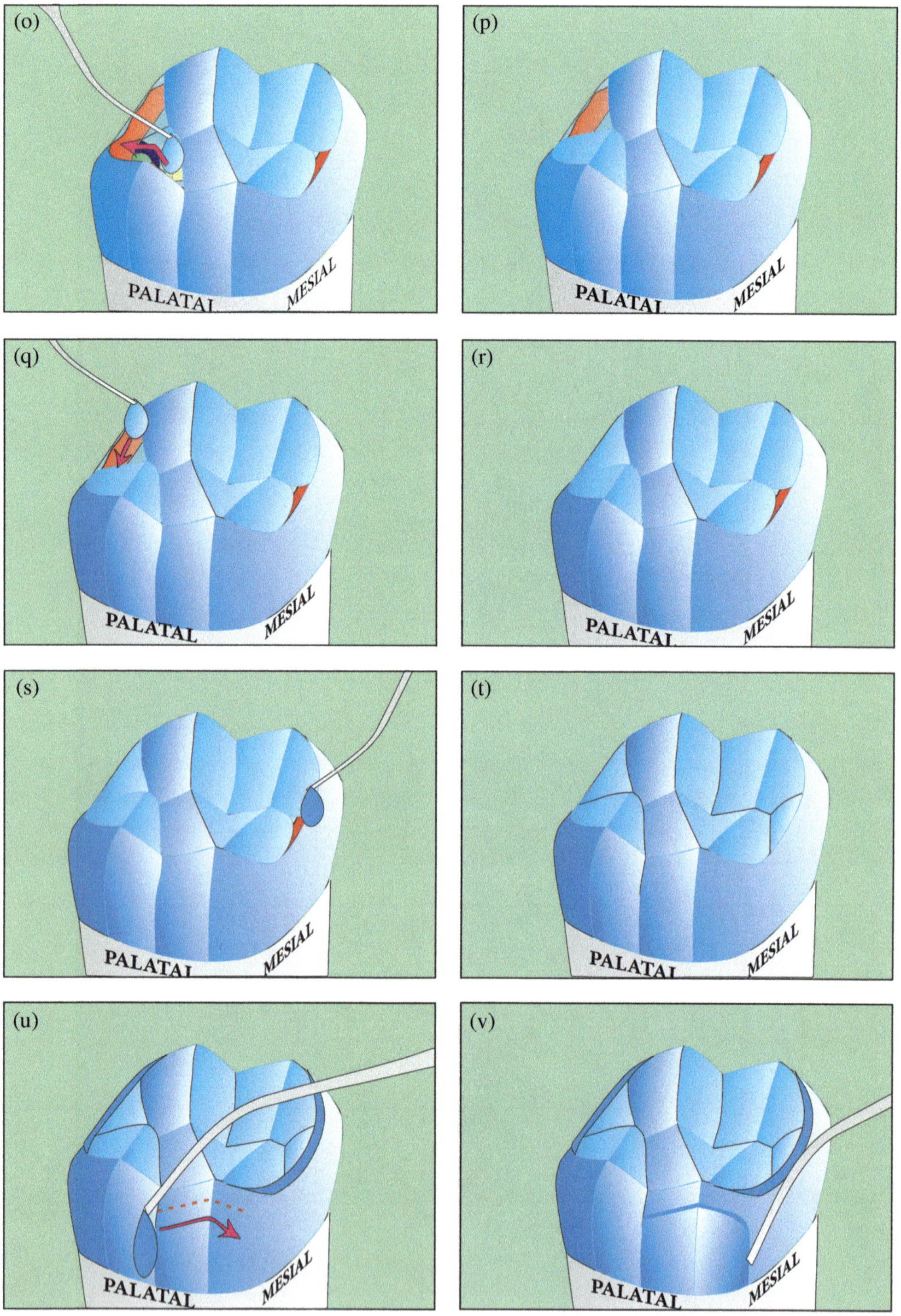

Figure 23.2 (Cont'd) (g–v)

References

1 Stephen, F.R., Martin, F.L., and Junhei, F. (2016). *Contemporary Fixed Prosthodontics*, 5e. St. Louis, MO: Elsevier.

2 Rowida, A. (2019). *The Art of Occlusal and Esthetic Waxing*. Kindle Edition. Batavia, IL: Quintessence Publishing Co Inc.

24

Waxing of the Permanent Mandibular Right First Molar

LEARNING OBJECTIVE
At the end of the chapter, the student should be able to wax up the permanent mandibular right first molar.

Exercise: Initial Layer of Wax Application

After the tooth preparation, multiple coats of the die lubricant are applied to get a smooth surface. Using the P. K. Thomas (PKT) no. 2 waxing instrument, the initial layer of wax is applied on the prepared surfaces. The PKT instrument is moved from the distolingual line angle of the prepared tooth along the distal and buccal surfaces to the mesiobuccal line angle (Figure 24.1a–b). In a similar way, the initial layer of wax is applied starting from the distolingual line angle along mesial and lingual surfaces to the mesiobuccal line angle (Figure 24.1c–d) [1]. Using a spatula, wax is also applied on the occlusal surfaces (Figure 24.1e).

Exercise: Placing the Cones and Contour Bars

The wax cones are placed at the cusp tips of all five cusps (Figure 24.1f and g). The contour bars are placed at the line angles by placing the molten wax from the cervical preparation connected to the cone of the particular buccal cusps (Figure 24.1h–j). Contour bars for the two lingual cusps are placed in a similar way (Figure 24.1k–m).

An Illustrated Atlas of Tooth Carving and Wax-Up Techniques, First Edition. Anil Bangalore Shivappa.

Companion website: www.wiley.com/go/bangalore/toothcarving

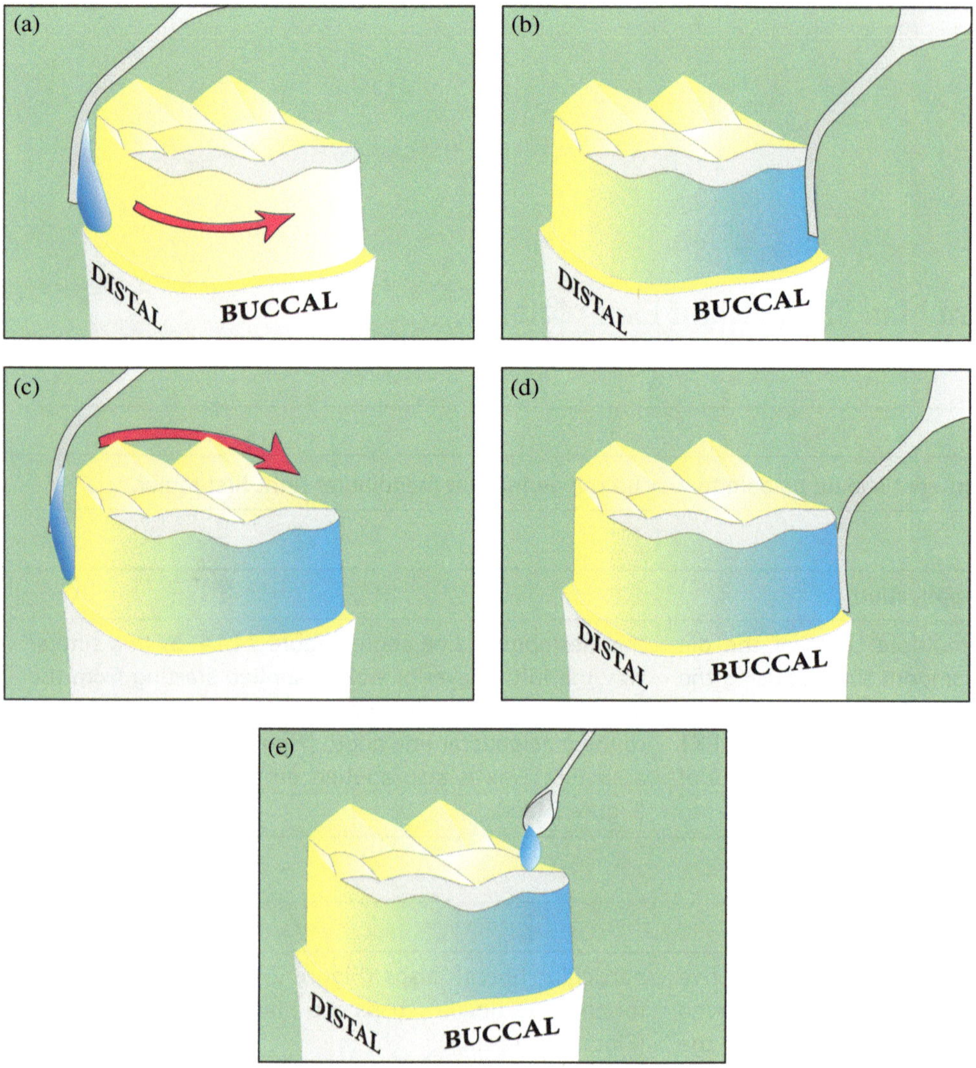

Figure 24.1 (a–e) Application of the initial layer of wax on all prepared tooth surfaces.

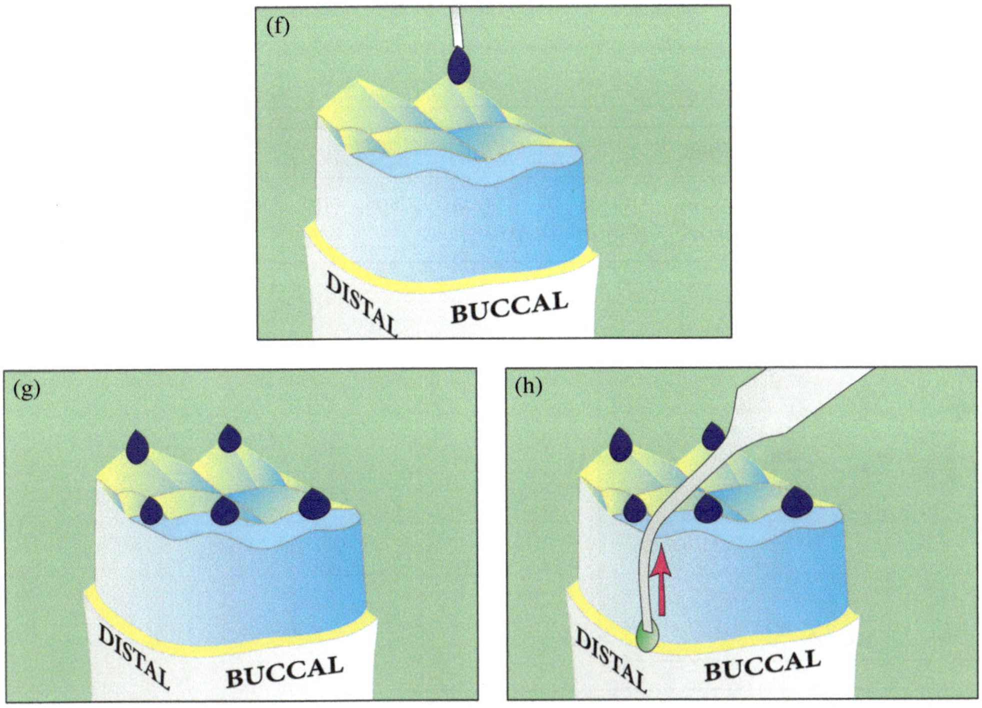

Figure 24.1 (f–h) Placing the molten wax cones at the tips of all five cusps.

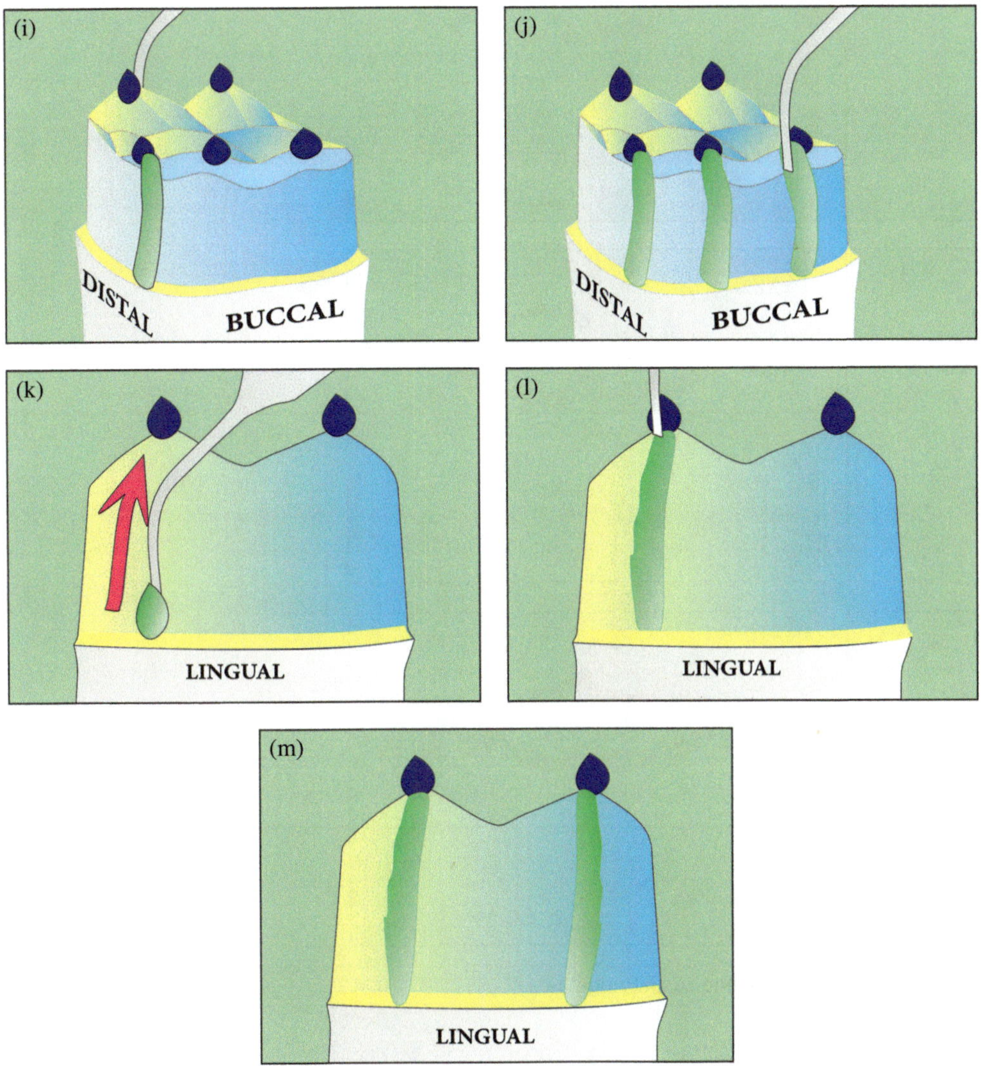

Figure 24.1 (i–m) Placing the contour bars on the buccal and lingual prepared surfaces, using the cones as a guide.

Exercise: Placing the Cuspal Ridges and Marginal Ridges
The cuspal ridge (red) bars are placed on the cuspal ridges of all buccal cusps, distal marginal ridges, cuspal ridges of lingual cusps, and mesial marginal ridge (Figure 24.1n–t).

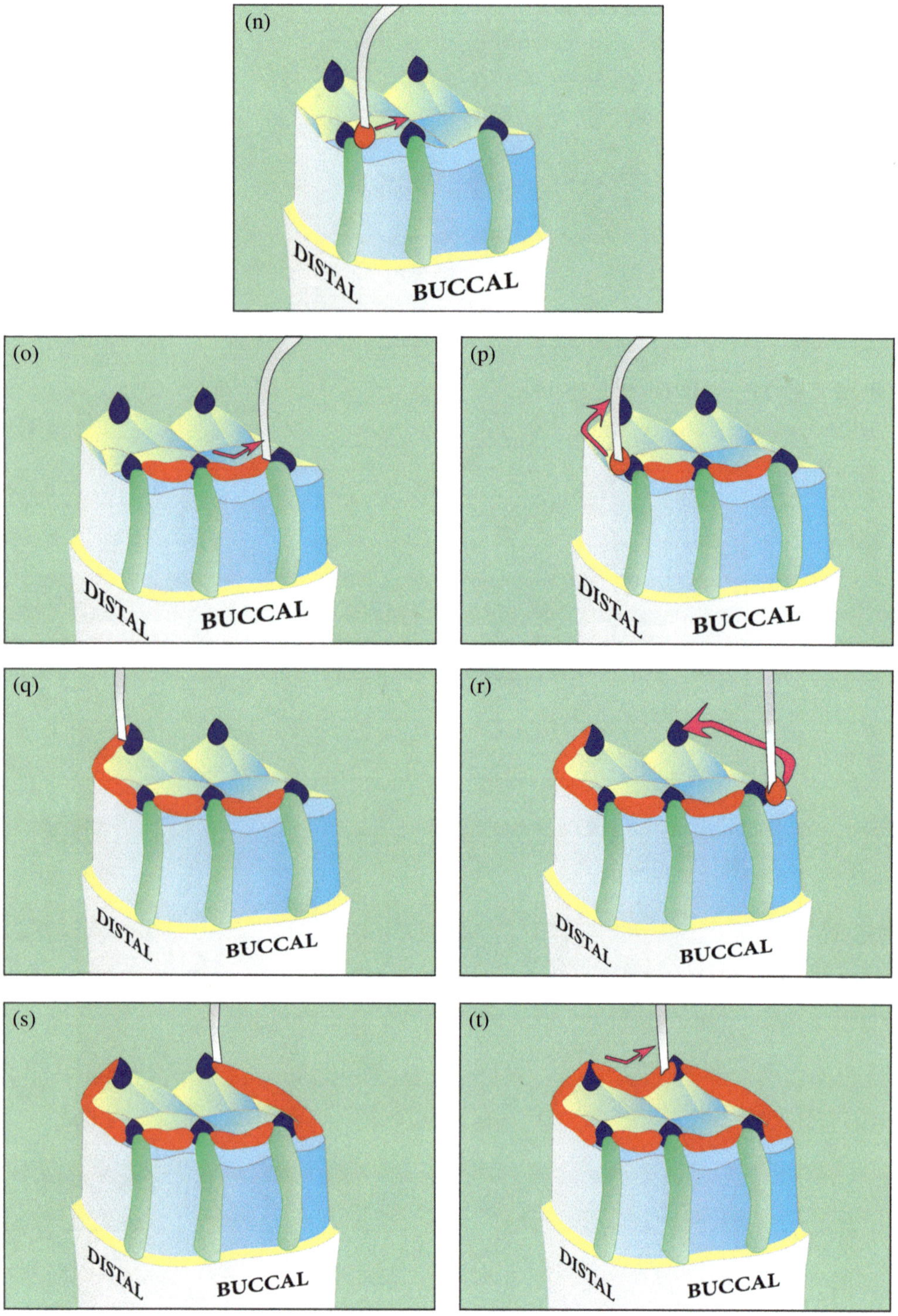

Figure 24.1 (n–t) Direction for placing the marginal ridge and cuspal ridge bars.

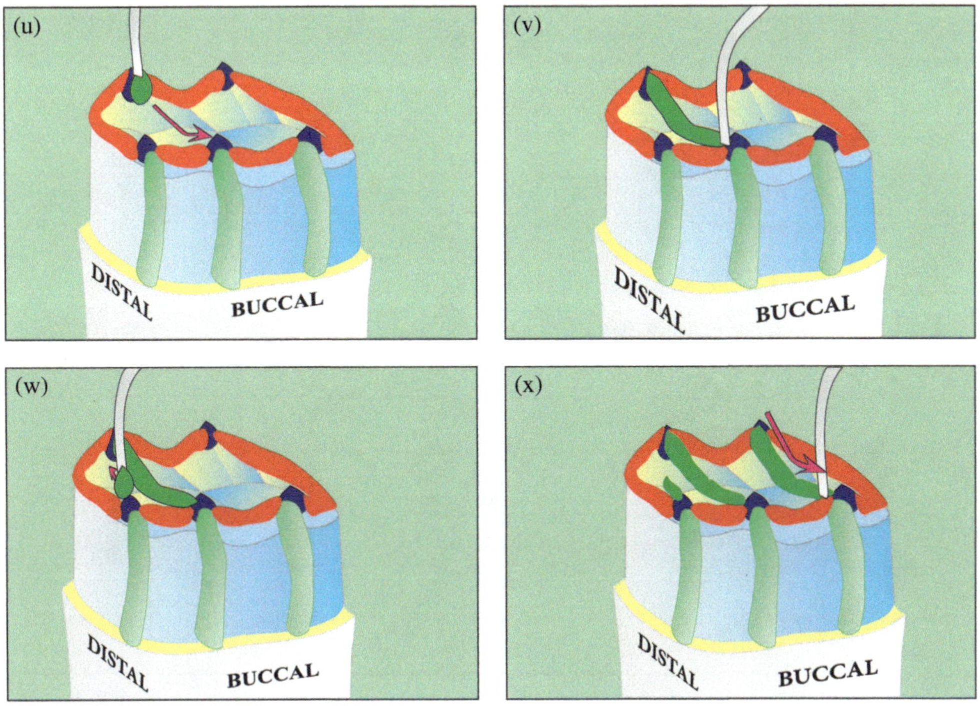

Figure 24.1 (u–x) Direction for placing the transverse ridge.

Exercise: Placing the Ridges of the Occlusal Surface

The triangular ridge bars (green) are placed on the distolingual and distobuccal ridges of the prepared tooth (Figure 24.1u and v). The ridge bar is also placed on the prepared distal cusp (Figure 24.1w). The transverse ridge bar is created along the mesiobuccal and mesiolingual triangular ridges of prepared tooth (Figure 24.1x) [1, 2].

Exercise: Bulk Waxing of the Buccal, lingual, and Proximal Surfaces

Molten wax is then applied on surfaces using the PKT no. 2 instrument to create the bulk of the surfaces. The instrument with molten wax is passed from the distolingual line angle along the buccal surface to the mesiobuccal line angle, while adding the bulk of wax in increments (Figure 24.2a–c). Bulk is added to the mesial and lingual surfaces in a similar way (Figure 24.2d and e) [1, 2].

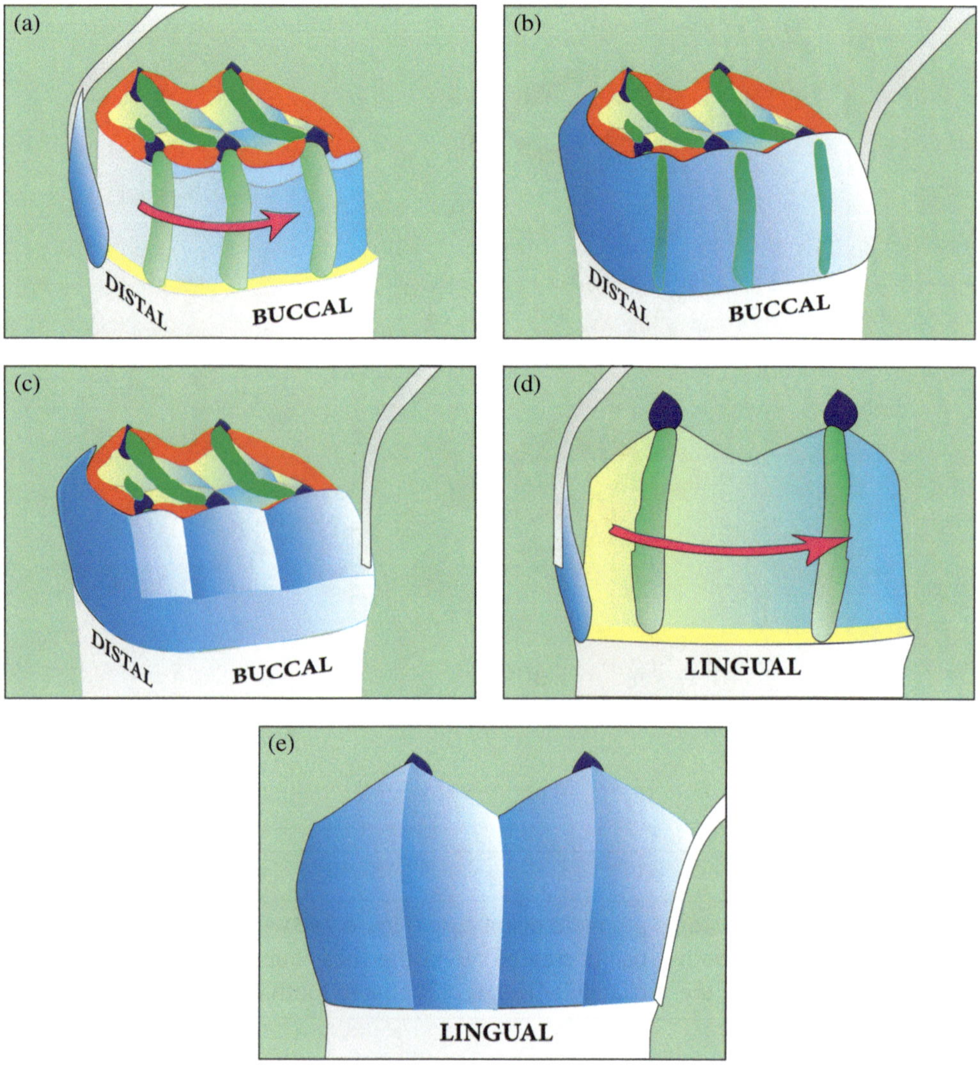

Figure 24.2 (a–e) Directions for placing the molten wax on the distobuccal and mesiolingual surfaces.

Exercise: Waxing the Slopes of the Triangular Ridges on the Occlusal Surface

The bulk of wax is added to create the slopes of the triangular ridges on the occlusal surface. The PKT no. 2 instrument carrying molten wax is applied to create the slopes of the mesiolingual cusp and mesiobuccal cusps (Figure 24.2f–j). In a similar way, molten wax is applied on the distolingual and distobuccal cuspal ridges (Figure 24.2k–o). The distal cusp is also created (Figure 24.2p). Finally, the mesial and distal fossae are created (Figure 24.2q and r). The entire crown is carved for any excess wax and polished to get a smooth surface (Figure 24.2s) [1, 2].

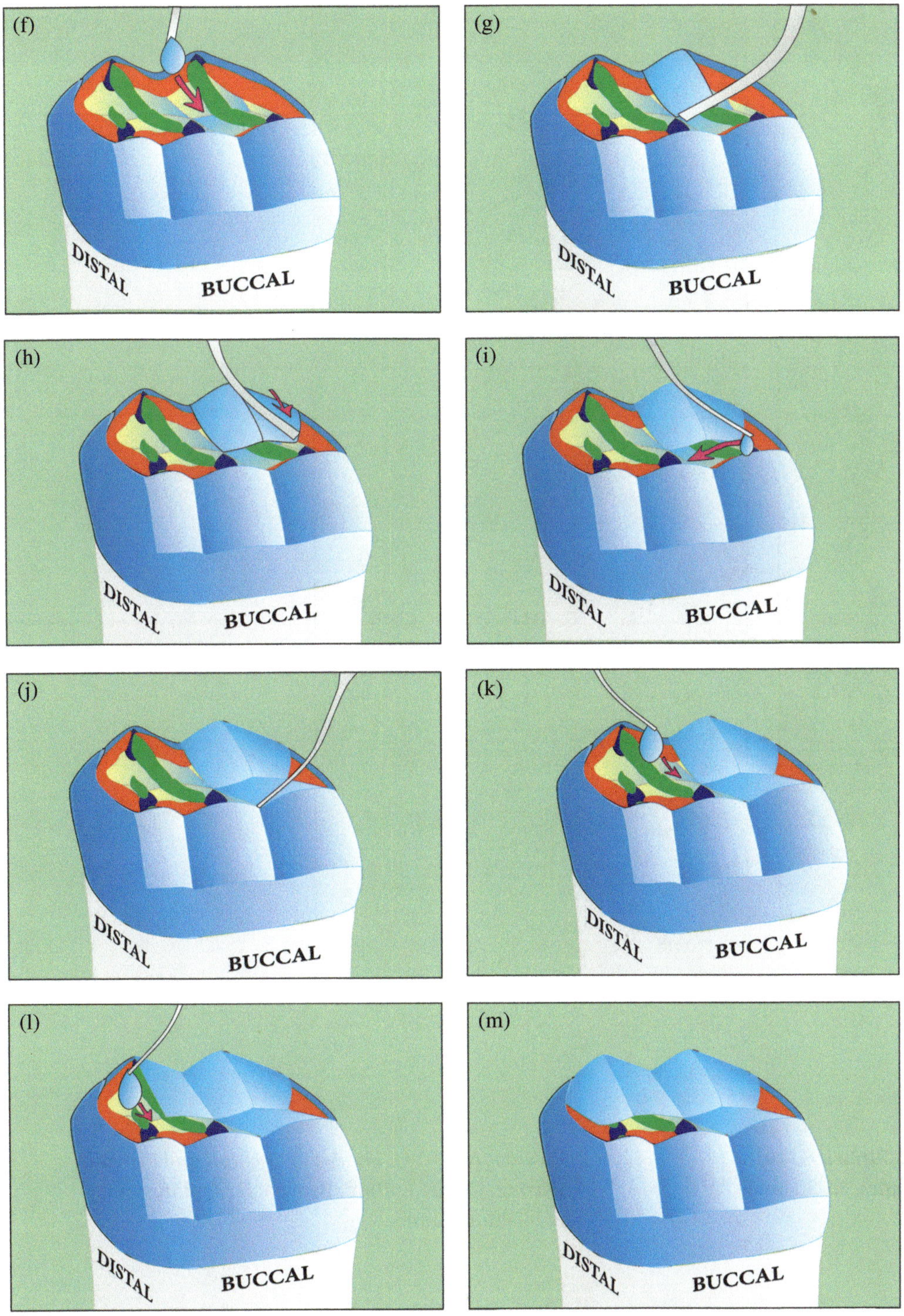

Figure 24.2 (f–s) Directions for placing the bulk of molten wax to create the slopes of the ridges of the occlusal surface.

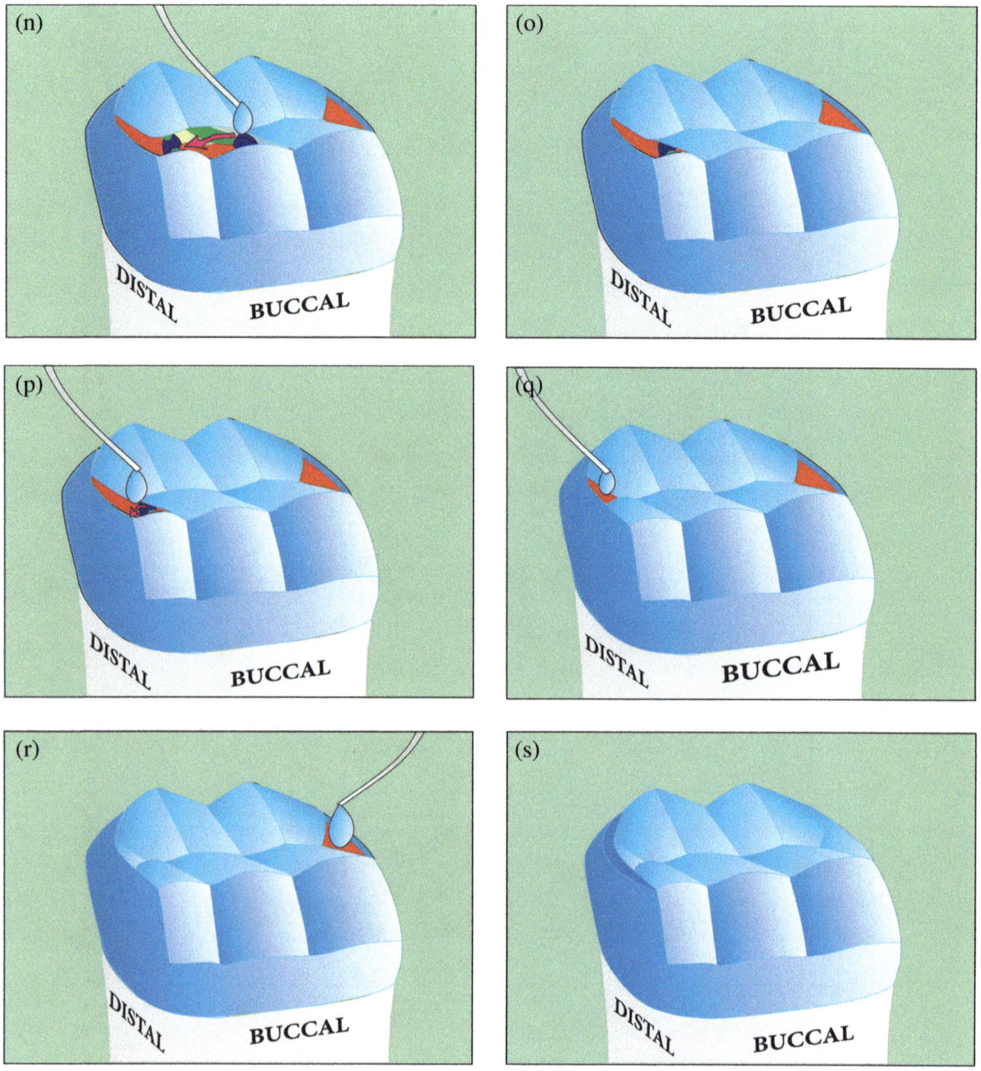

Figure 24.2 (Cont'd) (f–s)

References

1 Stephen, F.R., Martin, F.L., and Junhei, F. (2016). *Contemporary Fixed Prosthodontics*, 5e. St. Louis, MO: Elsevier.

2 Rowida, A. (2019). *The Art of Occlusal and Esthetic Waxing*. Kindle Edition. Batavia, IL: Quintessence Publishing Co Inc.

Index

An Illustrated Atlas of Tooth Carving and Wax-Up Techniques, First Edition. Anil Bangalore Shivappa.

Companion website: www.wiley.com/go/bangalore/toothcarving

d

Printed in the USA/Agawam, MA
September 16, 2026
910661.197